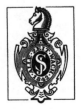

Assessment of Depression

Edited by
Norman Sartorius and Thomas A. Ban

Published on Behalf
of the World Health Organization

With 9 Figures

Springer-Verlag
Berlin Heidelberg New York Tokyo

Dr. NORMAN SARTORIUS
Director, Division of Mental Health
World Health Organization, CH-1211 Geneva 27
Professor of Psychiatry, University of Zagreb
Professeur invité à charge partielle, Université de Genève

Dr. THOMAS A. BAN
Professor of Psychiatry
Vanderbilt University, 242 Medical Arts Building
1211 21st Avenue, South, Nashville, TN 37212, USA

Library of Congress Cataloging-in-Publication Data. Main entry under title: Assessment of depression. Bibliography: p. Includes index. 1. Depression, Mental – Diagnosis. I. Sartorius, N. II. Ban, Thomas A. RC537.A87 1985 616.85'27075 85-20784
ISBN-13: 978-3-642-70488-8   e-ISBN-13: 978-3-642-70486-4
DOI:10.1007/978-3-642-70486-4

This work is subject to copyright. All rights are reserved, whether the whole or part of the material is concerned, specifically those of translation, reprinting, re-use of illustrations, broadcasting, reproduction by photocopying machine or similar means, and storage in data banks. Under § 54 of the German Copyright Law where copies are made for other than private use, a fee is payable to "Verwertungsgesellschaft Wort", Munich.

© by Springer-Verlag Berlin Heidelberg 1986
Softcover reprint of the Hardcover 1st edition 1986

The use of registered names, trademarks, etc. in this publication does not imply, even in the absence of a specific statement, that such names are exempt from the relevant protective laws and regulations and therefore free for general use.

Product Liability: The publisher can give no guarantee for information about drug dosage and application thereof contained in this book. In every individual case the respective user must check its accuracy by consulting other pharmaceutical literature.

Typesetting, printing and binding: Druckerei Appl, Wemding
2125/3130-543210

Foreword

Depressive illnesses, as epidemiological studies have consistently shown, are among the most frequent psychic disorders encountered in hospital and everyday practice. Moreover, during the last few decades the prevalence of depression has definitely been increasing. Its alarming frequency – especially among women – has recently been confirmed once again by epidemiological findings published in the United States of America. The World Health Organization estimates the world-wide prevalence of depression at 3% to 5%.

Among the factors contributing to the current increase are excessively abrupt changes in social structures and living conditions, as well as a departure from traditional values which is often accompanied by disruption of the family unit and loss of religious faith. Further factors include the unfettered materialism of the modern age, the hectic pace of technological progress, and the loneliness to which elderly people in particular are exposed. Finally, the increasing life expectancy of the population in almost all countries of the world raises the incidence of cardiovascular disorders, brain disease, and malignant tumors, thus inevitably adding to the risk of depressive illness in old age.

The prominent position occupied by the diagnosis and treatment of depression in everyday medical practice is apparent from the results of an enquiry conducted among some 15 000 doctors in Austria, the Federal Republic of Germany, France, Italy, Spain, and Switzerland. This enquiry disclosed that of all patients consulting a doctor, up to 10% – and sometimes more – could be classified as depressed, and that in more than one-half of the patients a so-called masked form of depression was found.

During the last 15 years, biological psychiatric research focusing on depression has made more significant progress than ever before. Thanks to interdisciplinary research, new modalities of biological therapy have been opened up whose effectiveness now awaits closer investigation.

The comparison of cross-cultural studies will continue to pose difficult problems until such time as world wide agreement is reached on a uniform system for classifying diagnoses and quantifying the symptomatology of the various forms of depression. Only then will it become possible to compare on an international scale the results obtained in studies on depression and its treatment.

In *The Assessment of Depression,* Professors Sartorius and Ban have assembled a unique collection of papers, in which authors of different and widely used instruments for assessing depression describe the methods they have developed. Papers reviewing the use of these instruments in different parts of the world are also included, so that the book presents both a cogent review of knowledge about the assessment of depression and a comprehensive account of methods used for the purpose. This material merits the attention of a wide readership, and I have no doubt that the book will be useful for the practitioner as well as for the scientist and the teacher interested in making a contribution to the prevention and treatment of depression, so righthy called "la maladie du siècle".

Psychiatric Clinic, University of Basle   Professor P. KIELHOLZ

Preface

It is estimated that there are 100 million people in the world who are suffering from some form of clinically recognizable depression and who could benefit from qualified help. What is more, there is every likelihood that this number will increase. Life expectancy is increasing in most countries, and the number and percentage of people running a higher risk of developing depression are accordingly also increasing. The rapidly changing psychosocial environment of man often gives rise to situations of acute and/or prolonged environmental stress, which may lead to depressive reactions. At a time when more and more individuals are suffering from the unsettling effects of uprooting, family disintegration, and social isolation, for example, it is likely that the prevalence of psychiatric disorders, which will often be of a depressive nature, will increase.

The current increase in morbidity from chronic diseases is also likely to contribute to the number of those with depression. Cardiovascular disease, collagen diseases such as rheumatism, gastroenterological diseases, and cerebrovascular and other neurological disorders have been shown to be associated with depressive illness in as many as 20% of all cases. If the prevalence of these diseases continues its present upward trend, an increase in the occurrence of somatogenic depressions must also be expected. To what extent this increase will be offset by a decrease in somatogenic depression associated with more acute forms of physical illness – such as communicable diseases – cannot be determined at this stage. Excessive medicament consumption may also contribute to the problem. Certain drugs whose consumption is now steadily increasing have been demonstrated to cause depression; among them are some antihypertensives and various hormone preparations.

There are thus several reasons to justify the prediction of a genuine increase in the prevalence of depressive illness. Planning in health investment, however, is often affected less by true prevalence than by impressions about the prevalence ("apparent prevalence") of an illness; in the case of depression there are also good grounds for believing that the apparent prevalence will likewise show an increase. A possible reason for this is that it is now possible to discern a change in doctors' diagnosing habits, in that they are showing a greater readiness to diagnose depression. This tendency is undoubtedly connected with the fact that in cases of depression the prospects for successful treatment, and hence the prognosis, have improved, as well as with the fact that, thanks to better standards of living and to higher incomes, more patients are now able to afford treatment. Second, new diagnostic concepts, such as that of masked depression, are gaining wider acceptance. Third, in many of the developing countries that are becoming increasingly "Westernized," more patients now tend – when faced with the problem of describing their symptoms to the doctor – to adopt a language which enables them to verbalize their experience of depression more accurately. Fourth, the increased emphasis now being placed on the quality of life, the waning influence of religions that put a premium on suffering, and the greater efforts being devoted to health education are prompting many patients who until recently would have considered their feelings of depression, misery, and unhappiness as being perfectly normal to seek medical advice. Improved health services, on the other hand, are also providing an opportunity and an inducement to patients to come forward and obtain treatment.

Recent advances in our knowledge concerning the biological correlates of the depressive syndrome would appear to promise early and important scientific breakthroughs in the realm of depression, and many institutions and individuals are now focusing their attention on the problem of depression. Although the efforts and resources being invested in this problem are steadily growing, there is a certain chaotic quality to this growth. True multidisciplinary work is still the exception, and those engaged in research are often far removed from their colleagues in clinical practice. Multicentric research is also still rare, although in studying a condition such as depression there are numerous obvious gains in such ventures.

Some of these obstacles to further improvement of our knowledge (and its application!) about depression are related to the diverse methodology employed in the assessment of depression by different investigators and by clinicians. A variety of instruments have been developed and are widely used, but there is little information on the availability and usage of these instruments in different languages; even less is known about the advantages and disadvantages of the various assessment instruments in different depressive populations.

These were the reasons which led to the production of this book. There is a serious need to bring together authoritative descriptions of the most frequently used and recommended assessment instruments. It is also hoped that this assembly of descriptions will facilitate the choice and use of such instruments, and there is a high probability that a more appropriate use of the measurement tools will facilitate research by providing systematically gathered data about the condition and its treatment.

The first part of the book gives a series of reviews on the use of instruments in different parts of the world; the second provides detailed descriptions of each instrument, providing information about its applicability, psychometric characteristics, advantages, and purpose. The third part deals with some special issues, such as the use of scales in children and the elderly, and differences in assessments which are attributable to the assessor's background.

We are indebted to the contributors to this volume for their collaboration and contribution. Thanks are also due to Mrs Charlton for her handling of the many administrative aspects of the preparation of this book, and to Mrs Vetsch for her tireless attention to the many tasks – from correspondence to proofreading – that had to be done to bring the manuscript to completion.

NORMAN SARTORIUS
THOMAS A. BAN

Contents

Chapter 1 Standardized Instruments Used in the Assessment
of Depression in German-Speaking Countries
E. FÄHNDRICH, H. HELMCHEN, and M. LINDEN 1

Chapter 2 Systems and Scales for the Assessment
of Depression in French-Speaking Countries
D. BOBON 9

Chapter 3 Standardized Instruments for the Evaluation
of Affective Disturbances in Spain and Spanish-Speaking
Countries
J. J. LÓPEZ-IBOR Jr. and J. M. LÓPEZ-IBOR 19

Chapter 4 The Area of the Bulgarian People's Republic,
Czechoslovak Socialist Republic, Polish People's Republic,
Union of Soviet Socialist Republics and Socialist Federative
Republic of Yugoslavia
C. ŠKODA and O. VINAŘ (With 1 Figure) 23

Chapter 5 Standardized Instruments Used in the Assessment
of Depression in the Scandinavian Countries
O. LINGJAERDE 30

Chapter 6 Instruments Used in the Assessment of Depression
in Japan
R. TAKAHASHI 36

Chapter 7 Rating Scales for Depression in Italy
G. B. CASSANO, P. CASTROGIOVANNI, and E. RAMPELLO 46

Chapter 8 Standard Instruments Used in the Assessment
of Depression in Africa
A. O. ODEJIDE 55

Chapter 9 The WHO Instruments for the Assessment
of Depressive Disorders
A. JABLENSKY, N. SARTORIUS, W. GULBINAT, and G. ERNBERG
(With 2 Figures) 61

Chapter 10 AMDP-III in the Assessment of Depression
B. WOGGON (With 1 Figure) 82

Chapter 11 Rating of Depression with a Subscale
of the CPRS
C. PERRIS 90

Chapter 12 A Self-Report Inventory on Depressive
Symptomatology (QD2) and Its Abridged Form (QD2A)
P. PICHOT 108

Chapter 13 Applications of the Beck Depression Inventory
R. A. STEER, A. T. BECK, and B. GARRISON 123

Chapter 14 The Hamilton Rating Scale for Depression
M. HAMILTON 143

Chapter 15 The Development of Four Self-Assessment
Depression Scales
R. P. SNAITH 153

Chapter 16 Assessment of Depression Using the Brief
Psychiatric Rating Scale
J. E. OVERALL and L. E. HOLLISTER (With 4 Figures) 159

Chapter 17 The Brief Depression Rating Scale
R. KELLNER 179

Chapter 18 The Carroll Rating Scale for Depression
M. FEINBERG and B. J. CARROLL (With 2 Figures) 188

Chapter 19 The Newcastle Scale
M. W. P. CARNEY 201

Chapter 20 The Symptom-Rating Test
R. KELLNER 213

Chapter 21 Zung Self-Rating Depression Scale and
Depression Status Inventory
W. W. K. ZUNG 221

Chapter 22 Depression Scales Derived from the Hopkins
Symptom Checklist
R. S. LIPMAN 232

Chapter 23 The Wittenborn Psychiatric Rating Scale
J. R. WITTENBORN 249

Chapter 24 The Melancholia Scale: Development,
Consistency, Validity, and Utility
P. BECH and O. J. RAFAELSEN 259

Chapter 25 Clinical Self-Rating Scales (CSRS)
of the Munich Psychiatric Information System
(PSYCHIS München)
D. VON ZERSSEN (With 2 Figures) 270

Chapter 26   The Clinical Interview for Depression
E. S. PAYKEL 304

Chapter 27   Schedule for Affective Disorders and
Schizophrenia: Regular and Change Versions
J. ENDICOTT 316

Chapter 28   The Assessment of Depression in Children and
Adolescents
M. STROBER and J. S. WERRY 324

Chapter 29   Instruments Used in the Assessment
of Depression in Psychogeriatric Patients
T. HOVAGUIMIAN 343

Chapter 30   Self-Report and Clinical Interview
in the Assessment of Depression
E. S. PAYKEL and K. R. W. NORTON 356

Chapter 31   Sensitivity to Treatment Effects of Evaluation
Instruments Completed by Psychiatrists, Psychologists,
Nurses, and Patients
A. RASKIN 367

List of Contributors

BECH, P., Institute of Psychochemistry, Rigshospitalet, 9 Blegdamsvej, DK-2100 Copenhagen Ø

BECK, A.T., Department of Psychiatry, University of Pennsylvania, 133 South 36th Street, Philadelphia, PA 19104, USA

BOBON, D., Clinique Psychiatrique, Université de Liège, 58 rue Saint Laurent, B-4000 Liège

CARNEY, M.W.P., Department of Psychiatry, Northwick Park Hospital and Clinical Research Centre, Watford Road, Harrow, Middlesex HA1 3UJ, Great Britain

CARROLL, B.J., Department of Psychiatry, Duke University Medical Center, Durham, NC 27710, USA

CASSANO, G.B., Centro per la Prevenzione e la Terapia della Depressione, Istituto di Clinica Psichiatrica, Ospedale Riuniti S. Chiara, Via Roma 67, I-56100 Pisa

CASTROGIOVANNI, P., Centro per la Prevenzione e la Terapia della Depressione, Istituto di Clinica Psichiatrica, Ospedale Riuniti S. Chiara, Via Roma 67, I-56100 Pisa

ENDICOTT, J., Department of Psychiatry, College of Physicians and Surgeons, Columbia University, New York, NY 10032, USA

ERNBERG, G., Division of Mental Health, World Health Organization, CH-1211 Geneva 27

FÄHNDRICH, E., Psychiatrische Klinik und Poliklinik, Freie Universität Berlin, Eschenallee 3, D-1000 Berlin 19

FEINBERG, M., The University of Michigan, 205 Washtenaw Place, Ann Arbor, MI 48109, USA

GARRISON, B., Center for Cognitive Therapy, Department of Psychiatry, University of Pennsylvania Medical School, Philadelphia, PA 19104, USA

GULBINAT, W., Division of Mental Health, World Health Organization, CH-1211 Geneva 27

HAMILTON, M., The University of Leeds School of Medicine, Psychiatry Annexe, 30 Clarendon Road, Leeds LS2 9NZ, Great Britain

HELMCHEN, H., Psychiatrische Klinik und Poliklinik, Freie Universität Berlin, Eschenallee 3, D-1000 Berlin 19

HOLLISTER, L. E., Veterans Administration Medical Center, Palo Alto, CA 94304, USA

HOVAGUIMIAN, T., University of Geneva, Geriatric Institution's Psychogeriatric Liaison-Consultation, University Cantonal Hospital, CH-1211 Geneva 4

KELLNER, R., Department of Psychiatry, University of New Mexico Mental Health Programs, Albuquerque, NM 87131, USA

LINDEN, M., Psychiatrische Klinik und Poliklinik, Freie Universität Berlin, Eschenallee, 3, D-1000 Berlin 19

LINGJAERDE, O., Gaustad Hospital, N-Oslo

LIPMAN, R. S., Friends Hospital, Roosevelt Boulevard and Adams Avenue, Philadelphia, PA 19124, USA

LÓPEZ-IBOR Jr., J. J., Av. Nueva Zelanda 78, Madrid 35, Spain

LÓPEZ-IBOR, J. M., Av. Nueva Zelanda 78, Madrid 35, Spain

NORTON, K. R. W., St. George's Hospital Medical School, London SW17 ORE, Great Britain

ODEJIDE, A. O., Department of Psychiatry, University College Hospital, Ibadan, Nigeria

OVERALL, J. E., Department of Psychiatry and Behavioral Sciences, University of Texas Medical School, P.O. Box 20708, Houston TX 77225, USA

PAYKEL, E. S., Department of Psychiatry, St. George's Hospital Medical School, University of London, Jenner Wing, Cranmer Terrace, Tooting, London SW17 ORE, Great Britain

PERRIS, C., Department of Psychiatry, University of Umeå, S-901 85 Umeå

PICHOT, P., Cliniques des Maladies mentales et de l'Encéphale, 100 rue de la Santé, F-75674 Paris

RAFAELSEN, O. J., Institute of Psychochemistry, Rigshospitalet, 9 Blegdamsvej, DK-2100 Copenhagen Ø

RAMPELLO, E., Centro per la Prevenzione e la Terapia della Depressione, Istituto di Clinica Psichiatrica, Ospedale Riuniti S. Chiari, Via Roma 67, I-56100 Pisa

List of Contributors

RASKIN, A., Anxiety Disorders Section, Pharmacological and Somatic Treatments Research Branch, National Institute of Mental Health, Rockville, MD 20857, USA

SARTORIUS, N., Division of Mental Health, World Health Organization, CH-1211 Geneva 27

ŠKODA, C., Psychiatric Research Institute, Bohnice, Prague 8, Czechoslovakia

SNAITH, R. P., Department of Psychiatry, The University of Leeds, 15 Hyde Terrace, Leeds LS2 9LT, Great Britain

STEER, R. A., Center for Cognitive Therapy, Department of Psychiatry, University of Pennsylvania Medical School, Philadelphia, PA 19104, USA

STROBER, M., Neuropsychiatric Institute, Center for the Health Sciences, 760 Westwood Plaza, Los Angeles, CA 90024, USA

TAKAHASHI, R., Department of Neuropsychiatry, Tokyo Medical and Dental University, 5-45 Yushima, 1-chome Bunkyo-ku, Tokyo, Japan

VINAŘ, O., Psychiatric Research Institute, Bohnice, Prague 8, Czechoslovakia

WERRY, J. S., Department of Psychiatry, University of Auckland School of Medicine, Auckland, New Zealand

WITTENBORN, J. R., The Interdisciplinary Research Centre, The State University of New Jersey, New Brunswick, NJ 08903, USA

WOGGON, B., Research Department, Psychiatric University Hospital Zürich, P. O. Box 68, CH-8029 Zürich 8

ZERSSEN, D. VON, Max-Planck-Institut für Psychiatrie, Kraepelinstraße 10, D-8000 München 40

ZUNG, W. W. K., Veterans Administration Hospital, Duke University Medical Center, Durham, NC 27705, USA

Chapter 1 Standardized Instruments Used in the Assessment of Depression in German-Speaking Countries

E. FÄHNDRICH, H. HELMCHEN, and M. LINDEN

Historical Perspective

Standardized instruments for the quantitative and objective assessment of psychopathology have been developed in German-speaking countries since the late fifties. This development has been stimulated by the need to objectify characteristics of psychiatric disorders in clinical trials of psychotropic drugs. Interests in nosological and pathogenetic problems and in empirical therapy research further prompted the development of psychopathometric scales. The anthropological and phenomenological schools prevailing in German psychiatry in the fifties presented an inhibiting influence whereas stimulating influence came from Anglo-American work in the field as well as from psychologists and statisticians, who stressed the importance of objectivity, reliability, and validity. The existing well-differentiated system of descriptive clinical psychopathology also helped to promote the need for the standardization of instruments and became one of the triggers for the foundation in 1965 of the *Arbeitsgemeinschaft für Methodik und Dokumentation in der Psychiatrie* (Association for Methodology and Documentation in Psychiatry) – AMDP – which devoted itself to the development of standardized instruments (see Woggon, Chap. 10, this volume). Since then several rating scales, observational instruments, tests, and experimental settings for the evaluation of depressive states have been published by psychiatrists, psychologists, clinicians, and experimental workers. Besides these instruments originally developed in German, there have been many translations of international scales, mostly English or American, some from Scandinavian countries. As will be pointed out later, these scales are now as important in German publications as those originally developed in German.

We will only refer here to instruments which may be used for the assessment of the depressive syndrome. We will not list methods which only focus on special aspects of depressive states such as anxiety, hopelessness, social interaction, or physiological phenomena.

A Survey of the Use of Scales

In order to obtain an estimate of which scales are used most often, the leading German-speaking journals *[Archiv für Psychiatrie und Nervenkrankheiten; Fortschritte der Neurologie und Psychiatrie; International Pharmacopsychiatry* (this journal is an exception because it has published contributions in English by German authors which are relevant to our topic); *Nervenarzt; Pharmacopsychiatria; Psychiatrie, Neurologie, Medizinische Psychologie; Psychiatrische Praxis; Schweizer Archiv für Neurologie, Neurochirurgie und Psychiatrie; Wiener Zeitschrift für Nervenheilkunde]* were screened from 1975 to 1980 for publications reporting the use of standardized instruments for the assessment of depression. A total of 85 papers listed 53 different instruments: some listed only one; many listed several in combination. Table 1.1 lists the most important instruments and gives the percentage of papers in which each scale was used. Among the nine scales mentioned more than once are six self-rating scales and three observer-rating scales. Four are originally German. Only the first four are used so often that they may contribute to a standardization and comparability of research between different researchers. These are the *Befindlichkeits-Skala* (BfS) [41], the Hamilton Depression Scale (HAM-D) [13], the AMDP System [1], and the Clinical-Global Impression (CGI) [9] rating.

Table 1.1. Depression scales used in German-speaking publications from 1975 to 1980 (figures indicate number of papers). Final column shows percentage of papers in which the scales were mentioned.

Scale	1975	1976	1977	1978	1979	1980	%
Befindlichkeits-Skala (BfS) (von Zerssen)	3		3	2	10	7	29.4
Hamilton Depression Scale (HAM-D)	3	2	5	2	6	4	25.9
Dokumentationssysteme der Arbeitsgemeinschaft für Methodik und Dokumentation in der Psychiatrie (AMP/AMDP)	4	2	5		5	1	20
Clinical Global Impression (CGI)	2		2		2	2	9.4
Beschwerde-Liste (BL) (von Zerssen)			1	1		2	4.7
Depressions-Skala (DBC-Skala) Bojanovski-Chloupkova			1	1	1	1	4.7
Freiburger Persönlichkeits-Inventar (FPI) (Fahrenberg et al.)		2	1			1	4.7
Beck *Depressions Inventar* (BDI)	1					2	3.5
Visuelle Analog Skala (VAS)					1	1	2.4

This selection of instruments poses some serious questions. There is no special depression self-rating scale among the instruments used most often. The BfS measures general distress rather than depression specifically. The problem with regard to the HAM-D is that there are several different translations; several forms with 17, 21, and 24 items; and almost no psychometric evaluations of the German version [3,

25]. The AMDP System is a comprehensive system for assessment and documentation of overall psychopathology. It was originally developed by German, Swiss, and Austrian psychiatrists with a strong bias toward schizophrenic psychopathology. It may also be used for depressive disorders, though it lacks some sensitivity in minor depressive states. Nevertheless data of good quality are available from the use of this instrument, which has been translated into several languages (see Woggon, Chap. 10, this volume).

Finally, although the CGI rating may give a lot of information, its reliability and differentiation are doubtful.

In general it seems that recommendations for assessment batteries for depression, as given in several German reviews, were not followed through at least up to 1980 [9, 12, 15, 19, 25]. The authors of these recommendations stressed the importance of reliability, validity, and international comparability, criteria which are not ideally fulfilled by the instruments used most often. Besides these psychometric problems there are questions with regard to the application of scales and the interpretation of scores. Most researchers use these instruments for analyses of changes over time and differences between groups: yet there are no generally agreed upon criteria for the interpretation of what represents change. Information about the training of raters is rarely reported and the training probably rarely adequate. The recommendation that rating scales should be complemented by performance tests and by systematic behavioral observation had no resonance in study designs [22, 25].

The application of standardized instruments for the assessment of depression is thus still a developing field in German-speaking countries and will undoubtedly expand and improve over the coming years.

Standardized Instruments in German

In the following pages we will briefly describe some instruments developed by German-speaking authors. (Some of the important ones are listed in Table 1.2.) AMDP and KSbS are discussed in separate chapters in this volume (see Woggon and von Zerssen) and will therefore not be dealt with here. There are of course many more scales. The scales discussed here were selected either because they are psychometrically well elaborated or well known among interested scientists or innovative in character.

The *Hamburger-Depressions-Skala* (HDS) [19] is a specific self-rating scale for depression consisting of 50 items. The patient answers "I agree," "I don't agree," or "I don't know." A manual is not available. Some data of good quality have been published [12, 15, 21, 32]. Retest reliability ranges from 0.86 to 0.87 and split-half-reliability from 0.90 to 0.92. Correlations with other depression scales and with clinical judgments range from 0.72 to 0.83. Factor analysis yields three factors called energy-loss, anxiety/hypochondriasis, and dysthymia. The total score range is from 0 to 50. The threshold score for depression is 26.

The *Eppendorfer-Stimmungs-Antriebs-Skala* (ESTA) [34] is a self-rating depression scale with 18 items which are each presented in a bipolar manner such as

Table 1.2. Some standardized instruments for the assessment of depression available in German

	Abbreviation	Reference
1. Original German instruments		
Observer rating		
Psychopathologie-System der Arbeitsgemeinschaft für Methodik und Dokumentation in der Psychiatrie	AMDP	[1]
Quantitative Video-Analyse	QVA	[38]
Zeitblinde Video-Analyse	ZVA	[31]
Self-rating		
Klinische Selbstbeurteilungs-Skalen	KsbS	[41]
Befindlichkeits-Skala	BfS	
Beschwerde-Listen	BL	
Paranoid Depressivitäts-Skala	PDS	
Depressivitäts-Skala	DS	
Hamburger Depressions-Skala	HDS	[19]
Depressions-Skala-Bojanovski-Chloupkova	DBC	[7]
Giessen-Test	GT	[4]
Freiburger Persönlichkeits-Inventar	FPI	[11]
Eppendorfer Stimmungs- und Antriebs-Scala	ESTA	[34]
Eigenschafts-Wörter-Liste	EWL	[17]
Hamburg-Erlanger-Stimmungs-Barometer	HESTIBAR	[8]
Erlanger-Depressions-Skala	EDS	[22]
Emotionalitäts-Inventar	EMIB	[39]
Mehrdimensionaler Stimmungsfragebogen	MSF	[16]
Adjektiv-Skalen zur Einschätzung der Stimmung	SES	[14]
Kurz-Skala Stimmung/Aktivierung	KUSTA	[5]
Test zur Erfassung der Schwere einer Depression	TSD	[26]
2. Translated instruments		
Observer rating		
Hamilton Depression Scale	HAMD	[2]
Present State Examination	PSE	[40]
Forschungs-Diagnose-Kriterien	RDC	[33]
Self-rating		
Beck-Depressions-Inventar	BDI	[18]
McNair Profile of Mood States	POMS	[9]
Visuelle Analog-Skala	VAS	[10]
Marke-Nyman Temperament Scale	MNT	[3]
Minnesota Multiphasic Personality Inventory – Saarbrücken	MMPI-Saarbrücken	[6]
Zung Selbst-Rating-Depressions-Skala	SDS	[15]
Qualitatives Depressions Inventar	QDI	[27]

"good and refreshing sleep" versus "sleeplessness." In between there is either a 13-point (ESTA-I) or 18-point (ESTA-III) rating scale or a visual analogue scale (ESTA-II) which is marked by the patient depending on whether he or she agrees more with one or the other formulation. The scale allows to calculate an overall "depression" score, a subscore "mood," and a subscore "drive" and to present a profile of all items. Groups of patients may be described in a two-dimensional system "mood and drive." The scale is recommended by the author for time-course analyses in order to objectify mood fluctuation over time. A large variety of examples are given to show how to interpret results.

The *Eigenschaftswörter-Liste* (EWL) [17] is an adjective checklist to measure the overall emotional state. It consists of 161 items and is also available in a short form of 123 items. It has 14 subscales such as "activity," "concentration," "fatigue," and "extra-introversion." Reliability coefficients are hard to interpret because the scale is devised to measure actual and short-term mood fluctuations. For the subscales the Alpha-Cronbach index ranges from 0.75 to 0.94 and retest-reliability coefficients range from 0.54 to 0.91.

The *Giessen-Test* (GT) [4] consisting of 40 items is a personality inventory based on psychoanalytic theory. There are six subscales called "social resonance," "dominance," "control," "mood," "permeability," and "social potency." The test allows to compare real-self with ideal-self. Test-retest reliability for items is about 0.30, for profiles about 0.56, and for subscales about 0.65-0.76. Internal consistency for subscales is about 0.86. Norms are given for neurotic patients, psychosomatic patients, and juvenile delinquents by age group and social class.

The *Freiburger Persönlichkeits-Inventar* (FPI) [11] is a general personality inventory similar to the Minnesota Multiphasic Personality Inventory (MMPI). It has a long form of 212 items, two half forms, and a short form. There are nine factor-analytically derived subscales called "nervousness," "spontaneous aggression," "depression," "irritability," "sociability," "calmness," "reactive aggression and dominance," "inhibition," and "openness." There are satisfactory reliability data for all subscales and items available, e.g., split-half reliability data for depression of 0.79-0.85. Validity data and norms are established for different sociological and clinical groups. The FPI is at present the leading and best-elaborated German personality inventory with several subscales of clinical interest.

The use of video technology opens up a new approach to the assessment of depression. Ulrich et al. developed a Quantitative Video Analysis System (QVA) for the assessment of manual kinetics in depressed patients [35, 36, 37, 38]. Frequency of body-centered hand movements correlates positively with agitation. Frequency of object-focused and speech-related hand movements correlates negatively with retardation. Thus, frequency of both, even in a mutually opposite direction, is correlated with the intensity of the present depressive syndrome, i.e., it represents a state factor. Besides, the lateral preponderance of manual kinetics may be a trait factor in endogenous depression.

Another video methodology, the *Zeitblinde Video-Analyse* (ZVA), was developed by Renfordt et al. [28-31]. This may be specifically used to assess the time course of treatment responses. Segments of several consecutive videotaped interviews, each about 120 s long, are given in a random way to raters who are unaware of the real-time sequence of the recordings. The rater then has to give the real-time order of the recordings, judging from the intensity of the depressive syndrome to be seen. This procedure has been successfully applied to comparative drug trials and seems to have a higher discrimination power than conventional methods. The biggest advantage is that it allows the control of observer and patient bias with regard to time.

Other standardized instruments in German for the assessment of depression, which will only be mentioned briefly, are the *Hamburg-Erlanger Stimmungsbarometer* (HESTIBAR) [8], the *Erlanger Depressions-Skala* (EDS) [23], the *Emotionalitäts-Inventar* (EMI-B) [39], the *Mehrdimensionaler Stimmungsfragebogen* (MSF) [16], the *Adjective-Skalen zur Einschätzung der Stimmung* (SES) [14], the *Kurz-Skala Stim-*

mung/Aktivierung (KUSTA) [5], and the *Test zur Erfassung der Schwere einer Depression* (TSD) [26].

In talking about German scales, translations must be mentioned briefly. Scales developed in other languages must be tested again after they have been translated. This problem has already been discussed in relation to the widely used German version of the Hamilton Depression Scale. Other instruments, for which German test criteria have at least partly been established, are the Beck Depression Inventory [18, 24], the McNair Profile of Mood States [9], the Visual Analogue Scale [10], the Marke-Nyman Temperament Scale (MNT) [3], the Minnesota Multiphasic Personality Inventory – Saarbrücken [6], the Zung Self-Rating Depression Scale [15], the Qualitative Depression Inventory [27], the Present State Examination [40], and the Research Diagnostic Criteria [33].

Translations without German test criteria are available, e. g., for the Zung Depression Status Inventory, the Derogatis Hopkins Symptom Check List, and the Wittenborn Psychiatric Rating Scale [9].

Conclusion

In the opinion of the authors the *Depressions-Skala* (DS v. Zerssen), the Hamilton Depression Scale (HAM-D), and the AMDP System with its subscales for depression are best suited for investigations of depressive disorders in German-speaking countries because of the national and international comparability of data assembled with these instruments.

References

1. AMDP. 1981. Das AMDP-System. Manual zur Dokumentation psychiatrischer Befunde. 4th Ed. Springer, Berlin Heidelberg New York.
2. Baumann, U. 1976. Methodische Untersuchungen zur Hamilton-Depressions-Skala. Arch. Psychiatr. Nervenkr. 222: 359–375.
3. Baumann, U., and Angst, J. 1972. Die Marke-Nyman Temperament-Skala (MNT). Z. Klin. Psychol. Psychopathol. Psychother. 3: 189–212.
4. Beckmann, E., and Richter, H.-E. 1975. Giessen Test. 2nd Ed. Huber, Bern.
5. Binz, U., and Wendt, G. 1983. KUSTA, Kurz-Skala Stimmungs/Antrieb Manual. Unpublished manuscript. Ciba-Geigy, Frankfurt.
6. Blaser, P., and Gehring, A. 1972. MMPI. Ein programierter Kurs zur deutschsprachigen Ausgabe des Minnesota Multiphasic Personality Inventory von S. R. Hathaway and J. C. McKinley. Huber, Bern.
7. Bojanovski, J., and Chloupkova, K. 1966. Bewertungsskala der Depressionszustände. Psychiat. Neurol. (Basel) 151: 54–61.
8. Burkhard, G., Upmeyer, H.J., Weidenhammer, W., and Schmidt, A. 1982. Das Hamburg-Erlanger Stimmungsbarometer (HESTIBAR). Psycho 8: 690–696.
9. CIPS. 1981. Internationale Skalen für Psychiatrie. Beltz, Weinheim.
10. Fähndrich, E., and Linden, M. 1982. Zur Reliabilität und Validität der Stimmungsmessung mit der Visuellen Analog-Skala (VAS). Pharmacopsychiatria 15: 90–94.

11. Fahrenberg, J., Selg, H., and Hampel, R. 1978. Freiburger Persönlichkeitsinventar. Hogrefe, Göttingen.
12. Gebhardt, R., Helmchen, H., Hippius, H., Kerekjarto, M. v., Lienert, G. A., and Refordt, E. 1969. Beurteilungsskalen (rating scales) and Merkmalslisten für depressive Syndrome. In: H. Hippius and H. Selbach (eds.), Das depressive Syndrom, pp. 603–643. Urban & Schwarzenberg, Munich.
13. Hamilton, M. 1960. Ratingscale für Depression. J. Neurol. Neurosurg. Psychiatry 23: 56–62.
14. Hampel, R. 1977. Adjektiv-Skala zur Einschätzung der Stimmung, SES. Diagnostica 23: 43–61.
15. Hautzinger, M., and Herrmann, C. 1981. Erfassung von Depression: Ebenen, Möglichkeiten und Probleme. In: M. Hautzinger and S. Greif (eds.), Kognitionspsychologie der Depression. Kohlhammer, Stuttgart.
16. Hecheltjen, G., and Mertesdorf, F. 1973. Mehrdimensionaler Stimmungsfragebogen. MSF. Gruppendynamik 2: 110–122.
17. Janke, W., and Debus, G. 1978. Die Eigenschaftswörterliste EWL. Handanweisung. Hogrefe, Göttingen.
18. Kammer, D. 1983. Eine Untersuchung der psychometrischen Eigenschaften des deutschen Beck-Depressions-Inventars (BDI). Diagnostica 29: 48–60.
19. Kerekjarto, M. v. 1969. Die Hamburger Depressionsskala. In: H. Hippius and H. Selbach (eds.), Das depressive Syndrom. Urban & Schwarzenberg, Munich.
20. Kerekjarto, M. v., and Lienert, G. A. 1970. Depressionsskalen als Forschungsmittel in der Psychopathologie. Pharmakopsychiatria 3: 1–21.
21. Krautzig, E., and Linden, M. 1980. Depressionsdiagnostik bei Untersuchungen an Studenten. Theoretische Richtlinien und empirische Normen zur HDS. In: M. Hautzinger and W. Schulz (eds.), Klinische Psychologie und Psychotherapie. 3rd Ed. DGVT und GwG, Tübingen.
22. Lehrl, S., and Gallwitz, A. 1977. Erlanger Depressions-Skala (EDS) Manual. Kless, Munich.
23. Lehrl, S., Straub, R., and Straub, B. 1976. Ein Vergleich von Beurteilungsskalen und Leistungsverfahren für die Schweregradmessung zyklothymer Depressionen. Pharmakopsychiatria 9: 247–256.
24. Lukesch, H. 1974. Testgütekriterien für das Depressions-Inventar von A. T. Beck. Psychologie und Praxis 18: 60–78.
25. Möller, H. J., and Zerssen, D. v. 1983. Psychopathometrische Verfahren: II. Standardisierte Beurteilungsverfahren. Nervenarzt 54: 1–16.
26. Obermair, W., Rickels, K., and Stoll, K.-D. 1981. Test zur Erfassung der Schwere der Depression. In: CIPS (ed.), Internationale Skalen für Psychiatrie. Beltz, Weinheim.
27. Perris, C. 1972. Ein für Längsschnittstudien geeignetes Untersuchungsinstrument zur qualitativen Charakterisierung von depressiven Syndromen. (Qualitatives Depressions-Inventorium - QDI). Pharmakopsychiatria 5: 269–282.
28. Renfordt, E. 1978. Fortschritte in der klinisch-psychopharmakologischen Forschung durch fernsehtechnische Hilfsmittel. Pharmakopsychiatria 11: 266–284.
29. Renfordt, E., and Busch, H. 1976. Time-Blind-Analysis of TV-Stored Interview: An Objective Method of Study Antidepressive Drug-Effects. Int. Pharmacophsychiatry 11: 129–134.
30. Renfordt, E., and Busch, H. 1976. Neue Strategien psychiatrischer Urteilsbildung durch Anwendung audiovisueller Techniken. Pharmakopsychiatria 9: 67–75.
31. Renfordt, E., Busch, H., Fähndrich, E., and Müller-Oerlinghausen, B. 1976. Untersuchung einer neuen antidepressiven Substanz (Viloxazin) mit Hilfe der Zeit-Reihen-Analyse TV-gespeicherter Interviews. Arzneim.-Forsch. (Drug Res.) 26: 1114–1116.
32. Schmidtchen, S., Kerekjarto, M. v., and Heim, H. 1972. Quantitative assessment of the development of depressions. Diagnostica 19: 49–62.
33. Spitzer, R. L., Endicott, J., Robins, E., and Klein, H. E. 1982. Forschungs-Diagnose Kriterien (RDC). Beltz, Weinheim.
34. Supprian, U. 1975. Die Eppendorfer Stimmung-Antriebs-Skala (ESTA). Pharmakopsychiatria 1: 8–25.
35. Ulrich, G. 1977. Video-analytische Methoden zur Erfassung averbaler Verhaltensparameter bei depressiven Syndromen. Pharmakopsychiatria 10: 176–182.
36. Ulrich, G. 1980. Verhaltensphysiologische und vigilanztheoretische Aspekte des Handbewegungsverhaltens Depressiver in einer Interviewsituation. Nervenarzt 51: 294–301.

37. Ulrich, G., and Harms, K. 1979. Video-analytic study of manual kinetics and its lateralization in the course of treatment of depressive syndromes. Acta Psychiatr. Scand. 59: 481–492.
38. Ulrich, G., Harms, K., and Fleischhauer, J. 1976. Untersuchungen mit einer verhaltensorientierten Schätzskala für depressive Hemmung und Agitation. Arzneim.-Forsch. (Drug Res.) 26: 1117–1119.
39. Ulrich, R., and Ulrich, R. 1978. Das Emotionalitätsinventar Testmanual EMI-B. Pfeiffer, Munich.
40. Wing, J. K., Cooper, J. E., Sartorius, N., and Cranach, M. v. 1982. Die Erfassung und Klassifikation psychiatrischer Symptome. Beltz, Weinheim.
41. Zerssen, D. v. 1976. Klinische Selbstbeurteilungsskalen (KSb-S) aus dem Münchner Psychiatrischen Informationssystem (PSYCHIS München) Manual a) allgemeiner Teil, b) Paranoid-Depressionsskala, c) Befindlichkeitsskala, d) Beschwerdeliste. Beltz, Weinheim.
42. Zerssen, D. v., Koeller, D. M., and Rey, E. R. 1970. Die Befindlichkeitsskala (B-S) – ein einfaches Instrument zur Objektivierung von Befindlichkeitsstörungen, insbesondere im Rahmen von Längsschnitt-Untersuchungen. Arzneim.-Forsch. 20: 915–918.

Chapter 2 Systems and Scales for the Assessment of Depression in French-Speaking Countries

D. BOBON

Introduction

Recent surveys of psychometric instruments in French, especially on depression, are to be found in a 235-page report on therapeutic trials in psychiatry at the 76th Annual Congress of French-Speaking Psychiatrists in Charleroi/Belgium in June 1978 [23], in the proceedings of a symposium on depressive symptomatology held in November 1978 in Paris [37], in a chapter of a Canadian textbook of psychiatry published in French [20] and in Mendlewicz's treatise of biological psychiatry [7a]. Ruillon [46] reviewed the use of depression rating scales by French general practitioners.

This survey begins by discussing briefly ICD, DSM, and PSE systems. Reviews follow of rating scales that have been developed in France (Widlöcher's Retardation Scale, AMDP Syndromic Scale) or substantially modified (Beck Depression Inventory) for use in French. The most frequently used observer scales and self-rating scales translated into French are mentioned. Finally, less-applied or less-validated scales are referred to.

The present survey leaves out applications of performance tests and projective techniques in the assessment of depression but the potential usefulness of these techniques in quantitative psychopathology should not be underestimated. For example, performance tests contribute to the understanding of electrodermal responses [30], whereas Rorschach variables are related to endocrinological subgroups in patients with impotence [31], or to low 5-hydroxyindole-acetic acid levels in the CSF [47].

Diagnostic Instruments

International Classification of Diseases (ICD-9)

The ninth revision of this classification has been literally translated into French by the WHO [32] whereas Bobon [5] adapted its diagnostic headings to the usual French terminology. Contrary to the previous revision [26], the INSERM has not published an official French classification more or less compatible with ICD.

Despite the fact that ICD-9 allows a clinically logical classification of mental disorders, its application has been superseded in research by the RDC and quite recently by DSM-III (see below).

Research Diagnostic Criteria (RDC)
Diagnostic and Statistical Manual (DSM-III)

The initial St. Louis criteria were translated by Plantey and Pringuey [44]. The derived Spitzer RDC have been rapidly adopted for selecting and describing depressed patients; their official translation [2] has been delayed until the publication of DSM-III [43].

As regards depression, the RDC categories are more comprehensive than the DSM; their interrater reliability is high but at an untested risk of a loss of validity (e.g., in the case of "dysthymic disorders" versus "neurotic depression").

ICD-9 and DSM-III have been compared by Bobon [5], more recently by Cosyns et al. [16], and by Dongier and Lehmann [19]. The latter authors express a common wish that ICD-10 and DSM-IV will come closer to one another and benefit from their respective advantages.

Present State Examination (PSE)

The PSE and the CATEGO computer classification have only recently been translated into French [58]. The 140 items lead to 38 syndrome scores – calculated in percentages on the basis of 1–15 items and derived from clinical factors instead of empirical factors – and to categories to an extent corresponding to ICD-8 diagnoses.

The usefulness of the PSE in the measurement of change appears limited.

Original French Scales

Retardation Scale (Echelle de ralentissement dépressif, ERD)

A team of psychiatrists and biometricians headed by Daniel Widlöcher at the Salpêtrière Hospital have elaborated a 15-item scale sensitive to depressive retardation and to changes under treatment with antidepressants. All items are graded from 0 to 4 with precise severity criteria. They evaluate gait, slowness versus paucity of movements (limbs, trunk), slowness versus paucity of movements (head, mimic), language and verbal flow, modulation of speech, brevity of responses, poverty of ideas, richness of associations, subjective experience of ruminations, fatigability, interest in habitual activities, patient's perception of the flow of time, memory, and concentration (official English translation by Michael Stone).

The original publication describes the careful construction and validation of two experimental versions of the scale, i.e., as regards its sensitivity to changes under treatment with antidepressants [27]. Principal component factor analyses of the final version with and without the items of the Hamilton Rating Scale for Depression demonstrate the unidimensional character of the Widlöcher scale and its validity for the measurement of depressive retardation, in inpatients [57] as well as outpatients [28].

AMDP Syndromic Scale (AMDP-SY)

The 1979 revision of the Psychopathology Scale developed by the Association for Methodology and Documentation in Psychiatry is made of 100 items + 15 write-in items (see p. 13). In anticipation of the validation of the factors which would be generated by factor analyses of results obtained in a group of Belgian and French patients with different diagnoses, a 12-item scale corresponding to the AMDP factors found in previously published analyses of the former German version was filled in for 388 patients along with the complete AMDP scale, and in 58 of these patients along with the Brief Psychiatric Rating Scale (BPRS). The results point to the superiority of this brief AMDP scale over the BPRS [13].

The final 17-item version of the AMDP Syndromic Scale evaluates the following functions: obsessions, hypochondriasis, exaggeration of affects, anxiety, depression, retardation, agitation, manic mood, hostility, delusions-hallucinations, syndrome of alien influence, dissociation-depersonalization, disorders of consciousness-orientation-memory, somatic complaints, vegetative symptoms, insomnia, and extrapyramidal symptoms. It has been elaborated and validated in Liège, later adopted by the AMDP French-speaking group, but still has to be officialized by other AMDP sections; in other words, it does not belong to the basic AMDP System yet.

Beck-Pichot Depression Inventory (BDI)

The Beck Depression Inventory (BDI) was translated by Delay et al. [17]. In 1966, Pichot et al. [38] added 12 items aimed at a better evaluation of endogenous and melancholic ideas of poverty, tension, lack of concentration, retardation, early insomnia, obsessions, monoideism, anxiety, restlessness, affective anesthesia, irrecoverability, and increased appetite. The sensitivity to change of this 33-item combined Beck-Pichot Inventory is illustrated by Agius et al. [1] and by Pichot [36].

In order to shorten the procedure, a 25-item version combining the 13 items of the BDI short form [3] and the 12 French items [38] was put to the test in Liège on 136 subjects. Total scores of this BP-25 version are significantly different in manic, euthymic, and depressed patients; they are significantly correlated with BfS/BfS'-self ratings (details on this scale below) and with self-rated as well as observer-rated Visual Analogue Scales [49]. Factor analyses of the 25 items and of the first 13 items from the BDI indicate that the variance amounts to 66% in both cases, that all items have a high positive loading in the first principal component, and that the short form of the BDI contains three factors like in the American analysis (retardation, guilt, somatic disturbances), whereas the Beck-Pichot combination contains a fourth factor on anxiety [12].

On the same sample, a reparametrization method for optimal scaling shows that there are differences between the a priori scaling of some items and the empirical data; these differences do not influence the item loadings in the first principal component but do modify the factor structure after orthogonal rotation [55]. A further weakness of the BDI lies in its multiple-choice questions which often worsen the patient's perplexity. Despite the fact that it is primarily a mood scale and not only a depression scale, the BfS/BfS' has definite advantages over the BDI (see below).

Most Frequently Used Observer Scales Translated from Other Languages into French

Hamilton Rating Scale for Depression (HAM-D)

A first translation of the 24-item version of the HAM-D was done by Pichot in 1969; it was called the DH69 (unpublished). This translation was used in the great majority of antidepressant trials in the French-speaking countries.

A slightly modified version, giving the same total score as the DH69, was put forward in 1978 by the Psychometric Commission of the Belgian College of Neuropsychopharmacology and Biological Psychiatry. Von Frenckell and Lottin [54] demonstrated that the last three items on helplessness, hopelessness, and worthlessness - the so-called Klerman items - reach high mean scores in depressed patients and account for an upper cutoff score for depression at 32; the authors found a lower cutoff score at 23 in a Belgian sample (with the 24-item version) against 20 in a Canadian sample (with the 21-item version).

Montgomery and Åsberg Depression Rating Scale (MADRS)

The back-translated official adaptation by Bobon of the ten-item Montgomery and Åsberg Depression Scale extracted from the 67-item Comprehensive Psychopathological Rating Scale, or CPRS (see below), was presented at the Paris symposium on depressive symptomatology [50].

Results of a pilot study on 44 patients from St. Etienne [34] speak for the scale's validity and sensitivity: its correlation coefficients are 0.88 with the HAM-D and 0.55 with the BfS ($P < 0.001$); its mean scores for three degrees of severity of depression evaluated by an external criterion are significantly different from each other.

In a larger sample of 103 depressed patients from Liège and St. Etienne, the correlation coefficients reach a higher level of significance: 0.89 with HAM-D, 0.78 with BfS', and 0.74 with BfS' (unpublished data presented at the Third World Congress of Biological Psychiatry, Stockholm, 1981). According to the same method as for the HAM-D there seems to be cutoff scores for depression at 20 and 33. In 36 patients before and after antidepressants, the t-value for paired samples was 7.77 for the MADRS and 7.45 for the HAM-D ($P<0.0001$), against 3.46 and 3.10 for the BfS and BfS' self-ratings ($P<0.004$) (same unpublished data).

Brief Psychiatric Rating Scale (BPRS)

The French version of the 18-item BPRS was published by Pichot et al. in 1967 [39]. Comparing 12 American and French factor analyses, Pichot et al. [40] put forward five factors (delusional-hallucinatory, hebephrenic, paranoid, depressive, and acute psychotic) which by and large correspond to the factors recommended by the ECDEU Manual [24]. Overall [33] reviewed the application of the BPRS in antidepressant trials. The excessive number of categories of severity, namely eight, probably weakens the interrater reliability. In a doctoral thesis, von Frenckell [52] applied a reparametrization technique for optimal scaling to Overall's eight-point depression scale, demonstrating that the maximum number of severity grades should be five.

Association for Methodology and Documentation in Psychiatry (AMDP)

The system elaborated by this association is detailed in Chap. 10. The second French edition [6] is fully compatible with the German revision.

The French-speaking section of the AMDP, composed of Belgian, Canadian, French, and Swiss psychiatrists and psychologists who met on 16 occasions in 8 years from 1975 to 1982, took several initiatives within the frame of the international system. Among others it (a) elaborated a semistructured interview [10] which was applied to the time-blind evaluation of antidepressants [4, 7]; (b) added items on anxiety to the standard psychopathological items, generating a ten-factor solution similar to the German nine-factor solution plus an anxiety factor (the other nine factors of the French solution evaluate obsessions, dramatization, depression, retardation, organicity, dissociation-incoherence, delusions, mania, and dysphoria [13]); and (c) made a preliminary validation of the Zurich Mania-Depression Subscale [6, 59] and applied the separate scoring of manic and depressive subscores for the longitudinal study of manic and depressive mood swings.

Most Frequently Used Self-Rating Scales Translated from Other Languages into French

Minnesota Multiphasic Personality Inventory (MMPI)

The French adaptation of the MMPI and the calculation of French norms was done by Perse [35], and its first computerized analysis by Lewi and Pinchard [29]. The very first factor analysis of all 550 items was accomplished by von Frenckell [53]; it showed, among other findings, that HS and HY clinical scales belong to the same factor, as well as the PT and SC scales, whereas the D scale is heterogeneous. This heterogeneity of the MMPI depression scale was also criticized by Heimann et al. [25]. Glatt [22] compared the French, German, and Spanish translations of the MMPI in an experimental design and concluded that there are "gross deficiencies in the French translation."

The MMPI questions refer to traits and states. The sensitivity of MMPI to change is therefore limited. However, Delay et al. [18], in Chaps. V–VII of their textbook on psychometric methods, as well as a recent study on stress and blood platelets by the Mertens group [51] show that the scale has sensitivity to change. Nevertheless, administration of the full MMPI is time-consuming and seldom feasible for depressed patients; its short forms have not been sufficiently validated.

BfS/BfS' Mood Scales (Zerssen's Befindlichkeits-Skala)
AMS (Affective Mood Scales)

Elaborated in 1970, the BfS and BfS' self-rating mood scales were surveyed in 1974 by von Zerssen et al. [56 and Chap. 25]. They consist of two equivalent forms of 28 pairs of antonymic adjectives, such as "right now, I am feeling rather alert (= 0 pt), rather listless (= 2 pts), or neither nor (= 1 pt)," the total score ranging from zero in manic patients to 56 in severe depressives.

The validation of the BfS/BfS' in French [8, 9, 11, 25] confirmed the excellent psychometric properties of the instrument:

1. The two equivalent forms have, in all samples, a correlation coefficient of over 0.90; they can therefore be alternated in case of frequent administrations.
2. They correlate with instruments validated for the quantitative evaluation of depression (HAM-D, MADRS, etc.).
3. The mean scores for manic patients, normals, neurotic depressives, and endogenous depressives are almost identical in the original samples (Munich) and in the French validation samples (Liège); they constitute normative data for the classification of a single patient on a manic-depression continuum.
4. Bimodal results suggest that a cutoff score of 26 for depression holds for both forms.
5. Both forms are sensitive to drug induced changes [11]; they reflect manic and depressive swings.

Miscellaneous

Ad hoc 100-mm Visual Analogue Scales (VASs) are widely used for measuring intraindividual changes in short intervals; it should be named the Scott scale according to its originator (see the history of the VAS in [8]).

Among observer's scales, the comprehensive behavioral scales such as the Inpatient Multidimensional Psychiatric Scale (IMPS) and the Wittenborn scales have almost been abandoned in favor of the psychopathological-phenomenological scales AMDP and PSE. Overall's depression scale [45, 52] and the WHO Schedule for Standardized Assessment of Depressive Disorders (SADD) [48] have not yet been able to compete with the HAM-D or the MADRS. In contrast, the Newcastle Anxiety-Depression Scale raises increasing interest but has not yet been published in French. The Nurses' Observation Scale for Inpatient Evaluation (NOSIE 30) is not uncommon in drug trials [41].

As for self-rating scales, Zung's Self-rating Depression Scale is occasionally used but it has not been validated in French. Heimann et al. [25] have pointed to its frequently reported lack of sensitivity; the Canadian study by Bobon et al. [11] reaches the same negative conclusion. As for the more promising Profile of Mood States (POMS), it exists in draft form but has not yet been published in French. Cattell's anxiety scale (ASQ, sometimes known as the IPAT anxiety scale in reference to the Institute for Personality and Ability Testing) is characterized by a subscore on depressive guilt which is sensitive to drug induced changes, but the other subscores are not related to depression and are less sensitive; moreover, the French translations differ in France [14] and Canada [15]. On the other hand, the ASQ/IPAT is recommended for measuring depressive traits.

The Stockton Geriatric Scale (SGRS) has been translated by Pichot et al. [42] and applied by Freyens and others [21].

Conclusions

The ICD, RDC, DSM, and the Newcastle Scale can help in making the nosological diagnosis of depression.

The severity of depression and its therapeutic responsiveness can be best evaluated with the HAM-D and MADRS observer scales, not forgetting the AMDP Mania-Depression Scale; with the BfS/BfS' self-rating scales, the AMDP-MD is the only depression scale at present that allows the longitudinal visualization of mood swings. Another specific scale, the Widlöcher Retardation Scale, is a valuable measure too, but its differences with the HAM-D and MADRS scales should be further explored. In order to describe a sample before treatment and to detect syndromatic shifts after treatment which cannot be achieved by a specific scale (e. g., a worsening of dysphoria and anxiety) a multifactorial scale such as the full AMDP can be applied before and after treatment.

The Cattell and MMPI questionnaires can be used for the assessment of depressive traits.

The number of adequately translated and validated diagnostic systems and rating scales has considerably increased in French-speaking countries in the past decade.

Acknowledgments. Drs P. Dick (Geneva), A. Gérard, and J. D. Guelfi (Paris) and Y. D. Lapierre (Ottawa) have kindly contributed to documenting the present survey.

References

1. Agius, S., Eisert, H. G., and Heimann, H. 1970. Essai de classification psychologique et physiologique du syndrome dépressif. Schweiz. Arch. Neurol. Neurochir. Psychiatr. 106: 105–120.
2. Ansseau, M. 1985. Critères de diagnostic pour la recherche en psychiatrie développés par Spitzer, Endicott et Robins (research diagnostic criteria). Acta Psychiatr. Belg. 85: 253–324.
3. Beck, A. T., and Beck, R. W. 1972. Screening depressed patients in family practice: a rapid technique. Postgrad. Med. 52: 81–85.
4. Bobon, D. P. 1978. Time-blind evaluation of psychopathology in drug research. Acta Psychiatr. Belg. 78: 635–645.
5. Bobon, D. P. 1980. Description et comparaison de la révision de deux classifications des maladies mentales: la CIM-9 (ICD-9) et la DSM-III. Acta Psychiatr. Belg. 80: 846–863.
6. Bobon, D. P. (ed.). 1981. Le Système AMDP. 2nd Ed. Mardaga, Bruxelles.
7. Bobon, D. P. 1983. Foreign adaptations of the AMDP-System. In: D. P. Bobon et al. (eds.), The AMDP System in Psychopharmacology, pp 19–34. Karger, Basel.
7a. Bobon, D. P. 1985. Psychopathologie quantitative et mesure du changement. In: J. Mendlewicz (ed.) Traité de psychiatrie biologique. Masson, Paris (in press).
8. Bobon, D. P., and Bobon-Schrod H. 1974. Les listes d'adjectifs BS/BS' de Zerssen et la ligne de Scott: Deux auto-évaluations de l'humeur. Feuille Psychiatr. Liège 7: 492–508.
9. Bobon, D. P., and von Frenckell, R. 1981. Validation française de la "Befindlichkeits-Skala" (BfS/BfS'), échelle d'auto-évaluation de l'humeur de Zerssen. In: P. Pichot and C. Pull (eds.), La symptomatologie dépressive: enregistrement et évaluation, pp. 31–44. Ciba-Geigy, Paris.
10. Bobon, D. P., Mormont, C., and Mirel, J. 1978. Un entretien psychopathologique semi-structuré adapté à l'échelle AMDP et à l'évaluation vidéo en temps aveugle. Acta Psychiatr. Belg. 78: 606–618.
11. Bobon, D. P., Lapierre, Y. D., and Lottin, T. 1981. Validity and sensitivity of the French version of the Zerssen BfS/BfS' self-rating mood scale during treatment with Trazodone and Amitriptyline. Progr. Neuropsychopharmacol. 5: 519–522.
12. Bobon, D. P., Sanchez-Blanque, A., and von Frenckell, R. 1981. Comparison between the short form of the Beck Depression Inventory and the combined Beck-Pichot Inventory. A factor-analytic study. J. Psychiatr. Biol. Thér. 1: 23–26.
13. Bobon, D. P., Mormont, C., Doumont, A., Mirel, J., Bonhomme, P., Ansseau, M., Pellet, J., Pull, C., De Buck, R., Gernay, P., Mormont, I., Lang, F., Lejeune, J., Bronckart, C., and von Frenckell, R. 1982. Analyse factorielle de la révision française de l'échelle AMDP. Résultats d'une étude internationale de 388 cas. Acta Psychiatr. Belg. 82: 371–389.
14. Cattell, R. B. 1962. Manuel de l'échelle d'anxiété de Cattell. Centre de Psychologie Appliquée, Paris.
15. Cormier, D. 1962. L'échelle d'anxiété IPAT: Manuel. Institut de Recherches Psychologiques, Montréal.
16. Cosyns, P., Ansseau, M., and Bobon, D. 1983. The use of DSM-III in Belgium. In: R. L. Spitzer et al. (eds.), International perspectives on DSM-III, pp. 127–133. American Psychiatric Association, Washington.
17. Delay, J., Pichot, P., Lemperiere, T., and Mirouze, R. 1963. La nosologie des états dépressifs. Rapports entre l'étiologie et la sémiologie. Résultats du questionnaire de Beck. Encéphale 52: 497–505.

18. Delay, J., Pichot, P., and Perse, J. 1966. Méthodes psychométriques en clinique. 2nd Ed. Masson, Paris.
19. Dongier, M., and Lehmann, H. 1982. Nouveaux systèmes de classification diagnostique (DSM-III et ICD-9). Encyclopédie Médico-chirurgicale. Psychiatrie 37065: A10.
20. Duguay, R. and Ellenberger, H.F., (eds.). 1981. Précis pratique de psychiatrie. Chenelière, Montreal.
21. Freyens, R. 1976. Application d'une échelle d'appréciation gériatrique aux patients d'un hôpital psychiatrique fermé. Acta Psychiatr. Belg. 76: 586-598.
22. Glatt, K.M. 1969. An evaluation of the French, Spanish and German translations of the MMPI. Acta Psychol. (Amst) 29: 65-84.
23. Guelfi, J.D., Dreyfus, J.F., and Pull, C.B. 1978. Les essais thérapeutiques en psychiatrie: méthodologie, éthique et législation. Masson, Paris.
24. Guy, W. (ed.). 1976. ECDEU Assessment Manual for Psychopharmacology. National Institute of Mental Health, Rockville.
25. Heimann, H., Bobon-Schrod, H., Schmocker, A.M., and Bobon, D.P. 1975. Auto-évaluation de l'humeur par une liste d'adjectifs, la "Befindlichkeits-Skala" (BS) de Zerssen. Encéphale 1: 165-183.
26. Institut national de la santé et de la recherche médicale. 1969. Classification française des troubles mentaux. Bull INSERM 24 (suppl. 2).
27. Jouvent, R., Frechette, D., Binoux, F., Lancrenon, S., and des Lauriers, A. 1980. Le ralentissement psychomoteur dans les états dépressifs: construction d'une échelle d'évaluation quantitative. Encéphale 6: 41-58.
28. Jouvent, R., Lecrubier, Y., Steru, L., Lancrenon, S., and Widlöcher, D. 1981. Analyse multifactorielle de l'échelle de ralentissement dépressif utilisée chez les déprimés ambulatoires. Psychol. Méd. 13: 97-107.
29. Lewi, P.J., and Pinchard, A. 1967. An automated Minnesota Multiphasic Personality Inventory Test. Acta Psychol. (Amst) 27: 397-399.
30. Mormont, C. 1978. Relations et corrélations entre électrodermogramme et données psychométriques. Psychol. Méd. 10: 117-126.
31. Mormont, C., Legros, J.J., Servais, J., and von Frenckell, R. 1980. Mise en évidence de profils psychologiques différents dans un échantillon d'impuissants érectifs. Acta Psychiatr. Belg. 80: 476-486.
32. Organisation Mondiale de la Santé. 1979. Troubles mentaux: glossaire et guide de classification en concordance avec la neuvième révision de la Classification Internationale des Maladies. OMS, Genève.
33. Overall, J.E. 1981. Des critères pour le diagnostic de dépression. In: P. Pichot and C. Pull (eds.), La symptomatologie dépressive: enregistrement et évaluation, pp. 15-26. Ciba-Geigy, Paris.
34. Pellet, J., Bobon, D.P., Mormont, I., Lang, F., and Massardie, R. 1981. Etude princeps de validation française de la MADRS, sous-échelle Dépression de la CPRS. In: P. Sizaret (ed.), Comptes rendus du 78e Congrès de Psychiatrie et de Neurologie de Langue Française, pp. 297-301. Masson, Paris.
35. Perse, J. 1966. Manuel de l'Inventaire Multiphasique de Personnalité du Minnesota (MMPI). Centre de Psychologie Appliquée, Paris.
36. Pichot, P. 1971. Etude comparative de l'action de l'amitriptyline et d'une association amitriptyline-chlordiazepoxide. In: O. Vinar, Z. Votava, and P. Bradley (eds.) Advances in Neuropsychopharmacology, pp. 433-445. North-Holland, Amsterdam.
37. Pichot, P., and Pull, C. (eds.). 1981. La symptomatologie dépressive: enregistrement et évaluation. Ciba-Geigy, Paris.
38. Pichot, P., Piret, J., and Clyde, D.J. 1966. Analyse de la symptomatologie dépressive subjective. Rev. Psychol. Appl. 16: 105-115.
39. Pichot, P., Overall, J.E., and Gorham, D.R. 1967. Echelle abrégée d'appréciation psychiatrique. Centre de Psychologie Appliquée, Paris.
40. Pichot, P., Overall, J.E., Samuel-Lajeunesse, B., and Dreyfus, J.F. 1969. Structure factorielle de l'échelle abrégée d'appréciation psychiatrique BPRS. Rev. Psychol. Appl. 19: 217-232.
41. Pichot, P., Samuel-Lajeuness, B., Blanc, J., Galopin, D., and Selva, G. 1969. Une échelle d'observation du comportement en salle des malades mentaux hospitalisés: la NOSIE 30. Rev. Psychol. Appl. 19: 35-43.

42. Pichot, P., Girard, B., and Dreyfus, J.C. 1970. L'échelle d'appréciation gériatrique de Stockton (SGRS) Etude de sa version française. Rev. Psychol. Appl. 20: 245–254.
43. Pichot, P., and Guelfi, G.D., (eds.). 1983. DSM-III, manuel diagnostique et statistique des troubles mentaux. Masson, Paris.
44. Plantey, F., and Pringuey, D. 1978. Présentation et traduction des critères diagnostiques de l'Ecole de St Louis. Encéphale 4: 323–339.
45. Pull, C.B., Pichot, P., Pull, M.C., and von Frenckell, R. 1979. The principal dimensions of manifest depression. A factor analysis of manifest depressive symptomatology. Neuropsychobiology 5: 207–212.
46. Rouillon, F. 1981. Les applications de la psychopathologie quantitative à la dépression en médecine générale. Psychol. Méd. 13: 2139–2152.
47. Rydin, E., Schalling, D., and Åsberg, M. 1982. Rorschach ratings in depressed and suicidal patients with low levels of 5-hydroxyindoleacetic acid in cerebrospinal fluid. Psychiatry Res. 7: 229–243.
48. Sartorius, N., and Jablensky, A. 1981. Recherche multicentrique coordonnée par l'OMS sur l'évaluation des états dépressifs dans différentes cultures. In: P. Pichot and C. Pull (eds.), La symptomatologie dépressive: enregistrement et évaluation, pp 151–165. Ciba-Geigy, Paris.
49. Sanchez-Blanque, A., Bobon, D.P., and von Frenckell, R. 1980. Analyse factorielle d'une échelle d'auto-évaluation de Beck-Pichot abrégée ou BP-25. In: P. Sizaret (ed.), Comptes rendus 77e Congrès de Psychiatrie et de Neurologie de Langue Française, pp. 527–532. Masson, Paris.
50. Schalling, D., Åsberg, M., and Montgomery, S. 1981. CPRS et dépression: construction d'une nouvelle échelle d'appréciation de la psychopathologie et d'une sous-échelle de dépression. In: P. Pichot and C. Pull (eds.), La symptomatologie dépressive: enregistrement et évaluation, pp 107–117. Ciba-Geigy, Paris.
51. Van Imschoot, K., Liesse, M., Mertens, C., and Lauwers, P. 1982. La triade névrotique et la modification du nombre de plaquettes sanguines en réaction au stress. Encéphale 8: 501–510.
52. von Frenckell, R. 1979. Première application de la méthode de reparamétrisation Prinqual en psychopathologie quantitative. Thèse de doctorat en sciences biomédicales expérimentales. Clinique psychiatrique Universitaire, Liège.
53. von Frenckell, R. 1982. Analyse factorielle du Minnesota Multiphasic Personality Inventory (MMPI). Une étude de 2500 passations par l'analyse des correspondances. Thèse d'agrégation. Clinique psychiatrique Universitaire, Liège.
54. von Frenckell, R., and Lottin, T. 1982. Validation d'un seuil de la dépression: l'échelle d'Hamilton. Encéphale 8: 349–354.
55. von Frenckell, R., Sanchez-Blanque, A., and Bobon, D.P. 1981. Reparametrisation of the Beck-Pichot Depression Inventory. A contribution to optimal scaling. J Psychiatr. Biol. Thér. 1: 34–37.
56. von Zerssen, D., Strian, F., and Schwarz, D. 1974. Evaluation of depressive states, especially in longitudinal studies. In: P. Pichot and R. Olivier-Martin (eds.), Psychological Measurements in Psychopharmacology, pp 189–202. Karger, Basel.
57. Widlöcher, D. 1981. L'échelle de ralentissement dépressif: fondements théoriques et premières applications. Psychol. Méd. 13: 53–60.
58. Wing, J.K., Cooper, J.E., and Sartorius, N. 1980. Guide pour un examen psychiatrique. Traduit de l'anglais par M. Timsit-Berthie et A. Bragard-Ledent. Mardaga, Bruxelles.
59. Woggon, B., and Dittrich, A. 1979. Konstruktion übergeordneter AMP-Skalen: "manisch-depressives" und "schizophrenes Syndrom" Int. Pharmacopsychiatry 14: 325–337.

Chapter 3 Standardized Instruments for the Evaluation of Affective Disturbances in Spain and Spanish-Speaking Countries

J. J. LÓPEZ-IBOR JR. and J. M. LÓPEZ-IBOR

In Spain, as in other countries, the instruments for the evaluation of psychiatric conditions proliferated first as a consequence of the need to evaluate psychopathological changes after the introduction of psychopharmacological treatments, and later because of the interest in the epidemiology of psychiatric conditions.

Spanish psychiatry over the past decades has had its scientific roots in phenomenological orientations, and has as a common denominator an eclectic attitude to the schools of other countries (German-, French-, and English-speaking). Therefore it has had no difficulty in adopting the basic concepts which underlie the majority of the systems of evaluation. These principles are valid for psychiatry in the rest of the Spanish-speaking countries, although during the last few decades the social, cultural and political situation in them has led to the rise of a social psychiatry, too politically involved and in which the evaluative research has had very low priority. This trend is changing now, owing to the changing political situation in many countries and to the influence of psychiatrists trained abroad (in Spain, the United States, United Kingdom, Federal Republic of Germany, France, and Canada).

There are two approaches, more often complementary than not, for the evaluation of affective disturbances: the specific partial scales and the comprehensive systems. The former are more suitable for the measurement of changes induced by therapy or for epidemiological surveys; the latter can provide information for diagnosis or psychopathological classification, although both approaches have been used for various purposes. In addition, personality measurement instruments are sometimes used for the evaluation of affective disorders. Three of them have been thoroughly investigated for reliability and validity: MMPI (Minnesota Multiphasic Personality Inventory: TEA, [25]), 16PF [24] and CEP ("Control, Extroversión, Paranoidismo," [21]).

Regarding the specific partial scales and questionnaires, Conde [10] has made a major contribution by translating them into Spanish and in standardizing and validating them in Spain. He has done field reliability studies and proposed some modifications of the original scales. The following scales have been validated and standardized by Conde:

– Hamilton Rating Scale for Depression in different configurations (21 items, 17 items, 24 items, melancholia subscale of 6 items by Beck) and forms of application (individual, for small groups, for large groups) [10]

– Zung's Self-Rating Depression Scale. The Spanish version, which bears the name Zung-Conde [3], is the most widely used in epidemiological surveys, owing to its validation [6] and standardization [5] in Spanish. There are versions for general application, and Conde has been able to describe a fourth factor besides the three described by Zung (depressive factor, biological factor, and psychological factor), the psychosocial factor [4].

Conde has also published studies on the Beck depression inventory and the Beck-Pichot depression and anxiety inventory [7-9] in its different versions, which are correctly validated and standardized. Other instruments have been translated and are more or less widely used, although no validation or standardization studies have yet been carried out. The most common are: the Montgomery-Åsberg depression scale, the Carroll Rating Scale for Depression, the Hamilton Anxiety Rating Scale, Zung's Anxiety State Inventory, the Taylor Manifest Anxiety Scale or Iowa Manifest Anxiety Scale, the Raskin Depression Screen, the Covi Anxiety Scale, and the Anxiety and Depression Scale (ADS) by Hassanyeh, et al. [10]. Some scales are used for specific measurements in affective patients: López-Ibor Jr. has translated the von Zerssen Scale (unpublished), which measures premorbid personality of depressive patients (typus melancholichus Tellenbach), and Ramos and Irala [22] have developed an original scale for the measurement of obsessive personality traits that can be used for the same purpose. Ledesma's scale of aggressivity [13] is in the developing stage. Until now the "Test miokinético" of Mira y López [18] has been used for the evaluation of aggressivity in affective disorders [19].

For surveys with nonpsychiatric patients and with the general population, Goldberg's questionnaire has been widely studied and applied [20].

The use in Spain of the Diagnostic and Statistical Manual of Mental Disorder (DSM-III) has introduced the study of "life events", translated into Spanish as *acontecimientos* or *sucesos vitales,"* validating the original questionnaires [11], using parts of comprehensive systems (AMDP [23]) or developing original item lists [2].

The trend toward the use and development of comprehensive documentation systems of psychopathology has been very significant in Spain. Several of them have been translated and adapted by Barcia, such as Perris' Multiaspect Classification Model (MACM) and Overall's Factor Construct Rating Scale (FCRS) [1]. The system of the *Arbeitsgemeinschaft für Methodologie und Dokumentation in der Psychiatrie* (AMDP) has been translated by J.J. López-Ibor Jr. [14, 17] in Spain and Heinze [12] in Mexico. A section of Spanish-speaking countries of the working group has been created (chairman, J.J. López-Ibor Jr.), and basic studies have been carried out by Sánchez Blanqué [23].

The Computerized Unified Psychiatric Clinical Record (Historia Clínica Unificada, HCU) [15, 16] presents an original approach. It is an attempt to overcome the problem that traditional clinical records and case histories do not contain data suitable for use in research, and that data collected by a specific research method usually do not find their way into present-day management records. The HCU tries to combine both approaches, research and everyday clinical practice. It is a conventional clinical record, with three kinds of data in the same folder: (a) ordinary clinical texts, (b) well-defined items to be processed by computer, and (c) short texts, also to be processed by computer. The definition of the items in (b) is provided in every folder, making the use of complementary booklets unnecessary. These data can be used in research because of their clear definition. The free texts in (c) provide flexibility of the computerized data which is important in everyday practice. Both (b) and (c) are a summary of the ordinary texts in (a), that is, of the case history. In addition, the computer is programmed to provide a summary of the clinical report written in plain language, by combining the items in (b) and the texts in (c). In other words, the computer not only stores information for research purposes, but also provides the clinician with information of immediate practical usefulness. The whole system works with microcomputers [15], and its use is spreading in Spain and Spanish-speaking countries. The system can be supplemented with the usual instruments designed for more specific research. An English version is being developed at present.

References

1. Barcia, D. and López-Ibor Jr., J.J. 1982. Documentación e información en psiquiatría. In: C. Ruíz Ogara, D. Barcia, and J.J. López-Ibor Jr (eds), Psiquiatría, Vol. 2. Toray, Barcelona, p. 1268.
2. Castillon Zazurca, J.J., Campo, C., Linares, J.L., Pericay, J.M. and Tejedor, M.C. 1984. Elaboración de un cuestionario de cambios vitales adaptado a la población española. Actas Luso Esp. Neurol. Psiquiatr. 12: 17-26.
3. Conde, V. 1969. La Escala Heteroaplicada y Heterovalorada para la depresión de Zung-Conde. Facultad de Medicina de Salamanca. Cervantes, Salamanca.
4. Conde, V. and Esteban, T. 1974. Contribución al estudio de la SDS de Zung en una muestra estratificada de población normal. Revista de Psicología General y Aplicada 29: 515-553.
5. Conde, V. and Esteban, T. 1975. Fiabilidad de la SDS de Zung. Revista de Psicología General y Aplicada 30: 903-913.
6. Conde, V. and Esteban, T. 1975. Validez de la SDS de Zung. Arch. Neurobiol. 38: 225-246.
7. Conde, V. and Useros, E. 1975. Adaptación castellana a la escala de evaluación conductal para la depresión de Beck. Revista de Psiquiatría y Psicología Médica de Europa y América 12: 217-236.
8. Conde, V., Esteban, T. and Useros, E. 1976. Revisión crítica de la adaptación castellana del cuestionario de Beck. Revista de Psicología General y Aplicada 31: 469-417.
9. Conde, V., Esteban, T. and Useros, E. 1976. Estudio crítico de la fiabilidad y validez de la EEC para la medida de depresión de Beck. Arch. Neurobiol. 39: 313-338.
10. Conde, V. and Franch, J.I. 1984. Escalas de evaluación comportamental para la cuantificación de la sintomatología psicopatológica en los trastornos angustiosos y depresivos. Upjohn Farmaquímica, Madrid.
11. Gonzalez de Rivera, J.L. 1983. Diferencias objetivas y subjetivas en la puntuación de una escala de sucesos vitales. Actas Luso Esp. Neurol. Psiquiatr. 11: 152-159.
12. Heinze, G. 1982. La versión española del Sistema AMDP en la enseñanza e investigación en México. Actas Luso Esp. Neurol. Psiquiatr. 6: 427-429.
13. Ledesma Jimeno, M.A. 1964. Fundamentos teóricos para la exploración de la agresividad. Revista de Psicología General y Aplicada 73, 608-614.
14. Lopez-Ibor Jr., J.J. 1980. El sistema A.M.D.P. Manual para la documentación de los hallazgos psiquiátricos de la Asociación para la Metodología y Documentación en Psiquiatría. Garsi, Madrid.
15. López-Ibor Jr., J.J. 1981. Historia Clínica Unificada. Garsi, Madrid.
16. López-Ibor Jr. J.J., Abad, R., Rey, G. and J. López-Ibor. 1985. The Unified Clinical Record (HCU). In: P. Berner et al. (eds.), Psychiatry: The State of the Art, pp. 147-152, Vol. 1. Plenum, New York.
17. López-Ibor Jr, J.J., Sánchez Blanqué, A. and Sansebastian, J. 1985. Spanish adaptation of the AMDP System. In: P. Berner et al. (eds.), Psychiatry: The State of the Art, pp. 167-172, Vol. 1. Plenum, New York.
18. Mira López, E. 1982. Psicodiagnóstico miokinético. Paidos, Buenos Aires.
19. Moriñigo Dominguez, A. 1981. Agresividad y psicosis maníaco-depresiva. Un estudio con el test miokinético de E. Mira y López. Actas Luso Esp. Neurol. Psiquiatr. 9: 125-136.

20. Muñoz, P. E., Vazquez Barquero, J. L., Rodriguez Insausti, F., Pastrana, E. and Varo, J. 1979. Adaptación española del General Health Questionnaire de D. P. Goldberg. Arch. Neurobiol. 42: 139-158.
21. Pinillos, J. L. 1960. Consistencia y validez del cuestionario de personalidad C. E. P. Revista de Psicología General y Aplicada 155: 65-76.
22. Ramos Brieva, J. A. and Irala San-Jose, M. V. 1983. Mini-inventario de rasgos anancásticos de personalidad (MIRAP). Actas Luso Esp. Neurol. Psiquiatr. 11: 219-230.
23. Sánchez Blanqué, A. 1982. La notation des événements pathogènes en psychiatrie par le System AMDP. Différences entre malades déprimés et non déprimés. Acta Psychiatr. Belg. 82: 390-397.
24. Seisdedos Cubero, M. 1968. 16PF, Monografía técnica. TEA, Madrid.
25. TEA 1967. Adaptación española del cuestionario de personalidad MMPI. TEA, Madrid.

Chapter 4 The Area of the Bulgarian People's Republic, Czechoslovak Socialist Republic, Polish People's Republic, Union of Soviet Socialist Republics and Socialist Federative Republic of Yugoslavia

C. ŠKODA and O. VINAŘ

The Slavic language area is located in central and eastern Europe. Slavic languages are spoken in Bulgaria, Czechoslovakia, Poland, the Soviet Union, and Yugoslavia. These countries have had different histories and have developed their cultures under different influences. Therefore, psychiatry also went through a different evolution, and only in the past 2-3 decades have common features become more important. Similar political atmosphere with the official acceptance of Marxist materialism has had a determinant role in this development.

In the Soviet Union, the development of a standardized assessment of psychopathology has been hindered by the view held by several influential psychiatrists that one could not express in figures the fine aspects of the mental state of psychiatric patients. Well-known Russian psychiatrists of the classical era (Korsakov, Kandinski) put great emphasis on a subtle description of symptoms of individual patients, and this tradition helped to prolong the discussion among younger, statistically-minded doctors and those who maintained that any attempt to translate a sensitive description into figures was condemned to failure. Therefore, only in recent years can papers be found in Soviet psychiatric journals using standardized rating scales, inventories, or questionnaires. The majority of these instruments were not published at all; they are a part of instructions or methodological directives issued by health authorities, or, in the minority of cases, they were published in proceedings of local psychiatric meetings or annual reports of psychiatric institutions. Data on validity or reliability of instruments are lacking in these publications.

There are several systems for registration of all psychiatric symptoms, which also enables their intensity or frequency to be estimated. Items on depressive symptoms are an integral part of such systems:

1. A comprehensive system was elaborated by Zharikov, Rudenko, and Zaitsev [41] which became obligatory with the organization of clinical drug trials approved by the Pharmacological Committee of the Ministry of Health of the USSR. The system represents an inventory of 92 productive ("plus" signed) psychiatric symptoms or syndromes and a similar list of 13 ("minus") symptoms or syndromes of mental defect. A rating of the intensity of all these symptoms is possible. A part of instructions on how to perform clinical trials for psychotropic drugs is devoted to antidepressants. Nevertheless, no special rating scale for the evaluation of depression was proposed for clinical investigators apart from the general inventory. Similar situations can be found with other systems used in the Soviet Union, e.g.,
2. Evaluation of the clinical state of psychiatric patients developed in the Psychiatric Department of the University of Tartu (J. Saarma, unpublished).

3. The system used in the Institute of Clinical Psychiatry of the Academy of Medical Sciences of the USSR (unpublished).
4. The system used in the Institute of Psychiatry of the Ministry of Health of the Russian SSR, etc.
5. A special chart (status praesens, variant 2) is a part of the last system developed by Zaitsev and Prochorova. It was designed for evaluation of affective disorders (and consequently not only for depressions). It consists of 71 items which can be rated according to the intensity of a symptom on a scale from 0 to 3.

Few attempts to develop a special rating scale for depression or anxiety can be found. In his dissertation Nuller [22] stated that an attempt should be made to assess Kraepelin's triads of depressive syndromes in research on effects of antidepressant drugs. He finds that Hamilton's [14] rating scale could serve the purpose. Using as a point of departure his and his wife's work [18, 21] he defines a rating scale (depressive patient's chart). Seven main syndromes are rated to be absent (0) or present to a described degree (1-3 or 4 or 5) and a symptom inversion scoring (−1) is provided for: mood, anxiety-fear, sociability, interests, quantitative psychomotor disturbance, thought disturbance [various kinds of delusion − self-deprecation, hypochondriac, persecutory; anancastic syndrome; bradypsychia (slowing of thought and speech)], and depersonalization [auto- (anesthesia dolorosa) somato- and time perception]. In addition seven somatic syndromes of depressions are defined: changes in weight, arterial tension, pulse, stool, urination, appetite, and sleep disturbances. In the same dissertation a short review of foreign and Soviet publications is included. Among the Soviet publications the reviews by Zaitsev [40] and Sopozjenin [24] document the interest of Soviet psychiatrists in this problem area. Improving the validity of the measurements by means of operational definition of each score and the problem of equidistance of separate scores on each item's ordinate scales are mentioned in the discussion of the topic.

Alexandrovski [1] developed a system to evaluate the clinical effects of anxiolytic drugs. Forty-eight symptoms grouped in eight syndromes can be rated as present or absent. Depression and anxiety are among the syndromes.

In Yugoslavia Bohaček and Sartorius [6] have developed a method for standardized assessment of psychopathological symptoms and their change over time. The Hamilton, Beck, Zung, and occasionally the Vinař scales, have been used in clinical research of depression. Recently the WHO Standardized Assessment of Depressive Disorders (SADD) scale (WHO, 1982) has been translated into Serbocroatian by Bohaček.

In Bulgaria, a rating scale for depressive illness was constructed by Tashev et al. [30]. Fifty symptoms can be evaluated with the help of this scale. The same author used an inventory for self-evaluation of patients with neurotic depressions where 53 symptoms and five syndromes can be quantitatively described. Other authors (e.g., Milev et al.) use a rating scale of Bojanovsky and Chloupkova [7].

In evident contrast to a more pragmatic use of various methods of assessment of information in psychiatry in other Slavic language areas, a substantial amount of theoretical and psychometric work has been done in Czechoslovakia, where a complex of new methods, covering the assessment of psychotic (FKP, [38]), and depressive (FKD, [31]) conditions, treatment of emergent symptomatology (DVP, [34];

previously a scale for assessing side-effects – VP, [32]) has come into general use in the clinical testing of psychotropic drugs [33, 36]. From the historical point of view it may be interesting to note that as early as the turn of the century the medical students of Prague's Charles University had been instructed to use a standardized psychiatric micro-interview during the lectures in psychiatry given by Heveroch [16]. Twenty simple questions learnt by heart were put by the students to patients, whose responses were recorded in short-hand reports. Based on a thoughtful comparative analysis of this unique material, "Diagnostics of Mental Illness" was published in 1906, and remains a classic example of the utilization of methodology, to which so much attention has been paid in recent years.

Much psychological, pedagogical, and behavioural research since World War II in Czechoslovakia has been based on stimulus standardization. Summarizing monographs have been published recently about measurement in general [5], and psychological scaling procedures [8] in particular. In psychiatry, the use of scaling techniques had already begun before the psychopharmacological era. Škoda has formalized the changes of process and defect psychopathology [26] by means of original rank order scales. These were used in the evaluation of the effects of outpatient administration of electroconvulsive therapy (ECT) and electronarcosis [25].

Psychopharmacology has given the greatest impetus to the standardized use of assessment scaling procedures in psychiatry. In the very beginning foreign global rating scales were translated and widely used [15]. The idiosyncrasies of foreign definitions of psychopathology were very soon recognized and efforts to develop national scales begun. A monograph about psychiatric rating scales and scaling methods has summarized the results of the attempt to standardize the Czech translations of foreign scales and the domestic developments [9]. All important rating scales in world-wide use have been tested on domestic samples of patients and healthy controls, and the dimensions of psychopathology derived by factor analysis compared transculturally. Most recently the methods of psychiatric information processing, psychiatric information systems, and computer diagnostic classification software have been reviewed [27] with authorized Czech translations of PSE (Present State Examination) and CAPPS (Current and Past Psychopathology Scales) schedules published as an Appendix. Original results of tests of the validity and reliability both of different scales and different computer programmes in cross-sectional and longitudinal experiments have been published [29]. Filip et al. [11] have announced the publication of the outlines of a brief manual of psychiatric rating scales, including six scales for the assessment of schizophrenia, seven for endogenous depression, two for anxiety neurosis, and three for all nosographic groups mentioned. For all scales there are unified coding sheets and punching instructions, and FORTRAN subroutines for checking for error, treating the missing data, and performing transformations and other treatments of the data, including the creation of a data base for biomedical data packages (BMDP).

An important publication in Czech was a monograph [9] describing the following methods for the assessment of depression: Hamilton's Rating Scale for depression; Grinker et al.'s Phenomena of depression; Vinař's FKD scale for the assessment of psychopharmacological treatment of depression; Overall et al.'s Psychiatric Judgment Depression Scale; Cutter R. P., Kurland H. D.'s Clinical Quantification of Depressive Reactions; Greenblatt et al.'s MMHC (Massachusetts Mental Health Center) Depression Rating Scale; Clyde's Mood Scale; Beck's Subjective Rating Scale of depression (introduced by Vinař in 1962); and Zung's Self-Rating Depression Scale.

Of these, the Czech translations of the Hamilton, Beck, and Zung scales are still used in various psychopharmacological and clinical research projects. Under the influence of nationwide-accepted multicentric research work organized by the Psychopharmacological Department of Psychiatric Research Institute in Prague, Vinař's FKD scale has become a nearly obligatory rating scale used in formalized research in depression in Czechoslovakia. Since the 1960's it has been used occasionally in Yugoslavia, the German Democratic Republic, and Poland. After the English translation [31] a Russian, a German, and a Serbian translation were prepared.

FKD is an abbreviation for "Quantification of Depressive Symptomatology for the Measurement of Pharmacotherapeutic Effects". The scale, constructed on the basis of experiments with Hamilton's [14] and Bojanovský's and Chloupková's [7] scales, covers 20 depressive symptoms rated in four degrees of severity (0, not present; 1-3, mild to severe; degrees 1-3 are defined in operational terms). The sensitivity, interrater agreement expressed by intraclass correlation coefficient, intercorrelations of FKD items, and results of factor analysis based on three different samples has been demonstrated [35]. In all samples two basic factors could be interpreted ("retarded depression with anhedonia" and "intrapunitive depression"), with additional minor factors in two of the samples examined.

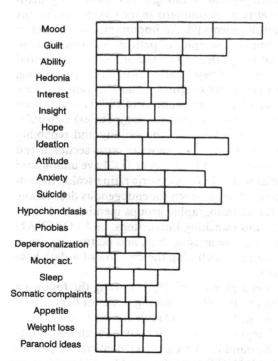

Fig. 4.1. FKD scale: weights of items and scores for degrees of severity

The intercorrelations of the FKD items have been compared with those of the items in Beck's inventory rated on the same sample. The intercorrelations of the items of the latter rating scale were found to be considerably higher than those found in a sample of French patients by Delay and co-workers [37]. Factors different from those found by Pichot and Lempérière [22 a] were identified. In order to allow for the unevenness of the intervals of an ordinal scale, relative weights of single FKD items and weights of within-item scores have been calculated by the analysis of responses of 70 psychiatrists well acquainted with the method (Fig. 4.1).

By employing the weights defined, the ordinal scale (FKD) ratings can be converted into interval scale ratings.

A recent publication, the brief manual of psychiatric rating scales by Filip et al. [11], induced the following scales for assessing the clinical effects of endogenous depression treatment: Feighner's diagnostic criteria [10]; Hamilton's HAM-D [13]; Vinař's FKD [31]; Montgomery and Åsberg's MADS [20]; Widlocher's SRS [12]; Beck's inventory [13]; and Zung's SDS [13].

References

1. Aleksandrovskii, Ya. A. 1976. Sostoyaniya psichicheskoi dezadaptacii i ikh kompensacii (States of mental maladaptation and their compensation). Izd. Nauka, Moscow.
2. Aleksandrovskii, Ya. A., and Neznamov, G. G. 1982. O metodicheskikh podkhodakh k otsenke deistviya psichotropnykh preparatov u bolnykh s pogranichnymi sostoyaniyami (Methodical approach to evaluation of the effects of psychotropic substances in borderline states). In: Problems of clinical and experimental pharmacology and side-effects of pharmacological substances. Proceedings of second conference, Tbilisi.
3. Avruckii, G. Ya., and Zaitsev, S. G. (eds.). 1975. Standartizovannaya registraciya klinicheskikh dannykh o techenii endogennykh psichozov i pogranichnykh sostoyanii pod vliyaniem psichofarmakoterapii (Standardization and registration of clinical data about the course of psychoses and borderline states under the influence of psychopharmacotherapy). Ministry of Health Research Institutes and Coordination of Research Division, Moscow.
4. Beck, A. T., Ward, C. H., Mendelson, M., Mock, J., and Erbaugh, J. 1961. An inventory for measuring depression. Arch. Gen. Psychiatry 4: 561-571.
5. Berka, K. 1977. Měření. Pojmy, teorie, problémy (Measurement - concepts, theory, problems). Academia, Prague.
6. Boháček, N., and Sartorius, N. 1964. Über objektive Beurteilung der Psychopharmaka: die Methode der standardisierten Protokolle. Neuropsychopharmacology 3: 85-89.
7. Bojanovský, J., and Chloupková, K. 1966. Bewertungsskala der Depressionszustände. Psychiatr. Neurol. (Basel) 151: 54-61.
8. Břicháček, V. 1978. Úvod do psychologického škálování (Introduction to psychological scaling). Psychodiagnostic and didactic tests, Bratislava.
9. Engelsmann, F. 1967. Psychiatric rating scales and scaling methods (in Czech). Reports of the Psychiatric Research Institute no. 11, PRI Prague.
10. Feighner, J. P., Robins, E., Guze, S. B., Woodruff, R. A., Winokur, G., and Munoz, R. 1972. Diagnostic criteria for use in psychiatric research. Arch. Gen. Psychiatry 26: 57-63.
11. Filip, V., Pošmurová, M., Provazníková, R., and David, I. 1982. A Brief Manual of Psychiatric Rating Scales (in Czech). Čsl. Psychiat. 78: 226-231.
12. Frenchette, D., Jouve, T. R., Allinaire, J. F., Le-Crubier, Y., Lauriers, A., and des. Widlocher, D. 1980. A depressive retardation rating scale. Paper presented at the 12th Congress of the Collegium Internationale Neuropsychopharmacologicum (CINP), Göteborg.
13. Guy, W. 1976. ECDEU Assessment Manual for Psychopharmacology. National Institute for Mental Health, Rockville.

14. Hamilton, M. A. 1960. A rating scale for depression. J. Neurol. Neurosurg. Psychiatry 23: 56-62.
15. Hanzlíček, L. 1960. Experience with quantification of case notes (use of Malamud Sands rating scale) (in Czech). Čs Psychiat. 56 (3): 188-195.
16. Heveroch, A. 1906. Diagnostika chorob duševních (Diagnostics of Mental Illness). Hejda, Tuček, Prague.
17. Lapin, I. P., and Khvilivickii, I. Ya. (eds.). 1966. Antidepressanty i lechenie depressivnykh sostoyanii (Antidepressants and treatment of depressive states). Reports of Institute of Neurology and Psychiatry V. M. Bekhterew, Leningrad, Vol. 34.
18. Mikhailenko, Ts. N., and Nuller, Yu. L. 1966. Isspol'zovanie novoi otsenochnoi graduirovannoi shkaly v klinicheskoi ispitanii antidepressantov (Use of new home-made evaluation scale in clinical research of antidepressants). In: Lapin, I. P., Khvilivickii, I. Ya. (eds.), Reports of Institute of Neurology and Psychiatry V. M. Bekhterew, Leningrad, pp. 143-153, Vol. 34.
19. Milev, V., Tanchev, O., and Masheva, S. 1982. Terapevticheskii effekt antidepressivnoi kombinacii psichoforina i piramena. Mediko-biologicheskaya informaciya MBI 1982, no. 4, pp 22-24. Pharmakhim, Sofia.
20. Montgomery, S. A., and Åsberg, M. 1979. A new depression scale designed to be sensitive to change. Br. J. Psychiatry 134: 302-309.
21. Nuller, Yu. L. 1964. Isspol'zovanie graduirovannykh ocenochnykh chkal dlya kolicheskvennogo opredeleniya terapevticheskoi effektivnosti antidepressantov (in Russian). Zh. Nevropatol. Psikhiatr. Korsakov. 64/3: 449-452.
22. Nuller, Yu. L. 1973. Klinicheskie issledovaniya antidepressantov (Clinical research of antidepressants). Doctoral dissertation, Institute of Neurology and Psychiatry V. M. Bekhterew, Leningrad.
22a. Pichot, P., and Lempérière, T. 1964. Rev. Psychol. Appl. 16: 105.
23. Pichot, P., Piret, J., and Clyde, D. J. 1966. Analyse de la symptomatologie dépressive subjective. Revue de Psychologie appliquée 16: 105-115.
24. Sopozjenin, V. V. 1967. O primenenii ocenochnykh shkal v psikhiatrii (Use of evaluation scales in psychiatry). In: Clinical and Therapeutic Problems in Psychoses, pp. 180-186.
25. Škoda, C. 1953, 1954, 1955, 1957. In Škoda 1963, pp. 21-23.
26. Škoda, C. 1963. Psychotic Process and Postpsychotic Defect. A Study of the Possibilities of Their Differentiation in Schizophrenia (in Czech). Edition Medical Papers Vol. 6, Series III, Slovak Academy of Sciences, Bratislava.
27. Škoda, C. 1976. Použití počítačů v psychiatrii (Use of computers in psychiatry). In: Škoda (ed.), Moderní přístupy k získávání a zpracovávání informací v psychiatrii (Modern Methods of Gaining and Processing the Information in Psychiatry). Reports of the Psychiatric Research Institute, no. 40, pp. 13-182. PRI, Prague.
28. Škoda, C. (ed.). 1976. Moderní přístupy k získávání a zpracovávání informací v psychiatrii (Modern Methods of Gaining and Processing the Information in Psychiatry). Reports of the Psychiatric Research Institute, no 40, PRI, Prague. Appendix No 1: PSE - Present State Examination, 9th Ed. Translation from: Wing, J. K., Cooper, J. E., and Sartorius, N. Measurement of Psychiatric Symptoms. Cambridge University Press, Cambridge, 1974.
29. Škoda, C. et al. 1978. Psychiatrická biometrie (Psychiatric biometry). 2 Vols. Reports of the Psychiatric Research Institute, no. 41. PRI, Prague.
30. Tashev, T., Roglev, M., Vlakhova, V., Balabanova, V., Moldovanska, P., Kukladzhiev, B., Bakalova, S., Ponchev, P., and Madzhirova, N. 1982. Antidepressivnaya terapiya, kombinirovannaya s preparatami piramen ili centrofenoxin (Antidepressive therapy in combination with piramen or centrophenoxin). Mediko-biologicheskaya informaciya MBI, no. 4, pp. 30-33. Pharmakhim, Sofia.
31. Vinař, O. 1966 a. Rating scale FKD (quantification of depressive symptomatology for evaluation of the results of psychopharmacotherapy). Act. Nerv. Super. (Praha) 8: 409-411.
32. Vinař, O. 1966 b. Scale for rating side-effects during psychiatric pharmacotherapy (VP). Act. Nerv. Super. (Praha) 8: 411.
33. Vinař, O. 1966 c. Zkoušení nových léků v psychiatrii (New pharmaca testing in psychiatry). In: Z. Modr (ed.), Clinical Testing of Drugs, pp. 3-28. Spofa, Prague.
34. Vinař, O. 1971. Scale for rating treatment emergent symptoms in psychiatry DVP. Act. Nerv. Super. (Praha) 13: 238-240.
35. Vinař, O. 1974. Clinical change as measured by the FKP and FKD rating scales. (pp. 48-67 in

Neuropsychopharmacology. Proceedings of the IX. Congress of the Collegium International Neuropsychopharmacologicum, Paris, 7-12 July, 1974. International Congress Series no. 359. Excerpta Medica, Amsterdam.
36. Vinař, O. 1976. Clinical testing of psychopharmaca. In: Z. Modr. (ed.), Clinical Testing of Drugs II (in Czech), pp. 107-129, Spofa, Prague.
37. Vinař, O., and Grof, P. 1969. Die depressive Symptomatologie im Lichte des Beckschen Fragebogens. In: H. Hippius and H. Selbach (eds.), Das depressive Syndrom. Urban und Schwarzenberg, Munich, pp. 327-332.
38. Vinař, O., Váňa, J., and Grof, S. 1966. Rating scale FKP (Quantification of psychiatric symptomatology for the evaluation of pharmacotherapy in psychoses). Act. Nerv. Super. 8/4: 405-408.
39. WHO. 1977. SADD - Schedule for a Standardized Assessment of Patients with Depressive Disorders, 5th Draft. Mental Health Division, WHO, Geneva.
40. Zaitsev, S. G. 1968. Quantitative evaluation of psychopathologic phenomena in present psychopharmacology (review) (in Russian). Zh. Nevropatol. Psikhiatr. 63/2: 270.
41. Zharikov, N. M., Rudenko, G. M., and Zaitsev, S. G. (eds.). 1980. Rukovodiashchie metodicheskie materialy po eksperimental'nomu i klinicheskomu izucheniyu novych eksperimental'nykh sredstev. Metodicheskie ukazaniya po klinicheskomu izucheniyu novych antidepressantov. Ministerstvo zdravookhraneniya SSSR, Moscow.

Chapter 5 Standardized Instruments Used in the Assessment of Depression in the Scandinavian Countries

O. LINGJAERDE

Use of Depression-Rating Scales in Scandinavia

In 1969 the Committee on Clinical Investigations of the Scandinavian Society of Psychopharmacology carried out a questionnaire survey on the use of psychiatric rating scales in all psychiatric institutions in Denmark, Sweden, Norway, and Finland [12]. Answers were received from 131 (44%) institutions, 36 of which had been employing rating scales. In half of these institutions, rating scales had been used in depressive states, in nine institutions in schizophrenia, in six institutions in neuroses, and in four institutions in psychogeriatric patients. Thus, depression was by far the predominant illness for which rating scales had been used. The most commonly used depression rating scales were Hamilton's (mentioned by eight), Beck or Beck-Pichot's (mentioned by four), and Cronholm-Ottosson's (mentioned by three). Only rarely were scales used routinely – in most instances they were used in connection with special research projects.

Ten years later, in 1979, a somewhat similar enquiry was carried out in Denmark by P. Bech, on behalf of the Danish Psychiatric Association [4]. A total of 85 psychiatric departments were asked about the use of psychiatric rating scales for scientific purpose during the period 1970–1979. The number of replies was 82, covering a total of 91 clinical studies in which rating scales had been used. Symptom-rating scales had been used in 65 studies, diagnostic scales in 15, and personality scales in 11. In 50 out of the 65 instances, symptom-rating scales had been used in affective disorders, again showing that standardized assessment instruments are used primarily in affective disorders.

In 37 of the 50 instances, the depression (or mania) scale used was an observer scale: Hamilton's depression-rating scale (22 times), Cronholm-Ottosson's depression scale (7 times), a depression subscale from the CPRS (Comprehensive Psychopathological Rating Scale) [3] (once), self-constructed rating scales (5 times), Bech-Rafaelsen's Melancholia Scale (once), and Bech-Rafaelsen's Mania Scale (once).

Self-rating scales for affective disorders had been used in ten studies: Beck's Depression Inventory in nine studies, and the Taylor Anxiety Scale in one study.

Similar surveys have not been carried out recently in other Scandinavian countries. However, it is reasonable to believe that the use of depression-rating scales in the rest of Scandinavia was rather similar to that shown in the Danish survey for the period 1970–1979.

During the past few years, a depression subscale from the CPRS has gained more widespread use. Thus, in both of the two Scandinavian trials with antidepressants that have been published in Acta Psychiatrica Scandinavica in 1982 (January to October, inclusive), a CPRS-D scale was used. In one study [7] it was used together with Hamilton's scale and the "Newcastle II" scale; in the other [1] it was used together with Hamilton's scale and Beck's self-rating scale. There are also several ongoing clinical studies in which a CPRS-D scale is being used.

Depression-Rating Scales Developed in Scandinavia

As appears from the foregoing, the most widely used depression-rating scales in Scandinavia have been Hamilton's Depression Rating Scale, and Beck's Depression Inventory, which have both been used in translation from the English.
However, there are at least three original depression-rating scales that have been developed in Scandinavia (and translated into English) and that deserve special discussion in this connection: the Cronholm-Ottosson rating scale, the Bech-Rafaelsen Melancholia Scale, and a depression subscale derived from the CPRS. All three are observer scales. The two last-mentioned are discussed in other chapters in this volume. In the following, we will concentrate on the Cronholm-Ottosson rating scale. A Swedish version of a nurses' rating scale for depression will also be mentioned.

Cronholm-Ottosson Rating Scale (CORS or CODS)

The original version of CORS was first described (in English) in a monograph on the mode of action of electroconvulsive treatment (ECT) [6]. The scale comprised the following ten items, each of them (except one) to be rated on a scale from 0 to 3: (I) depression of mood, (II) anxiety, (III) depressive ideas, (IV) suicidal tendencies, (V) disturbance of sleep, (VI) experience of intellectual and conative retardation, (VII) experience of emotional indifference, (VIII) psychomotor retardation, (IX) ability to carry out activities of work and daily life, and (X) general improvement (which, unlike the foregoing, is a variable pertaining to change). By adding up the scores on different variables, the following composite scores were obtained: a *total* score (sum or variables I-IX), a *depression* score (I-V), and a *retardation* score (VI-IX, or VI-VII). When adding the scores, the variables are automatically weighted in proportion to their standard deviation; this seemed justifiable since a large standard deviation may signal a good discriminative power.
No reliability studies were mentioned in this first presentation of CORS.
A slightly revised version of the CORS (in Swedish) was presented at a symposium on the treatment of depression in Lidingö, Sweden, in 1967 [15]. In this version, item IX (ability to carry out activities of work and daily life) from the first version was omitted and two new items added: agitation and diurnal variations. Item X (general improvement) of the original version was now designated "general change" (in Swedish: *Allmän förändring i tillståndet*), to be rated on a scale from -3 to $+3$.

At the same symposium, d'Elia et al. [9] presented two reliability studies of the CORS (first eight items). In both studies the ratings were performed by different raters before, during, and after treatment. In the first study, in which a total of eight doctors participated, two doctors rated the same patient independently on the same day, with so short an interval that possible diurnal variations in mood could not influence the result. The interrater reliability was calculated on the basis of Spearman's rank correlation, with correction for ties [13], between the two parallel ratings. The reliability for the single items varied from 0.22 (psychomotor retardation) to 0.71 (disturbance of sleep); for the total syndrome the reliability was 0.72.

In the second study, a total of 127 depressive patients were rated independently by two experienced psychiatrists who often discussed their results afterwards (without, of course, correcting the ratings). As might be expected, much higher reliability scores were obtained in this study: for the single items, the reliability varied from 0.66 (experience of retardation) to 0.95 (disturbance of sleep), and the reliability for the total syndrome score was 0.86.

In these studies each single patient was, as a rule, rated by the same two doctors before and during treatment. It was thus possible also to calculate the reliability of the *differences* between scores obtained at different times by different doctors. In the first study this reliability was generally found to be somewhat lower than for the single-time scores, whereas in the second study it was about equal to the reliability of the single-time scores.

The authors comment that the higher reliabilities in the second study were probably due to several factors, such as fewer raters, with diminished systematic and random errors, more favorable rating conditions (more severe depressions, more typical syndromes, etc.), and better training of the raters. It was concluded that the rating scale displayed a very satisfactory reliability.

CORS has been used in several clinical studies in depressive states, mainly in Sweden (e. g., [14]), but also in Denmark and some other countries.

A revised English version of the CORS was presented by Åsberg and co-workers in 1973 [2]. This version comprises nine items (one of them, however, being divided in two): (1) depressed mood, (2) anxiety, (3) death wishes – suicidal intent, (4) thought content, divided into (4a) depressive thoughts and (4b) hypochondriacal ideas, (5) sleep disturbance, (6) intellectual and conative retardation, (7) emotional retardation, (8) psychomotor retardation, and (9) agitation.

Each item is rated on a seven-point scale, with each scale step specified.

The authors stress that the scale is explicitly concerned with the measurement of change, i. e., therapeutic effect in the depressive syndrome, and argue that the sensitivity of the scale for this purpose can be increased if the selection of items is limited to those symptoms where change can reasonably be expected during treatment, since this will minimize the amount of "noise" in the scale. Therefore, "agitation," which may be a characteristic symptom, but only in a small number of patients, is not included in the total score, and "diurnal variation in mood" is not rated at all.

The explicit aims of the study reported by Åsberg and co-workers were as follows: (1) to modify the CORS so that it might be used by raters of different theoretical orientations, speaking different languages; (2) to study the reliability of the modified version of the scale between raters of different nationalities, and (3) to compare scores obtained on the modified scale with other measures of depression.

In a collaboration between Swedish, Danish, and English psychiatrists, the scale was translated from Swedish into Danish and English, and the interrater reliability tested in each country. One Swedish psychiatrist participated as co-rater in the Danish and English rating sessions. Two other measures of depression were also used: a slightly modified version of the Beck Self-Rating Scale, and a nurse-rating scale developed by Schildkraut (unpublished).

The reliabilities, expressed as Spearman's rank correlations corrected for ties, for the individual items ranged from 0.51 (anxiety, English data) to 1.00 (sleep disturbance, Danish data). The reliabilities of the summed scores were 0.86 in the English, 0.92 in the Danish, and 0.97 in the Swedish data. There was a high correlation ($r=0.87$) between the ratings on the CORS and the ratings on the nurse-rating scale by the nursing staff on the wards. There was a somewhat lower, but still significant, correlation between the ratings on the CORS and the patients' own rating on the Beck scale ($r=0.63$).

The authors comment that the interrater reliability found was surprisingly good in view of the differences in language, cultural background, and psychiatric training between the raters. It should be noted, however, that the reliabilities were assessed on the basis of conjoint interviews, with both raters present, but rating independently. This method is likely to yield somewhat higher correlations than repeated observations, which were used in the study by d'Elia et al. [9].

A modified version of the CORS was used by d'Elia and collaborators in a study on the combination of tryptophan and ECT in 1977 [10]. The scale, which is now called the Cronholm-Ottosson Depression Scale (CODS), comprises the following 12 items: (1) depression of mood, (2) psychic anxiety, (3) agitation, (4) muscular tension, (5) vegetative anxiety, (6) suicidal tendencies, (7) depressive ideas, (8) hypochondriasis, (9) sleeping disturbance, (10) intellectual and conative inhibition, (11) emotional inhibition, and (12) psychomotor retardation. Each item is scored on a seven-point scale. The sum of scores for items 1-9 assesses a "depression-anxiety syndrome," and the sum of scores for items 10-12 a "retardation syndrome." The interrater reliability coefficients for the single items, based on independent double ratings, varied from 0.55 (agitation) to 0.95 (hypochondriasis); for the total score the reliability coefficient was 0.94, whereas for the depression-anxiety syndrome it was 0.95 and for the retardation syndrome 0.85.

To this author's knowledge, CORS has not been compared directly with, for instance, the Hamilton scale. However, the reliability studies that have been mentioned seem to indicate that CORS may be as good as any other observer-rating scale for the assessment of improvement in a clinical study on depressive states.

A Nurse-Rating Scale of Depression (NRS)

The nurse-rating scale for depression originally constructed by Schildkraut (unpublished) has already been mentioned in connection with the study by Åsberg et al. [2]. This scale has been translated into Swedish by Åsberg, and later modified by d'Elia and collaborators [8]. In this revised version, it contains the following 13 items (here again translated into English, from the version of d'Elia et al.): (1) depressive outlook, (2) verbal expression of depression, (3) crying spells, (4) hopelessness, (5) worthlessness, (6) feelings of guilt, (7) suicidal tendencies, (8) loss of appetite, (9) sleep disturbance, (10) tension, anxiety, and agitation, (11) slowness of speech, (12) psychomotor retardation, and (13) inactivity. Each item is to be rated on a nine-point scale (except the insomnia item). Items 1-10 are assumed to indicate a depression-anxiety syndrome, and items 11-13 a retardation syndrome. Evaluating this scale [8] interrater reliability (correlation coefficients) was found to vary from 0.41 (feelings of guilt) to 0.90 (sleep disturbance); the reliability was 0.90 for the depression-anxiety syndrome, 0.79 for the retardation syndrome, and 0.89 for the total syndrome.

Patients were also rated by doctors on CODS, and this rating turned out to be more sensitive than the NRS rating. Furthermore, there was a rather low correlation between ratings on CODS and on NRS, which was thought to be due at least partly to the fact that the ratings referred to different times. The NRS ratings also correlated rather modestly with the patients' own rating on the Zung scale.

The authors conclude that CODS proved to be superior to other measurements of severity of depression and improvement. However, NRS showed good interrater reliability and a satisfactory sensitivity, and is therefore regarded as a valuable additional assessment, probably measuring partly different aspects of the patient's symptomatology.

The Translation of Rating Scales into Different Scandinavian Languages

Scandinavian psychiatrists usually prefer to use rating scales in their own language. Thus, the most commonly used depression scale, Hamilton's, exists in several translations into all Scandinavian languages. Likewise, the CPRS subscale for depression has been translated from Swedish (or from the English version) into Danish, Norwegian, Finnish, and Icelandic. (The Bech-Rafaelsen Melancholia Scale has not, as yet, been translated from Danish into the other Scandinavian languages.)

The Committee on Clinical Investigations, under the Scandinavian Society of Psychopharmacology, has seen it as an important task to coordinate the translation of good, standardized rating scales into the Scandinavian languages, and to keep the members of the society and other interested persons informed about the available scales and the proper use of them (without, of course, wanting to have a monopoly on such endeavors!). When translations have not been available, the Committee members (one each from Denmark, Sweden, Finland, and Norway, plus one representing the pharmaceutical industry) have made the necessary translations. In this connection, it may be mentioned that the Committee has available translations into all Scandinavian languages of Hamilton's Depression Rating Scale and the CPRS subscale for depression. Several other scales are also available, partly through collaboration with the Psychochemical Institute at the University of Copenhagen: the Newcastle diagnostic depression scales, the Beck and Zung self-rating scales, and the Bech-Rafaelsen Melancholia Scale.

The Committee on Clinical Investigations also have some videotaped interviews available especially made for the training of rating on the Hamilton Depression Scale and the CPRS Depression Subscale. Further information can be obtained from members of the Committee.

References

1. Åberg-Wistedt, A. 1982. A double-blind study of zimelidine, a serotonin uptake inhibitor, and desipramine, a noradrenaline uptake inhibitor, in endogenous depression. Acta Psychiatr. Scand. 66: 50-65.
2. Åsberg, M., Kragh-Sørensen, P., Mindham, R. H. S., and Tuck, J. R. 1973. International reliability and communicability of rating scale for depression. Psychol. Med. 3: 458-465.
3. Åsberg, M., Perris, C., Schalling, D., and Sedvall, G. 1978. The CPRS - Development and applications of a psychiatric rating scale. Acta Psychiatr. Scand. (suppl. 271).
4. Bech, P. 1979. Anvendelse av psykiatriske Rating Scales i Danmark. Paper presented at symposium organized by the Danish Psychiatric Society, November 9-10, Copenhagen, Denmark.
5. Cronholm, B. 1967. Metoder för depressionsskattning, applicerbara i läkemedelsprövningar. In: B. Cronholm and F. Sjökvist (eds.). Symposium om depressionsbehandling, pp. 125-130. Appelbergs boktryckeri AB, Uppsala.
6. Cronholm, B., and Ottosson, J. O. 1960. Experimental studies of the therapeutic action of electroconvulsive therapy in endogenous depression. In: J. O. Ottosson (ed.), Experimental Studies of the Mode of Action of Electroconvulsive Therapy, pp. 69-101. Acta Psychiatr. Neurol. Scand. 35 (suppl. 145).
7. Dahl, L. E., Lundin, L., Honoré, P., and Dencker, S. J. 1982. Antidepressant effect of femoxetine and desipramine and relationship to the concentration of amine metabolites in cerebrospinal fluid. Acta Psychiatr. Scand. 66: 9-17.
8. d'Elia, G., and Raotma, H. 1978. Reliability and validity of a nurses' rating scale of depression. Acta Psychiatr. Scand. 57: 269-278.
9. d'Elia, G., Isaksson, A., Larkander, O., Morsing, C., Ottosson, J. O., Perris, C., and Rapp, W. 1967. Reliabilitet vid skattning av depressionssymptom och läkemedelsbiverkningar. In: B. Cronholm and F. Sjöqvist (eds.), Symposium om depressionsbehandling, pp. 131-141. Appelbergs boktryckeri AB, Uppsala.
10. d'Elia, G., Lehmann, J., and Raotma, H. 1977. Evaluation of the combination of tryptophan and ECT in the treatment of depression. Acta Psychiatr. Scand. 56: 303-318.
11. Lindegaard Pedersen, O., Kragh-Sørensen, P., Bjerre, M., Fredrickson Overø, K., and Gram, L. F. 1982. Citalopram, a selective serotonin reuptake inhibitor: Clinical antidepressive and long-term effect - a Phase II study. Psychopharmacology (Berlin) 77: 199-204.
12. Lingjaerde, O. 1969. Bruk av rating scales ved psykiatriske institusjoner i Skandinavia. Nord. Psykiat. Tskr. 23: 275-281.
13. Siegel, S. 1956. Nonparametric Statistics for the Behavioural Sciences. McGraw-Hill, New York.
14. Wålinder, J., Scott, A., Carlsson, A., Nagy, A., and Roos, B. E. 1976. Potentiation of the antidepressant action of clomipramine by tryptophan. Arch. Gen. Psychiatry 44: 1384-1389.

Chapter 6 Instruments Used in the Assessment of Depression in Japan

R. TAKAHASHI

Introduction

Instruments used for the assessment of symptoms of mental disorders have already received adequate attention and were, in fact, developed in Japan in the 1960s. In particular a rating scale for schizophrenic and behavioral symptoms [5] was devised for the first time in 1961 for the purpose of evaluating the efficacy of pharmacotherapy in this disorder. This became the impetus for the subsequent developing symptom rating scales for schizophrenia [13] and manic-depressive illness [1] in the field of pharmacopsychiatry. Later, in 1966, the Clinical Psychopharmacology Research Group (CPRG) rating scales of depression were formulated by the group with which the author collaborates and tested in terms of validity, reliability, and sensitivity [4]. Since then, these scales have been widely used, especially for assessing efficacy of almost all new antidepressant drugs evaluated in Japan such as clomipramine, protriptyline, amoxapine, sulpiride, viloxazine, dothiepine, nomifensine, dimetacrine, maprotyline, carbamazepine, and others. These results have been reported in more than 20 papers so far. At the same time the Japanese version of the Beck Depression Inventory as well as Hamilton's Rating Scale for Depression have also been used in this country.

CPRG Rating Scales of Depression

CPRG rating scales consist of three mutually independent scales for use by the doctor, the patient, and nurse or family member respectively. These were developed in 1966 based on the conclusions of examinations made by group members on rating scales from all over the world as well as Japanese psychopathology for 2 years [7, 8].

The rating scale for the doctor's use covers the following depressive symptoms and signs: depressed mood, anxiety, psychomotor retardation, thought retardation, obsessive-compulsive ideas, depressive thought contents, depersonalization or derealization, lack of insight, diurnal fluctuation of mood, and somatic symptoms. The thought contents are assessed in terms of suicidal ideas, hypochondriasis, self-deprecation, and feelings of guilt. In addition to an overall assessment of somatic symptoms, each somatic symptom is rated. Insomnia, difficulty in falling asleep, restless sleep, early awakening, difficulty in awakening, and fearful dreams are assessed separately. Lack of appetite, decrease of libido, feeling of tiredness, headache or a sensation of pressure on the head, constipation, and dry mouth are also rated. Other somatic signs and symptoms not mentioned above, if present, are described and rated as well. In all, the CPRG Rating Scale of Depression for Doctor's Use [9, 10] consists of 26 variables of which the somatic symptoms item can be used for the overall assessment of all somatic symptoms and signs. Every item is rated according to a five-point scale:

5 present, extremely severe;
4 present, severe;
3 present, mild;
2 present, slight;
1 absent.

The rating scale for the doctor's use is shown in Table 6.1. The rating should be based on clinical judgment after an interview with the patient. The total score for the patient is calculated by adding up the item scores.

Table 6.1. Doctor's Rating Scale for Depression

| Name/initials (| |) | Date of interview (| / |) |
| Period of observation | (/ - / |) | Name of investigator (| |) |

	Extremely severe	Severe	Mild	Slight	None
Depressed mood	Apathetic	Severely depressed mood	Mildly depressed mood	Feeling of dullness or pleasurelessness	None
Anxiety (agitation, agony)	Agony	Overwhelmed with anxiety	Often has anxiety attack	Rarely has anxiety	None
Psychomotor retardation	Stupor	Always bedridden, no active movement	Slowness of active movement	Loss of nimble movement, decreased efficiency in work	None
Thought retardation	Stupor, complete inhibition of thinking	Thought does not come into mind, unable to make decision	Slow stream of thought, difficult to make decision	Slightly slow stream of thought, slow to reach decision	None
Suicidal idea	Strong suicidal drive	Repeatedly aware of suicidal thought	Wishes were dead	Feels life is not worth living	None
Hypochondriacal idea	Delusion		Idea		None
Self deprecatory idea	Delusion		Idea		None
Guilty idea	Delusion		Idea		None
Depersonalization, Derealization	Severe		Mild		None
Obsessive-compulsive ideas	Severe		Mild		None

Table 6.1 (continued)

Name/initials (	) Date of interview (/)
Period of observation (/ - /	) Name of investigator ( )

	Extremely severe	Severe	Mild	Slight	None
Loss of insight		Severe	Mild		None
Diurnal fluctuation of mood — worse in morning		Clearly present		Slight	None
Diurnal fluctuation of mood — worse in evening		Clearly present		Slight	None
Somatic symptoms		Severe	Mild		None
Difficulty falling asleep		Severe	Mild		None
Restless sleep		Severe	Mild		None
Early awakening		Severe	Mild		None
Difficulty awakening		Severe	Mild		None
Fearful dream		Severe	Mild		None
Lack of appetite		Severe	Mild		None
Decrease of libido		Severe	Mild		None
Feeling of tiredness		Severe	Mild		None
Headache, feeling of pressure on head		Severe	Mild		None
Constipation		Severe	Mild		None
Dry mouth		Severe	Mild		None
Other somatic symptoms		Severe	Mild		None

The rating scale for patient's use [9, 10] is a self-rating inventory as shown in Table 6.2. This scale contains 72 items of subjective experience of depression and three grade ratings: (5) clearly present, (3) slightly or occasionally present, and (1) absent. Most depressed patients are able to understand the directions and items and to answer correctly. When the patient cannot concentrate sufficiently to read the inventory the doctor or some other suitable person may read it for him or her.

The rating scale for nurse's use [9] is a behavioral rating scale with 57 items describing the patient's social behavior and adjustment in the hospital or at home. The scale is rated according to three grades as shown in Table 6.3. When the patient is not hospitalized a key member of his or her family may fill out the rating scale. The period of assessment for the CPRG rating scales is usually 1 week, subject to change according to the purpose of employing the scales.

Instruments Used in the Assessment of Depression in Japan

Table 6.2. Depression rating scale for patient's use

Answer the following items for the past week.
Place a circle in the column which you feel is most appropriate to yourself.

Date: _____
Name: _____
Hospital: _____

No.	Item	Clearly present	Slightly present	Absent
1.	I wake up early and cannot fall back to sleep			
2.	I feel like throwing things			
3.	I have difficulty concentrating			
4.	I always feel ill and miserable			
5.	I become concerned about everything that happens to me and around me			
6.	I am afraid I might become mentally ill			
7.	I cannot smile even when I hear jokes			
8.	I feel that I have lost weight recently			
9.	I feel very irritable			
10.	I feel hopeless and discouraged about the future			
11.	I always feel weak			
12.	I am taking days off from my job because of my illness			
13.	I wake up frequently during the night			
14.	I think my illness is a punishment			
15.	I feel I would be better off dead			
16.	I have had many failures in my life			
17.	I feel more depressed in the evening			
18.	My head is always heavy			
19.	My health is at its worst at the present			
20.	I feel very pessimistic about the future			
21.	I feel more depressed in the morning			
22.	I blame myself for failures			
23.	My comprehension of what I read has become less			
24.	My head feels as though it is empty			
25.	My appetite has become very poor			
26.	I have lost interest in everyday activities			
27.	I have lost interest in amusements and hobbies			
28.	I feel sad all the time			
29.	I plan on committing suicide			
30.	I become very concerned over trivial matters			
31.	I am always worried about illness			
32.	My judgment has become much worse			
33.	I often feel very exhausted			
34.	I think I have less endurance than before			
35.	I hate myself			
36.	I wish I could be as bright and happy as others			
37.	I dislike mingling with others			
38.	I find it difficult to begin work			
39.	My mind dwells on useless ideas			
40.	My desire for luxury articles (wine, tobacco, tea, cakes, etc.) has diminished			
41.	I have lost interest in the opposite sex			
42.	I often cry			
43.	I think my appearance has changed and that I have lost my attractiveness			
44.	I lack interest to do things			

Table 6.2 (continued)

No.	Item	Clearly present	Slightly present	Absent

Circle the column

45. I have only dark, pessimistic ideas
46. I am constantly worried about the future
47. I think I have less ability and lower intelligence than others
48. I am unable to think as rapidly as before
49. I have lost confidence in myself
50. I feel that people have malicious plots against me
51. I am unable to work
52. I think I am more nervous than others
53. I feel depressed with no particular cause or reason
54. I often suffer from constipation
55. I find it difficult to fall asleep
56. My impression of things around me has become vague
57. I find it difficult to concentrate
58. I always feel apathetic
59. I am unable to feel as happy as before
60. I think that my efficiency has dropped
61. I feel worthless and useless
62. I frequently dream
63. I think it is worthless to live
64. I work reluctantly
65. I feel very despondent
66. I always feel unbearably anxious
67. I feel continually sad and am unable to alter my mood
68. I have lost interest in my family and those around me
69. My mouth is often very dry
70. My memory has become very poor
71. My sexual desire has greatly decreased recently
72. I think I have done wrong to others

(Menstrual difficulties   (severe, mild, none)
(Hobbies: _____)
(Religion: _____)

Table 6.3. Depression-rating scale for nurse's use

No.	Item	Clearly present	Slightly present	Absent

1. The patient has become more uncommunicative
2. He speaks more slowly recently
3. He has become talkative and fidgety
4. He speaks so feebly that it is very difficult to understand him
5. He has become almost unable to sleep
6. He is very self-derogatory in his speech
7. He shows needless concern over financial matters
8. He expresses sorrow for those around him
9. He shows overconcern over the health of his family members
10. He speaks of his anxieties and fears

Table 6.3 (continued)

No.	Item	Clearly present	Slightly present	Absent
11. He speaks of feeling inferior				
12. He expresses a great deal of guilt about his past				
13. He frequently speaks about how sad he feels				
14. He speaks pessimistically about the future				
15. He states that he wants to die				
16. He says he has lost interest in things				
17. He says he is molested and talked about by others				
18. His movements have become very slow				
19. He has become very restless				
20. He appears to be very anxious and fearful				
21. His behavior and facial expression appear very depressed				
22. He no longer smiles				
23. He appears more uncomfortable in front of others				
24. His eyes are frequently filled with tears				
25. He is jittery				
26. He has become irritable				
27. He uses violence				
28. He frequently sighs				
29. He says he feels apathetic or easily fatigued				
30. He is often worried about his mental and physical condition				
31. He says he has a very severe illness or that his internal organs are rotten				
32. He says that his head is of no use				
33. He appears to be contemplating suicide				
34. He is no longer able to read the newspaper				
35. He no longer watches television				
36. He no longer speaks with others				
37. He dislikes eating with others				
38. He has difficulty rising in the morning				
39. He dislikes mingling with other people				
40. He dislikes going out of the house				
41. He goes to bed early				
42. He is unoccupied most of the day				
43. He is very hesitant in beginning work				
44. He is unable to stick to his work				
45. He has become completely unable to work				
46. He has difficulty falling asleep				
47. He awakens frequently during the night				
48. He states he is unable to sleep soundly				
49. He wakes up very early in the morning				
50. He is slow to fully awake in the morning				
51. He appears very uncomfortable when he arises				
52. He states he feels sleepy during the day				
53. His appetite has decreased				
54. He eats nothing at all				
55. He eats more than the average				
56. He has lost weight recently				
57. His complexion has become worse				

Comment and Conclusion

The validity, reliability, and sensitivity of each of the three rating scales were examined by using pretreatment scores of 123 patients with affective disorder of depressed type, and the results were found to be satisfactory [4, 6].

After Varimax rotation on factor analysis, ten independent group factors were extracted from the pretreatment scores on the doctor's rating scale of the cohort of patients mentioned above. Ten and nine factors respectively were determined from the nurse's and the patients' rating scales in the same way. These factors were tentatively interpreted as shown in Table 6.4.

Correlations among factors extracted from these three rating scales were examined. As shown in Table 6.5, in the great majority of group factors, no significant correlation was found, the confidence level being 99%. Therefore the group factors from three rating scales appear to show different aspects of manifestation of depression. Therefore it is likely that the simultaneous employment of the three rating

Table 6.4. Tentative interpretation of factors

From doctors' rating scale
- F1. Somatic symptoms
- F2. Depressive mood or retardation
- F3. Morbid thought content
- F4. Disturbance of sleep and appetite
- F5. Constipation
- F6. Sexual desire and potency
- F7. Loss of insight
- F8. Disturbance of awakening
- F9. Depersonalization and dry mouth
- F10. Hypochondriacal thoughts

From nurses' and/or family members' rating scale
- F1. Loss of interest and concern
- F2. Slowing of movement
- F3. Decline in working capacity
- F4. Decline in eating and speaking activity
- F5. Expression of fretfulness
- F6. Expression of hypochondriacal and depressed mood
- F7. Expression of morbid thought content
- F8. Disturbance of sleep
- F9. Disturbance of awakening, and unpleasant feeling
- F10. Expression of worry

From patients' rating scale
- F1. Pessimism and despair
- F2. Decline in vitality
- F3. Awareness of decline in working capacity
- F4. Envy of health
- F5. Disturbance of sleep
- F6. Hypochondriacal complaints
- F7. Worries
- F8. Conservative and withdrawn
- F9. Awareness of decline in intellectual faculties

Instruments Used in the Assessment of Depression in Japan 43

Table 6.5. Correlation matrix of three rating scale factor scores on 123 depressive patients

Dc	Nr	Pt	Doctors' rating	Nurses' rating	Patients' rating
GF	GF	GF	F1 F2 F3 F4 F5 F6 F7 F8 F9 F10	F1 F2 F3 F4 F5 F6 F7 F8 F9 F10	F1 F2 F3 F4 F5 F6 F7 F8 F9
GF	**	**	F1 **		**
GF		**	F2 **		** ** **
	GF		F3 **		** ** ** **
			F4		** **
			F5 **		
			F6 **		**
			F7		
			F8		
			F9		
			F10		
				F1 **	
				F2	
				F3 ** **	
				F4	
				F5 ** **	
				F6	
				F7	
				F8	
				F9	
				F10	
					F1
					F2
					F3
					F4 **
					F5 **
					F6
					F7
					F8
					F9

Significant correlation among factors: **, at the 1% level

scales for one patient could provide us with a comprehensive assessment of symptomatology of depression. However, it was indicated by weekly assessment of depression in our studies on the efficacy of drug treatments that general factor scores from three rating scales corresponding to overall severity of illness decreased at a similar rate throughout the treatment period. For this reason only the doctor's depression rating scale is normally used in evaluating the effects of drug therapy.

In comparison with Hamilton's Rating Scale for Depression [2] and Standardized Assessment of Depressive Disorders (SADD) schedules [12], the CPRG doctor's depression rating scale does not include the symptoms loss of bodyweight and ideas of reference or persecution which seem to be important for the classification of melancholia and psychotic types of depression. Change of bodyweight, however, can be recorded on items of other somatic symptoms should the doctor wish to assess it. Furthermore, the patient's and the nurse's rating scales contain questions concerning ideas of persecution and loss of body weight respectively. Nonetheless, these two important items must be incorporated into the CPRG doctor's rating scale. Although symptom items would seem to be self-explanatory for trained psychiatrists, recent studies on psychiatric diagnosis criteria suggest that variance in reliability of observations derives not only from unsatisfactory interviewing but also from insufficient definitions of symptoms. Therefore it may be necessary to provide a glossary of definitions of symptoms along with the doctor's CPRG rating scale for depression.

Since the introduction of the SADD schedule many psychiatrists have paid attention to this schedule in Japan. The Japanese version of this schedule has been used not only in the assessment of depressed patients in the WHO field centres in Tokyo and Nagasaki but also in the multiclinical trial of antidepressant drugs; this demonstrates the usefulness of the SADD schedule in clinical psychopharmacology [11]. The Japanese version of the Hamilton Rating Scale for Depression has been widely employed in the clinical trials of new antidepressant drugs for the past 20 years for the sake of international comparability of the results. Recent emphasis on the importance of diagnostic criteria lead to a combination of employment of Research Diagnostic Criteria (RDC) and Hamilton Rating Scale for Depression in pharmacopsychiatry [3, 11, 15] in Japan.

References

1. Akimoto, H., Kurihara, M., Fujiya, T., and Sasaki, K. 1964. The clinical evaluation of psychotropics and anticonvulsant-antidepressive drugs (in Japanese). Seishinigaku 6: 813–825.
2. Hamilton, M. 1960. A rating scale for depression. J. Neurol. Neurosurg. Psychiatry 23: 56–62.
3. Hiramatsu, K., Takahashi, R., Mori, A., Murasaki, M., Inoue, R., Kazamatsuri, H., and Sakuma, A. 1983. Comparison of clinical effects of zimelidine and imipramine on depression using multi-center double blind technique (in Japanese). Seishinigaku 25: 1341–1350.
4. Ichimaru, S., Itoh, H., Kudo, T., Kurihara, M., Kawakita, Y., Sato, Y., Takahashi, R., Tanimukai, H., Asano, C., and Sakamoto, T. 1966. A double blind controlled study of antidepressants with CPRG rating scales. In: Fourth World Congress of Psychiatry. 1956–1961, no. 150. Excerpta Medica International Congress Series.
5. Kawaguchi, S. 1961. A study of chlorpromazine therapy in cases of chronically disturbed schiz-

ophrenics: A quantitative evaluation according to behavioral rating sheet (in Japanese). Tokyo Ikadaigaku Zasshi 19: 1559–1591.
6. Kawakita, Y. 1966. Significance and limitation of rating scale for assessment of efficacy of antidepressants. Psychiatrica Neurologica Japonica 68: 122.
7. Kudo, Y., 1974. Problems in developing clinical rating scales (in Japanese). Japanese Medical Journal 2612: 28–34.
8. Kurihara, M. 1975. Evaluation of antidepressant drug-technical problems of symptom rating scale and a survey on double blind trials of antidepressants (in Japanese). Clinical Evaluation 3: 3–17.
9. Kurihara, M., Sato, Y., Ichimaru, S., Itoh, H., Kawakita, Y., Kudo, Y., Takahashi, R., and Tanimukai, H. (CPRG). 1973. Further analysis of the double-blind controlled study on the clinical efficacy of four antidepressant drugs – imipramine, trimipramine, safrazine and amitriptyline. Clinical Evaluation 2 (3): 147–165.
10. Kurihara, M., Itoh, H., Kawakita, Y., Kudo, Y., Sato, Y., Takahashi, R., and Tanimukai, H. (CPRG). 1972. A double-blind controlled study on the clinical efficacy of four antidepressant drugs – clomipramine, dimethacrine, nortriptyline and protriptyline (in Japanese). Clinical Evaluation 1: 1–25.
11. Murasaki, M., Takahashi, R., Kazamatsuri, H., Mori, A., Inoue, R., Okazaki, Y., Oguchi, T., Yamazumi, S., Yoshimoto, S., Hironaka, I., Takemura, M., Okazaki, K., Kasahara, H., Suzuki, M., Abe, T., Saito, E., Nakayasu, N., and Hiramatsu, K. 1982. Clinical evaluation of zimelidine, 5-HT. Uptake inhibiting antidepressant multiclinical study using RDC and Hamilton Rating Scale (in Japanese). Japanese Journal of Clinical Psychiatry 11: 1175–1187.
12. Sartorius, N., Davidian, H., Ernberg, G., Fenton, F. R., Fujii, I., Gastpar, M., Gulbinat, W., Jablensky, A., Kielholz, P., Lehmann, H. E., Naraghi, N., Shimizu, M., Shinfuku, N., and Takahashi, R., 1983. Depressive Disorders in Different Cultures, World Health Organization, Geneva.
13. Sato, Y., Nishimura, M., Kato, T., Takahashi, R., Kaneda, Y., Katada, A., Naruse, H., Kogi, M., and Kato, M. 1964. The clinical evaluation of psychotropics and anticonvulsants – schizophrenics (in Japanese). Seishinigaku 6: 827–837.
14. Takahashi, R., Sakuma, A., Hara, T., Kazamatsuri, H., Hori, A., Saito, Y., Murasaki, M., Oguchi, T., Sakurai, Y., Yuzuriha, T., Takemura, M., Kurokawa, H., and Kurita, H. 1979. Comparison of efficacy of amoxapine and imipramine in multiclinic double-blind study using the WHO schedule for a standard assessment of patients with depressive disorders. J. Int. Med. Res. 7: 1.
15. Takahashi, R., Kurihara, M., Miura, S., Sakurai, S., Noguchi, T., Hasue, I., Suzuki, K., Jinbo, M., Hada, H., Fujiya, Y., Shigeta, M., Yabuki, A., Matsudaira, J., Masuda, Y., Itoh, H., Kamishima, K., Kabeshima, Y., Narita, S., Komiya, H., Shikano, T., and Kaizawa, S. 1983. Comparison of clinical effect on depression of dosulepin and amitriptyline using double-blind technique (in Japanese). Clinical Evaluation 11: 201–228.

Chapter 7 Rating Scales for Depression in Italy

G. B. CASSANO, P. CASTROGIOVANNI, and E. RAMPELLO

General Considerations

In Italy, rating scales for depression, like other quantitative instruments and like psychodiagnostic techniques themselves, met a certain amount of initial resistance. They did, in fact spring from a need to standardize and to quantify what was out of line with the traditions of medicine – especially psychiatry – in Italy which in its early stages, tended to attach an absolute value to individual clinical judgments and intuitions.

Rating scales were criticized for both: the excessive subdivision of the clinical picture they were believed to impose and the incompleteness of the symptomatological pattern they were supposed to cover. It was believed that rating scales failed to reflect the specific features of individual cases. It was feared that the specialist's work would be made to conform to a preconceived scheme, and that the use of rating scales would disrupt the doctor-patient relationship, since it required the subject to be treated as an object.

It was also argued that the scores recorded on rating scales would successfully quantify the severity of a psychopathological syndrome, because it was thought that this could not be translated into numerical terms.

Nevertheless, the need that emerged from clinical trials and the earliest experiments with these rating scales weakened criticisms or made them irrelevant. Therefore, in the early 1960s the first attempts were made to use and adopt scales that had originated abroad, especially the Hamilton Rating Scale for Depression (HAM-D).

Once the early resistance had been overcome, the use of rating scales in the study of the psychopathological facets of depressive states and their evolution during treatment became at least as widespread as in other European countries, so much so that nowadays one or more rating scales are an invariable feature of clinical trials.

The specific characteristics of the population of Italian depressives soon made it clear that there was a need for new instruments suitable for Italian patients, who, especially in the case of self-rating, often found that their predicament was not reflected in self-rating scales invented by foreign investigators for foreign populations.

So far four scales for depression have been devised and tried out in Italy. The earliest was the Scale of Anxious-Depressive Symptomatology [*Scala di Sintomatologia Ansioso-Depressiva* (SSAD) by Gainotti and Cianchetti [10]]. It comprises 48 items, which are administered under guidance. The first group of items explores anxious symptomatology and the second depressive symptomatology. The patient is allowed to note down two symptomatological items in his or her words, since it was supposed that the questionnaire might have overlooked the corresponding disorders.

The second scale was developed at the Institute of Clinical Psychiatry, University of Pisa; it was the Self-Rating Scale for Depression, or *Scala di Autovalutazione per la Depressione* (SAD) by Cassano and Castrogiovanni [1] and Cassano et al. [5]. It comprises 31 items, each of them allowing for an assessment of symptoms on a quantitative scale scored from one to four. A wide symptomatological area is explored, including both strictly depressive symptoms and symptoms of psychic and somatic anxiety.

More recently, two new scales have been introduced. The first is the Rome Depression Inventory [12], and the second is the Observer-Rating Scales for the Assessment of Depression, or *Scala di Valutazione per la Depressione, forma di Eterovalutazione* (SVDE) by Faravelli [8] and Faravelli et al. [9]. This scale displays two special features: firstly, there is a 10-cm-long analogous scale for each of the 15 items, with reference points marked along it, and, secondly, on this rating scale, unlike the others mentioned here, the choice of items is not based on theoretical criteria, but on the results of a factorial analysis of six other commonly used scales. One set of items is used to assess the basic depressive nucleus, whereas the others identify the subsidiary symptomatology.

Inquiry About the Use of Rating Scales for Depression in Italy

The Questionnaire

In order to survey the opinions and judgments of Italian medical doctors and specialists on rating scales used to assess depression, we have drawn up a questionnaire divided into four parts. The first part deals with personal data (age, sex, educational qualification, title, profession, place of work). The second inquires into the extent of the subject's knowledge of rating scales, his or her opinion on their general usefulness, and preferences for other methods of inquiry. The third part collects information about the rating scales known to the subject (type and frequency of use, judgment on their worth, possible improvements). The fourth part elicits personal judgments on rating scales in general (acceptability, sectors where they can be applied, comparison between Italian and foreign rating scales, changes noted in frequency of use, and experience in automated processing).

The Sample

The questionnaire was randomly distributed to 65 MDs and specialists working in university clinics (47%), hospitals (46%), and local health organizations (21%). All of those who answered the questionnaire were aged between 25 and 60 years and 85% were male. Most of them (87%) were specialists in psychiatry or in nervous and mental illnesses, and nearly all of them (92%) were involved in outpatient care; many also lectured (38%) or carried out research (58%) and a clear majority worked and lived in central or northern Italy.

Results

The Most Commonly Used Rating Scales

The HAM-D was shown to be undoubtedly the most well-known and the most valued and widely used rating scale.

Answers to the questionnaire showed that 95% of those who answered had a knowledge of the scale; of these, 50% had a superficial knowledge of it and 50% knew it well: 77% of those answering had used it; of these, 57% had done so for research purposes and 43% for clinical purposes. This scale had been administered both to outpatients (40%) and, more often, to inpatients (60%).

The overall assessment of the HAM-D was positive. Only 5% of those answering the questionnaire considered the scale to have a low degree of reliability, whereas 47% considered it to be sufficiently reliable, and 26% to be very reliable. These results were confirmed by the data on the frequency of its use, which correspond quite clearly to those on its value, and show an increase in its use by 25% of those questioned.

Only 20% of those who had used the HAM-D did not consider it to be useful in current conditions. The reasons given were as follows: it restricts subjective evaluation (12.5%); the results are inconstant (12.5%); it cannot be applied in the appropriate working environment (12.5%); it is based on an arbitrary system (12.5%); it is superficial (12.5%); and it fails to account for the various aspects of clinical symptomatology (12.5%). A closer examination of the data recorded reveals that 65% of the subjects who expressed this negative evaluation had previously admitted that their knowledge of this instrument was superficial.

The subjects who had a knowledge of this scale but did not use it gave a variety of explanations: 5% of them admitted that they did not know it well; 25% reported that they did not use it because they were working in a different field of research; a further 25% stated that they preferred a traditional clinical interview; another 25% said that they did not use it because they considered it to be unsatisfactory; the remaining 20% complained that it was hard to use in a clinical setting.

Of those who had a knowledge of this scale, 62% considered that it could be improved; thus, of the 95% of those questioned who stated that they had a knowledge of this scale, only about half were really familiar with it, and there was a fairly clear consensus of opinion that it is more useful for research purposes than in aiding professional work. Most of the criticisms made of the scale were directed against what was thought to be its rather low degree of flexibility, which also, in the present form of the scale, was said to tend to impede the setting up of a satisfactory doctor-patient relationship.

The self-rating scales turned out to be less well-known and less commonly used.

Of these the Beck Depression Inventory (BDI) turned out to be best known, 25% of the whole sample stating that they had a knowledge of this instrument; half of these said they had a superficial knowledge and the other half a good knowledge of it. Of those questioned, 80% had used the scale; it had been most frequently used for research purposes (70%), but had also been used for clinical purposes (50%). The scale had mainly been administered to inpatients (70%).

In most cases the view regarding of its usefulness was that it was adequate (80%); it was thought to be very useful by 13% of the sample and insufficiently useful by 70%. At the moment of answering the questionnaire, 80% thought it was still valid.

Of those who stated that they did make use of it, 50% said they did so occasionally, 40% often, and 10% rarely. Only 30% of those who said they had used it recorded having done so to an increasing degree. Forty-five percent of the sample considered that the BDI could be improved.

The overall impression is that the BDI is fairly well-known, at least as a useful instrument in research. In addition, it is not denied a possible use in the assessment of changes in the treatment of inpatients in a clinical setting. There is a fairly good level of knowledge about the scale; the use made of it, as recorded by those questioned, is at a medium level.

The level of the sample's knowledge of the Zung Self-Rating Depression Scale turned out to be fairly good, although it was much lower than that of the HAM-D and slightly below that of the BDI. Twenty-three percent of the sample stated that they had a knowledge of this scale, even if only a superficial one. In this case no difference appeared as regards the type of use made of the scale; it had, in fact, been used to an equal degree for research purposes and for clinical purposes, mainly (85%) with outpatients, but also (50%) with inpatients still in hospital. The prevalent use of the scale for outpatients should probably be attributed to the fact that the Zung Self-Rating Scale can be applied quickly and easily.

Of those who stated that they had a knowledge of the scale, 85% said they considered it to be sufficiently useful, 7.5% very useful, and 7.5% insufficiently useful. The same percentages were recorded regarding the frequency of its use; 85% said they had used it occasionally, 7.5% often, and 7.5% rarely. Of those who had used it, 75% thought that it could be improved.

Thus, just over a fifth of the sample questioned had a knowledge of this scale, even if their knowledge was superficial in most cases. They considered that it could be applied both in research and in a clinical setting, and they had administered it more widely to outpatients than to inpatients. Of those who said they had used it, 25% did not believe that it was still a valid scale.

The other rating scales in the questionnaire were: Brief Psychiatric Rating Scale (BPRS, by Overall and Gorrham), Depression Rating Scale (DRS, by Wechsler and Coll), Mental Status Schedule (MSS, by Spitzer et al.), Rome Depression Inventory (RDI, by Pancheri and Carilli), Scale of Anxious-Depressive Symptomatology

(SSAD, by Gainotti and Cianchetti), Self-Report Symptom Inventory (SCL 90, by Derogatis, Lipman, and Covi), the Carrol Rating Scale for Depression (by Carrol et al.), and the Wittenborn Psychiatric Rating Scale (by Wittenborn et al.).

Opinions and Judgments on Rating Scales

Most of those questioned approved of the use of rating scales, above all as instruments of research (90%). Rating scales received a lower degree of approval as regards their clinical use (65%). Despite this mainly positive evaluation, quite a large percentage of the sample would prefer other methods of inquiry, such as biological parameters (30%) or traditional psychodiagnostic tests (24%).

Considered globally, the instruments available at the moment of sending out our questionnaire were not thought to be altogether satisfactory, especially the self-rating scales, which were said to meet the requirements of 22%–53% of the doctors. It must also be noted that, considered as a whole, the other rating scales were judged to be adequate by only 28%–41% of the sample, although evaluation of the HAM-D alone was much more positive.

Many (50%) recorded a lack of comprehension by the patient in using self-rating instruments, whereas the patient's acceptance of them is considerably better (60%). This discrepancy between levels of acceptance and comprehension should prompt changes in the form, the content, and the typographical layout of self-rating questionnaires, so as to overcome the difficulties encountered by the average members of the population to which these instruments are directed.

About one-third of those questioned expressed the opinion that rating scales tend to be refused by researchers themselves, and a small percentage of the sample considered rating scales to be hard to understand.

A refusal of rating scales by MDs or specialists may be attributed to personal or ideological views which inculcate a critical stance. Failure to understand scales can only be due to a lack of training in the use of such scales or to a lack of preliminary study of the problems and criteria involved in psychiatric assessment.

In any case, a clear majority of those questioned singled out the following research fields for the application of these instruments: psychopharmacological research (69%), clinical research (69%), and epidemiological research (49%). Other fields in which rating scales can be applied came far behind: in fact 60% of the sample used only one or two of these fields, since they far preferred the three research fields, and did not indicate any others.

One must point out the lack of appreciation of rating scales as a means of recording and assessing data that are standardized, and which, as a result, favor the transmission of information and hence communication not only between specialists, but also between specialists and nonspecialists.

Only one of those questioned, in fact, indicated among the possible applications of rating scales that of aiding communication in the domain of liaison psychiatry. A small but significant percentage (12%) referred to their possible application in university teaching.

One of the doubts originally raised about the introduction of rating scales was whether instruments developed in given cultural settings and in given spheres of application could be properly transferred to very different populations. The issue is still alive; in fact, 35% of the sample considered instruments devised abroad and translated into Italian to be inappropriate for use with an Italian population and 32% preferred the use of rating scales devised in Italy.

Despite these and other critical observations on rating scales, their use was generally estimated to be steadily increasing, even if some respondents referred to a decrease.

One of the advantages of rating scales is that they provide an assessment expressed in numerical terms that is suitable for automatic processing. In Italian psychiatry, the introduction of standardized recording scales began at the same time as the use of computers, and they developed in parallel in a situation providing mutual feedback. Even so, only a very small percentage of our sample stated that they had any first-hand experience of this kind; this is probably due to the limited spread of the application of computer techniques in psychiatry in this country. The commonest use of computers was in statistical analysis (30%), while between 1% and 23% of those questioned referred to an experience of automated psychodiagnostic processing (automated diagnosis, and the production of profiles and narrative descriptions).

The sample's overall views of the adequacy of rating scales in meeting the needs of clinicians and researchers was certainly not enthusiastic. All the rating scales mentioned, in fact, were, to a greater or lesser degree, judged to require improvement.

Experiences of Rating Scales for Depression at the Institute of Clinical Psychiatry of Pisa University

The data so far reported and the opinions, side by side with the conclusions to be drawn from the experience acquired by using the rating scales for depression, were collected at the Institute of Clinical Psychiatry at the University of Pisa. This institute was one of the first to take these instruments into consideration and apply them, and its competence in this field is based on about 20 years of research and practical application. That experience shows that, in centers or institutions with a specific interest in research or patient care in the field of depression, the use of rating scales has been more frequent and that it has been spread over a wider variety of sectors than one would imagine from the study just reported.

The frequency and continuity of the use of rating scales over the past 20 years bears witness to the favorable reception they have received, and it implies a globally positive judgment on the value of rating scales, which appear to be indispensable instruments in these centers. At the Institute of Clinical Psychiatry at the University of Pisa, for example, rating scales on depression have been used in the outpatients' department and in experimentation in the domain of clinical pharmacology.

After having surveyed the sample's reactions to Wechsler, BDI instruments such as the Zung Rating Scale and the HAM-D, it may be concluded that the HAM-D, as originally formulated, is considered to be quite satisfactory and to correspond quite well to the mentality of Italian researchers, whereas the self-rating scales are judged to be less satisfactory, not only as regards their content and the symptomatological pattern of depression they presuppose, but also as regards their conformity to the cultural and psychopathological characteristics of Italian patients. This is the reason why a self-rating instrument – the *Scala di Autovalutazione per la Depressione* (SAD), [1] – has been devised to allow the assessment of both nuclear depressive symptoms and of a wide range of anxious symptoms and forms of somatization which almost always form an integral part of the clinical profile of an Italian patient. The patient identifies his or her own disorders by using the list and the techniques for assessment provided by the SAD. Patients very often say they are glad that, among the items listed, they have discovered exactly those which express the symptoms they have noted; this immediately gives them the impression that their illness is known and, therefore, understood. It cannot, however, be excluded that as a result of a low cultural level or a mentality that is less accustomed to answering questionnaires than in other countries, or that is actually suspicious of them, a significant proportion of Italian patients may encounter difficulty or show reluctance in answering questionnaires.

Considered globally, the answers obtained from our questionnaire show an appreciation of the positive features and the potential value of rating scales in clinical, psychopathological, and, especially, psychopharmacological research. We would now like to mention some of the applications of rating scales devised so as to be useful in patient care.

Scales have been devised for general practitioners (GPs) to induce them to play their part in a type of psychopathological or psychopharmacological research that will mark an initial move towards their greater receptiveness and towards an acquisition of competence in a sector – that of the diagnosis and therapy of depression – in which the average Italian GP is not very willing to cooperate. It must also be said that while Italian GPs have declared their total willingness to cooperate, their often inadequate knowledge of psychiatry has made it difficult for them to fill in rating scales, so that the data obtained may be unreliable.

A more suitable way of arousing the GPs interest appears to be the use of self-rating scales. When used in epidemiological research on inpatients and outpatients, these scales have made doctors aware of the importance of the degree of depression, which may otherwise be underrated or scotomized by them [6].

The formulation in numerical terms of the psychopathological picture is, in many cases, in keeping with the mentality of GPs who are accustomed to attribute the meaning to quantitative parameters such as those of traditional hematochemical investigations, and facilitates communication with psychiatrists [3].

A self-rating scale for depression (SAD) has been used in an attempt to collaborate with GPs on the telephone.

The service allows GPs to get their outpatients to fill in a self-rating scale and send the scores so obtained, by telephone, to the Center for Prevention and Treatment of Depression at the Institute of Clinical Psychiatry in Pisa. Here the scores are fed into the computer, and the results of the analysis are telephoned back to the GP, after which strategies for treatment are jointly decided with him or her.

Special attention has been devoted in this center to the processing of SAD data. This is done on line by transmitting all the scores through the terminal to the computer center and obtaining the printout on a fast printer. This processing yields a total score, an index of the severity of the clinical picture, a graph showing the scores for single items, and a psychopathological profile obtained from factor scores derived from a previous factor analysis. The output also includes a narrative account clearly describing the distinctive features of the clinical picture composed of the scores for the single items, as well as an automated diagnostic assessment expressing the probability that the individual patient belongs to one or another of five symptomatological groups selected by cluster analysis [7].

Conclusions

Despite the limited size of our sample and its imperfectly representative nature, the data gathered allow us to put forward a series of observations on the use of rating scales for depression in Italy that should give a fairly accurate picture of the present situation.

Nowadays, these scales are known to most psychiatrists and are generally considered to be useful in attaining a standardized assessment of depressive symptomatology, especially in the research field. Even so, there is dissatisfaction with scales and a demand for alternative, more objective methodologies stemming from a still deeply rooted medicobiological mentality or from a belief in traditional psychodiagnostic techniques. In Italy, as elsewhere, by far the most commonly used instrument is the HAM-D, which is unanimously judged to be valuable and which is almost the only one scale rated by others to be used, especially with inpatients. Of self-rating scales, those most widely used are the Zung scale, and, to a lesser extent, the BDI; the first is mainly used for outpatients and the second for inpatients. Even if self-rating scales are less commonly used than the Hamilton Scale they too are considered to be quite useful. So far none of the instruments devised in Italy have been widely used outside the centers where they were devised, despite the fact that locally they are generally preferred to those developed abroad and then translated into Italian.

The most intensive use of rating scales and their application over the widest range of sectors is to be found in psychiatric institutions that are particularly interested in research and medical care in the field of depressive states. They have, in fact, often been utilized in psychopharmacological trials and also as an aid to diagnosis and treatment in patient care.

Satisfactory results have been obtained in patient care where rating scales have turned out to be a good means of communication between psychiatrists and nonspecialists. Lastly, rating scales have revealed their potential usefulness in university lecturing, since they appear to allow young doctors to get used to making a comprehensive description of depressive conditions, to using quantitative assessment in psychiatry, and to beeing accurate in expressing their judgments of psychopharmacological treatment.

References

1. Cassano, G. B., and Castrogiovanni, P. 1977. S.A.D. Scala di Autovalutazione per la Depressione. International Committee for Prevention and Treatment of Depression.
2. Cassano, G. B., Castrogiovanni, P., Conti, L., Nardini, A. G., and Viola, L. 1974. Recognition and treatment of depressive symptoms by non-psychiatrists. In: P. Kielholz (ed.), Depression in Everyday Practice. International Symposium, St. Moritz, 1974.
3. Cassano, G. B., Castrogiovanni, P., Maggini, C., and Mauri, M. 1975. An attempt to improve communication between psychiatrists and non-psychiatrists in order to achieve cooperation in the treatment of depression. In: Therapy in Psychosomatic Medicine. Atti del III Congresso Mondiale ICPM, Rome, 16–20 September 1975. Luigi Pozzi, Roma.
4. Cassano, G. B., Castrogiovanni, P., Conti, L., and Nardini, A. G. 1976. Depression as seen by non-psychiatrist physicians. Comprehen. Psychiatry 17: 315.
5. Cassano, G. B., Castrogiovanni, P., Ghiozzi, M., and Principe, S. 1977. Rilevazione standard dei dati socio-ambientali mediante un questionario di autovalutazione. Atti XXXIII Congresso S.I.P., Naples, 29 October – 1 November 1977. CLEUD, Verona.
6. Castrogiovanni, P., Brunori, F., Raggi, F., Raglianti, P., and Gianfranchi, C. 1980. L'indagine epidemiologica quale momento preliminare alla pianificazione della consulenza in ospedale generale. Arch. Psicol. Neurol. Psichiat. 41: 79.
7. Castrogiovanni, P., and Pasculli, E. L'automazione nei tests psicodiagnostici. In: Progressi e prospettive dell'automazione in psicologia e psichiatria, Milano, 20–21 November/Regione Lombardie 1982. In press.
8. Faravelli, C. Le scale di valutazione in psichiatria. Quad Ital Psichiatr. In press.
9. Faravelli, C., Poli, E., Rosati, E., Paoli, M., and Ambronetti, A. 1982. Costruzione e validazione di una nuova scala per la valutazione dei sintomi nucleari della depressione. Riv. Psichiatr. 17: 101.
10. Gainotti, G., and Cianchetti, C. 1968. Questionario di autovalutazione guidata per indagini di psicofarmacologia clinica nelle sindromi ansioso-depressive. Riv. Patol. Nerv. Ment. 89: 442.
11. Gainotti, G., Cianchetti, C., Taramelli, M., and Tiacci, C. 1971. Studio comparativo di 4 scale di sintomatologia ansioso-depressiva (correlazioni con i criteri clinici). Riv. Patol. Nerv. Ment. 92: 98–109.
12. Pancheri, P., and Carilli, L. 1982. Standardizzazione e validazione di una nuova self-rating scale per la valutazione della sintomatologia depressiva. Riv. Psichiat. 17: 22.

Chapter 8 Standard Instruments Used in the Assessment of Depression in Africa

A. O. ODEJIDE

Introduction

In the first half of this century, depression as a syndrome was thought to be rare in Africa. Gordon (1936; cited in [9]), in Kenya, saw no cases of depression in a series of 120 admissions while Smartt (1956; cited in [9]) found only 15 cases of depression in a series of 252 admissions in Tanganyika. Similarly, Carothers [8] in Kenya recorded 24 cases of depression in 1508 admissions. Most of these reports were based on clinical diagnosis of depression.

More recently, however, it has become evident that depression is a common psychiatric disorder in Africa. Collomb and Zwingelstein reported depressive features in 16.3% of 580 psychiatric admissions in Dakar [12]. Similarly, Leighton et al. [24] in a cross-cultural study, found neurotic depressive symptomatology to be as common in Nigeria as in Stirling County in North America. Though there is a paucity of objective studies of depression in Africa, indigenous African psychiatrists agree that depressive illnesses were commonly found among Africans [1, 2, 10, 13, 16, 21, 28].

Clinical Presentation of Depression in African Patients

In most of the African countries, depression was not recognized as a psychological illness until the advent of Western culture. Odejide et al. [29] studying traditional healers found that there was a term ("were") in the local language to describe schizophrenia, but no term for depression. This nonrecognition of depression as an illness might be responsible for the reports of the low incidence of depression across the African continent by the earlier authors who came to Africa with Western concepts of depression and did not sufficiently appreciate the influence of sociocultural values on the symptom presentation (especially psychic) of depression. On the other hand, Western-trained medical doctors are perceived by the population in many African countries as being particularly capable of treating physical illnesses: hence, patients are more likely to describe to them somatic rather than psychological symptoms.

The view expressed in the preceding paragraph is supported by well-documented observations that somatic and autonomic complaints are often present in depressed Africans [1, 4, 13, 14, 21]. At the same time, however, the conclusive evidence that psychophysiological symptoms in depressed patients are universal [3, 26, 33, 35] makes it unnecessary to employ separate terms such as "somatization" when describing depression among the Africans.

Recent cross-cultural studies tend to show that certain features of depression are culture-dependent and that others are culture-independent [3, 27, 34]. Angst [3] listed the following depressive symptoms as amenable to cultural influence: suicidal tendencies, apathy, inhibition, retardation, agitation, feelings of guilt, hypochondriasis, delusions, and hallucinations. The author also identified changes in mood and disorders of drive and initiative as culture-independent features of depression. Similarly, Lehmann [23] considered what he described as organismic features (reduced interest, reduced capacity to enjoy, and reduced productivity) as the invariant core of depression present in all cultures.

The views expressed by the authors in the preceding paragraph have been supported by studies of depression in Africa. Field [15], in her study of Accran rural women, reported that depressed patients went to shrines (religious healing centers) with spontaneous self-accusation of witchcraft. The cultural belief of such patients in the mystical power of the shrines might be responsible for the spontaneous emission of psychological symptoms similar to what is observed in western Europe. Claver [10] in the Ivory Coast identifies "symbolic anthropopagia" as one of the symptoms of self-accusation. Diop [13] from Senegal found a similar feature called "Jaafur" in which patients firmly believe, without foundation, that they have eaten human flesh. Also, in a symposium on the recognition of depression in the African, Gruter [16] argued "that while depressive illness as a group of nosological entities is in principle the same in African patients as in Europeans, the phenomenological patterns it assumes seem to be clearly different."

The implication of this observation of the influence of culture on the psychological symptoms of depression is that an instrument devised in western Europe for the study of depression might need to be modified to make it applicable in Africa. In support of this viewpoint, Collomb remarked that the well-known Hamilton scale used to assess the severity of depression is very difficult to apply in Africa in the form originally suggested by Hamilton himself [11]. Collomb admitted introducing certain modifications to the scale in order to adapt it to African conditions.

Standardized Instruments Used in the Assessment of Depression in Africa

In the very few objective studies of depression in Africa, the standardized instruments used were:

1. The Present State Examination (PSE) schedule;
2. Zung's Self-Rating Depression Scale;
3. Hamilton Rating Scale for Depression

The Present State Examination

The PSE is an interview technique which allows functional psychotic and neurotic symptoms to be elicited and rated in a standard way [38]. After rating, the symptoms can be grouped into syndromes in order to present a profile of the mental state of the population studied. Further classification of the symptoms can be done using the computer classification called CATEGO.

The Present State Examination schedule was used in Nigeria for the study of depression across cultures [6]. It was also used in Kenya for the study of "life events and depression in a Kenyan setting" [36].

Binitie's [6] study was a cross-cultural comparison of Nigerian depressed patients in Uselu, Nigeria, and London, United Kingdom. The author administered the 7th edition of the PSE to patients he diagnosed as depressed. He then compared his clinical diagnoses with those made on the bases of PSE ratings and the computer program (CATEGO). Binitie claimed that depression in African cultures presented principally depressed mood, somatic symptoms, and motor retardation, while in London depression presented depressed mood, guilt, suicidal ideas, motor retardation, or anxiety.

Recently, doubts have been expressed about Binitie's findings. Olatawura [31] noted that when the author's clinical diagnoses were compared with those derived from CATEGO, there were striking differences. Eleven of the 37 cases diagnosed as psychotic depression (ICD 296.2) by the author were diagnosed as definitely schizophrenic and another five as probably schizophrenic by CATEGO. Similarly, 21 of the 37 cases Binitie diagnosed clinically as Neurotic Depression (ICD 300.4) were identified according to CATEGO criteria as Retarded Depression. Binitie's explanation of the disparity and a possible "personal" diagnostic style notwithstanding, it is clear, that there is a need to examine further the applicability of the PSE in the assessment of depression in Africa.

Vadher and Ndetei [36] used the PSE to exclude depressed patients from the control group in a study of the association between life events and depression in a Kenyan setting. Though the authors claimed to have taken into consideration the cultural variation in the presentation of depressive symptoms in the use of the PSE, they failed to describe the modifications to the PSE schedule. It is my belief that the PSE schedule is not yet sufficiently tested for the study of depression in Africans.

Zung's Self-Rating Depression Scale

Zung's Self-Rating Depression Scale (SDS) was introduced in 1965 and revised in 1974. Its reliability and validity have been established in European societies [39–41]. The instrument has also been shown to be applicable in Nigeria [18].

Jegede [20] tested the psychometric characteristics of the Yoruba version of the SDS. In the responses to the English and Yoruba versions of the SDS by the respondents with formal education and the illiterates (no formal education) the author obtained low correlations between the populations in the following items: (2)

Morning is when I feel the best; (6) I enjoy looking at, talking to, and being with attractive women or men; (16) I find it easy to make decisions; and (18) My life is pretty full. For the Yoruba version of the scale, the author also obtained low correlations on item (1) I feel downhearted and blue; and (14) I feel hopeful about the future. Jegede [20] offered possible explanations for these low correlations. His view was that item (6) may have different implications to a well-educated person who reads it in English and a less-educated person who reads it (or has it read to him) in Yoruba. He states that "To many persons in the latter category (persons with little or no formal education), admission of enjoying looking at, talking to, and being with an attractive member of the opposite sex may signify immorality."

It is obvious from this and other explanations that societal cultures and values can affect the interpretation of some of the SDS items, especially those that are psychologically oriented. The author's appreciation of this viewpoint made him conclude that there is a need to modify some of the SDS items to reflect local peculiarities before its further use in Nigeria.

Hamilton Rating Scale for Depression

In the 1975 analysis [17] of the pretreatment ratings of 480 subjects with the diagnoses of neurotic depression, the six factors identified were:

Factor I: Anxiety/somatization
Factor II: Weight
Factor III: Cognitive disturbance
Factor IV: Diurnal variation
Factor V: Retardation
Factor VI: Sleep disturbance

In Nigeria the Hamilton Rating Scale for Depression (HAM-D) was used in the open trial of Motival on patients with the diagnosis of depressive neurosis [30] (Motival is a combination of fluphenazine hydrochloride and nortriptyline) and it was shown that the prevailing symptoms were loading factors I, II, and VI. Only a few of the patients had cognitive disturbances or psychomotor retardation since they were mostly neurotic patients. This study can therefore not be used to assess the psychometric attributes of the HAM-D. However, my observation is that the symptoms contributing to factor III (cognitive disturbance) are essentially those symptoms of severe depression which have been suggested to be culture-dependent [3, 34]. As in the PSE and SDS, the modifications of culturally influenced items under factors II and V seem desirable prior to the application of the HAM-D in the African culture. This supports Collomb's call for modifying the HAM-D in order to adapt it to African conditions [11].

In conclusion, it is now evident that the various subtypes of depressive illness are present among Africans. However, the present review of some of the studies of depression in Africa, where the Western-oriented instruments were used, suggests the need to modify such instruments for valid data collection. In particular, the psychological symptoms of depression such as self-reproach, guilt feelings, suicidal ideations, delusions, and hallucinations are usually not disclosed voluntarily by Africans to the Western-trained doctors. Therefore, information in these areas might be unobtainable or falsified if the existing depression scales are used in Africa without necessary modifications of these items which are particularly culture-dependent.

References

1. Adomakoh, C. 1975. The pattern of depressive illness in Africans. In: Recognition of Depression in the African: Proceedings of a Round-table Discussion, pp. 14-17. Ciba-Geigy, Basle.
2. Ammar, S. 1975. A review of the problem of depression in Africans with particular reference to the situation in Tunisia. In: Recognition of Depression in the African: Proceedings of a Round-table Discussion, pp. 9-13. Ciba-Geigy, Basle.
3. Angst, J. 1973. Masked depression viewed from the cross-cultural standpoint. In: P. Kielholz (ed.), Masked depression, pp. 269-274. Huber, Bern.
4. Asuni, T. 1962. Suicide in western Nigeria. Br. Med. J. 2: 1091-1097.
5. Asuni, T. 1966. Suicide in Western Nigeria. In: T. A. Lambo (ed.), First Pan-African Psychiatric Conference Report, pp. 164-175. Government Printer, Ibadan.
6. Binitie, A. 1975. A factor-analytical study of depression across cultures (African and European). Br. J. Psychiatry 127: 559-563.
7. Carothers, J. C. 1948. A study of mental derangement in Africans and an attempt to explain its peculiarities more especially in relation to the African attitude to life. Psychiatry 11: 47-85.
8. Carothers, J. C. 1951. Frontal lobe function and the African. Journal of Mental Science 97: 12-48.
9. Carothers, J. C. 1972. The mind of man in Africa. Stacey, London.
10. Claver, B. 1975. Two special types of depression. In: Recognition of Depression in the African: Proceedings of a Round-table discussion, pp. 19-21. Ciba-Geigy, Basle.
11. Collomb, H. 1975. Masks assumed by depressive states in Africa. In: Recognition of Depression in the African: Proceedings of a Round-table Discussion, pp. 22-25. Ciba-Geigy, Basle.
12. Collomb, H., and Zwingelstein. 1961. Depressive states in an African community (Dakar). In: T. A. Lambo (ed.), First Pan-African Psychiatric Conference Report, pp. 227-234. Government Printer, Ibadan.
13. Diop, B. 1975. Self-accusation as a symptom of depression. In: Recognition of Depression in the African: Proceedings of a Round-table Discussion, pp. 25-26. Ciba-Geigy, Basle.
14. Ebie, J. C. 1972. Some observations on depressive illness in Nigerians attending a psychiatric out-patient clinic. Afr. J. Med. Sci. 3: 149-155.
15. Field, M. J. 1960. Search for Security: an ethno-psychiatric Study of Rural Ghana, Faber and Faber, London.
16. Gruter, W. 1975. Cardinal symptoms of depression. In: Recognition of Depression in the African: Proceedings of a Round-table Discussion, pp. 27-30. Ciba-Geigy, Basle.
17. Guy, W. 1976. ECDEU Assessment manual for Psychopharmacology. NIMH Production, Rockville.
18. Jegede, R. O. 1976. Psychometric attributes of the self-rating depression scale. J. Psychol. 93: 27-30.
19. Jegede, R. O. 1978. Depressive symptomatology in patients attending a hospital-based general out-patient clinic. Afr. J. Med. Sci. 7: 207-210.
20. Jegede, R. O. 1979. Depression in Africans revisited. A critical review of the literature. Afr. J. Med. Sci. 8: 125-132.
21. Lambo, T. A. 1956. Neuropsychiatric observations in Western region of Nigeria. Br. Med. J. 2: 1388-1394.
22. Lambo, T. A. 1960. Further neuropsychiatric observations in Nigeria. Br. Med. J. 2: 1696-1704.

23. Lehmann, H. E. 1973. Definition of the term "Masked Depression." In: P. Kielholz (ed.), Masked Depression, pp. 283-285. Huber, Bern.
24. Leighton, A. H., Lambo, T. A., Hughes, C. C., Leighton, D. C., et al. 1963. Psychiatric Disorders Among the Yoruba. Cornell University Press, New York.
25. Lopez-Ibor, J. J. 1972. Masked depression and depressive equivalents. In: P. Kielholz (ed.), Depressive Illness, pp. 38-44. Huber, Bern.
26. Lopez-Ibor, J. J. 1973. Depressive equivalents. In: P. Kielholz (ed.), Masked Depression, pp. 97-112. Huber, Bern.
27. Murphy, J. M., and Leighton, A. H. 1963. Native conceptions of psychiatric disorders. In: J. Murphy and A. Leighton (eds.), Approaches to Cross-cultural Psychiatry, pp. 64-107. Cornell University Press, Ithaca, New York.
28. Muya, W. J. 1975. The influence of increasing sophistication on the nature of depressive symptoms. In: Recognition of Depression in the African: Proceedings of a Round-table Discussion, pp. 35-37. Ciba-Geigy, Basle.
29. Odejide, A. O., Olatawura, M. O., Sanda, A. O., and Oyeneye, A. O. 1978. Traditional healers and mental illness in the city of Ibadan. Journal of Black Studies 9 (2): 195-205.
30. Oheari, J. U., and Odejide, A. O. 1981. Drug trial on Motival. Journal of Pharmaceutical and Medical Sciences 5 (6): 393-414.
31. Olatawura, M. O. 1973. The problem of diagnosing depression in Nigeria. Psychopathologie Africaine 9: 389-403.
32. Pichot, P. 1972. The problem of quantifying the symptomatology of depression. In: P. Kielholz (ed.), Depressive Illness, pp. 74-81. Huber, Bern.
33. Pichot, P., and Hassan, J. 1973. Masked depression and depressive equivalents – problems of definition and diagnosis. In: P. Kielholz (ed.), Masked Depression, pp. 61-76. Huber, Bern.
34. Prince, R. H. 1968. The changing picture of depressive syndrome in Africa: Is it fact or diagnostic fashion. Canadian Journal of African Studies 1: 117-192.
35. Serry, D., and Serry, M. 1969. Masked depression and the use of antidepressants in general practice. Med. J. Aust. 56 (1): 334.
36. Vadher, A., and Ndetei, D. M. 1981. Life events and depression in a Kenyan setting. Br. J. Psychiatry 139: 134-137.
37. Wing, J. K. 1970. A standard form of Present State Examination. In: E. H. Hare and J. K. Wing (eds.), International Symposium on Psychiatric Epidemiology. Oxford University Press, London.
38. Wing, J. K., Cooper, J. E. and Sartorius, N. 1974. The Measurement and Classification of Psychiatric Symptoms. Cambridge University Press.
39. Zung, W. W. K. 1969. A cross-cultural survey of symptoms in depression. Am. J. Psychiatry 126: 116-121.
40. Zung, W. W. K. 1971. Depression in the normal adult population. Psychosomatics 12: 164-167.
41. Zung, W. W. K. 1973. From art to science: The diagnosis and treatment of depression. Arch. Gen. Psychiatry 29: 328-337.

Chapter 9 The WHO Instruments for the Assessment of Depressive Disorders

A. JABLENSKY, N. SARTORIUS, W. GULBINAT, and G. ERNBERG

Introduction

The instruments for the evaluation of patients with depressive symptoms produced by the World Health Organization in the 1970s occupy an intermediate position between selectively focused, brief rating scales like the Hamilton Depression Scale [5] and the comprehensive, semistructured interviews like the Present State Examination (PSE [17]) or the Schedule for Affective Disorders and Schizophrenia (SADS [14]). The WHO depression battery consists of a Screening Form, a Schedule for Standardized Assessment of Depressive Disorders (WHO-SADD) which is the core of the battery, and a follow-up version of the WHO-SADD. The WHO-SADD is a "dedicated" instrument, in the sense that it is designed for the rating of symptoms and recording of other relevant information in patients with depressive illnesses; symptomatology other than affective receives less coverage in it than in the PSE or SADS. However, the scope of psychopathology that can be rated in the WHO-SADD is considerably wider than that of the brief depression scales.

These characteristics, together with simplicity of use, have made the WHO-SADD attractive to investigators engaged in various kinds of research in the affective disorders. Originally, the instrument was drafted for a clinical study of depressive states in different cultures [6, 12, 13]. Subsequently, it has been used in studies of therapeutic response to antidepressants [1, 15]; general practice studies [8]; and service-based epidemiological studies [7]. In addition to the centers participating in the original WHO study – Basle (Switzerland), Montreal (Canada), Nagasaki and Tokyo (Japan), and Teheran (Iran), the WHO-SADD has research applications in Austria, Bulgaria, Denmark, Finland, France, Federal Republic of Germany, Ghana, India, Poland, and the United Kingdom. It is at present available in ten languages. Considering the total number of patients assessed and the countries where it has been introduced, the WHO-SADD certainly counts among the most widely used instruments for the study of depression.

This paper provides an overview of the development and of the most important features of the three interrelated WHO instruments.

History and Development

The first draft of the WHO-SADD was prepared in 1971 for the initial meeting of collaborating investigators, who agreed to carry out a comparative study of depressive disorders treated at psychiatric facilities in several countries.[1] The requirements which were laid down for the new instrument were:

Relative simplicity in application and economy in terms of time needed for completion

Comprehensiveness, in terms of coverage of all clinically relevant manifestations of depressive illnesses

Cross-cultural applicability

Standardized content of items and specified rating rules

Acceptability to clinicians, researchers, and patients

In order to meet these requirements, it was decided not to compile a fully structured interview with specified questions and probes to be asked verbatim, but rather to make a checklist of demographic, past history, symptomatological, and other items which were to be rated by the investigator in the course of an ordinary clinical interview. The rater was to be encouraged to use clinical judgment on the basis of all available information from the interview, case notes, informants, and other sources. The items of the draft schedule were selected by taking into consideration the literature on the phenomenology and course of depressive states in various populations and the expert opinion of the senior investigators. As distinct from other schedules for rating psychopathology, which are usually developed through the reduction and condensation of a large pool of initial items, the WHO-SADD was drafted as a core set of agreed items, to which open-ended items for "other" symptoms, particularly culture-specific ones, could be added as necessary. Standardization of item content and uniformity of rating were to be achieved by providing a glossary of definitions and by specifying the rules for making particular ratings on the individual items.

With these characteristics, the schedule was expected to be easy to master and adapt to a variety of individual interviewing styles. Two consecutive drafts of the WHO-SADD were pilot-tested in different research centers, and thoroughly re-

---

[1] The collaborating investigators in the study were:

Basle:	Dr P. Kielholz (chief collaborating investigator)
	Dr M. Gastpar and Dr. G. Hole
Montreal:	Dr H. E. Lehmann (chief collaborating investigator)
	Dr F. R. Fenton, Dr. R. Lajoie, Dr. S. Ang, and Dr. R. Yassa
Nagasaki:	Dr R. Takahashi (chief collaborating investigator)
	Dr I. Fujii, Dr. N. Hirota, Dr. Y. Sakurai, and Dr. T. Yuzuriha
Teheran:	Dr H. Davidian (chief collaborating investigator)
	Dr M. Naraghi
Tokyo:	Dr N. Shinfuku (chief collaborating investigator)
	Dr K. Hasegawa and Dr. M. Shimizu
WHO Headquarters:	Dr N. Sartorius (principal investigator)
	Dr A. Jablensky (chief Headquarters investigator)
	Mr W. Gulbinat (statistician)
	Mrs G. Ernberg (technical assistant)

viewed at meetings of the collaborating investigators. The prefinal, fourth draft was the version actually used in the multicenter study, which involved an initial clinical assessment of 573 patients and a 5-year follow-up.[2] In the course of this study, comments on the general framework and on individual items were systematically collected. Together with directions which emerged from the statistical analysis of the data, and from intercenter reliability exercises, they provided the input for the fifth, final draft of the schedule, which has been published as an annex to the WHO monograph on the results of the initial evaluation phase of the study [13] and is the one currently recommended for use.

The Screening Form was drafted at the same time as the schedule, as a simple checklist of inclusion/exclusion criteria for the selection of patients for the above-mentioned study.

The follow-up version of the schedule (FU-SADD) was designed in 1977. It has retained the basic format of the WHO-SADD, but includes supplementary sections for rating the course and outcome of the disorder.

Simultaneously with the development of the WHO-SADD, the collaborating investigators at the field research centers and at WHO headquarters in Geneva worked on consecutive versions of its accompanying glossary. Whereas the first draft of the glossary only contained brief descriptive notes on individual items, the final version, prepared after the completion of the field studies, included more detailed and explicit rating rules, notes on the culture-specific presentations of certain symptoms, and recommended probes, found in different centers to be particularly useful in eliciting symptoms.

The three instruments and the glossary were drafted in English. The schedules were translated, for the purposes of the WHO study, into German, Japanese, and Farsi by psychiatrists working with professional translators. Each translated version was retranslated into English by a person who had not been involved in the first translation. After comparing the retranslation into English with the original at the headquarters of the study, modifications of the local translation were made, sometimes after repeated retranslation into English, until satisfactory textual and semantic equivalence was attained. Similar translation procedures were adopted by other investigators and centers using the WHO instrument.

The Screening Form

The purpose of the screening procedure in the WHO study was to differentiate between patients who were probably depressive and other psychiatric in- and outpatients. The Screening Form was designed for the identification of eligible cases within already defined patient populations, but not for the detection of undiagnosed depressive illnesses in general population samples. However, it has since been applied also to consecutive attendances at general practices or general outpatient departments, and has proved effective in identifying patients with depressive disorders in such nonpsychiatric settings (report in preparation).

---

[2] Several of the research centers have now also completed a 10-year follow-up on the original cases

In principle, the Screening Form can be applied by a psychiatrist, a general practitioner, or a clinical psychologist familiar with the symptoms of depressive disorders, organic brain disease, schizophrenia, and other functional psychoses.

The Screening Form (Appendix A) specifies two sets of criteria. The first set has the following four exclusion items: (a) the presence of definite physical disease, toxic disorder, or cerebral damage or disease; (b) moderate or severe mental retardation (IQ 70 or less); (c) the presence of one or more symptoms characteristic of psychoses other than affective, and in particular of schizophrenia – thought withdrawal or intrusion, "echo" of thought, delusions of being controlled, elaborate systems of delusions (other than guilt, hypochondriasis, impoverishment, nihilism), and elaborate hallucinations with content other than depressive; and (d) the presence of severe language or hearing difficulties. A patient exhibiting none of these exclusion criteria could be considered to have a nonorganic depressive disorder if *at least two* of the following eight inclusion criteria were present: depressive mood, suicidal thoughts, hopelessness, feelings of worthlessness, hypochondriasis and/or anxiety, feelings of diminution of ability, self-reproach or guilt, and inability to feel or enjoy. Symptoms that would distinguish between forms or subtypes of depressive disorders are not included in the screen.

The method of application of the Screening Form is not rigidly prescribed, and can be adjusted to the particular context in which the screening is carried out. Case notes, informants, or a brief interview with the patient have been the principal sources of information in the WHO study. Professional experience is, in all instances, a prerequisite for making the judgments implied in several of the items.

Sensitivity and Specificity.[3] The validity criterion for the capacity of the Screening Form to distinguish depressive patients from other kinds of patients was the clinical diagnosis made independently by routine psychiatric assessment. Table 9.1 presents data on the sensitivity and specificity[3] of the Screening Form obtained in the process of selecting patients for the WHO multicenter clinical study. Taking as a validating variable the presence of a clinical diagnosis of a nonorganic depressive disorder [ICD (International Classification of Diseases) rubrics 296, 298.0 or 300.4], the sensitivity and specificity of the instrument, determined on the basis of a total of 1208 screened cases in five centers, were relatively high: 85.8% and 90.4%, respectively.

---

[3] Sensitivity is defined as the ability of a test to classify correctly as "positive" all those who have the disorder that is being investigated (the lower the rate of false-negative results, the more sensitive the procedure).

Specificity, by contrast, is the ability of the test to classify correctly as "negative" all those who do not have the disorder. Therefore, specificity is a measure of the rate of false-positive results of the screening procedure (the fewer false-positives, the more specific the test).

Sensitivity and specificity can be presented as proportions [16]:

$$\text{Sensitivity} = \frac{\text{Subjects who have the disorder and are classified as "positive" by the test}}{\text{All subjects in the population who have the disorder}} \times 100$$

$$\text{Specificity} = \frac{\text{Subjects who do not have the disorder and are classified as "negative" by the test}}{\text{All subjects in the population who do not have the disorder}} \times 100$$

Table 9.1. Sensitivity and specificity of the WHO Screening Form for depressive disorders in different centers

	Basle	Montreal	Nagasaki	Teheran	Tokyo	All centers
Number of patients screened	272	192	210	234	300	1208
Sensitivity (%)	91.2	81.8	78.7	83.3	89.6	85.8
Specificity (%)	91.8	84.1	88.3	93.8	92.6	90.4

Table 9.2. Patients in whom one or more Screening Form depressive symptoms were present on first contact (percentage of all patients in each diagnostic category)

	Men	Women	Total
Organic psychoses	4.9	11.1	7.6
Schizophrenia	11.3	8.5	10.2
Affective psychoses	98.0	99.4	98.9
Paranoid and other nonorganic psychoses	3.7	17.1	11.8
Neuroses	23.7	20.9	21.7
Personality disorders	22.7	25.5	23.8
Mental retardation	1.4	6.6	3.8
Other conditions	7.2	10.6	8.9

Since the specificity of the Screening Form is higher than its sensitivity, it can be expected that a screening procedure based on this instrument would tend to be somewhat underinclusive – i.e., it would select for study patients who are likely to be considered depressive by most psychiatrists, and exclude patients in whom a diagnosis of depression might still be considered but would command less agreement.

Frequency of Screening Symptoms in Different Diagnostic Categories. The above conclusion about the high specificity of the Screening Form was reinforced by the data from an epidemiological study [7], in which a total of 10 176 persons contacting for the first time any outpatient or inpatient psychiatric service in Bulgaria were screened with the WHO instrument. Table 9.2 shows the percentages of patients within each major ICD diagnostic category (assigned at the facility independently from the screening procedure) in whom at least one of the depressive symptoms listed in the Screening Form was present. While 98.9% of the patients who had received a clinical diagnosis of affective disorder were positive on one or more of the Screening Form items, the proportion of individuals with depressive symptoms in diagnostic categories such as mental retardation or organic psychoses was as low as 3.8% and 7.6%.

The Standardized Schedule for Assessment of Depressive Disorders (WHO-SADD)

The structure of the WHO-SADD is as follows: Part 1 contains data on the patient and the investigator(s) who completed the schedule, on the interview, and on other sources of information that were used. The data on the patient include name (optional), age and sex, marital status, socioeconomic status, employment, education, religion, and current treatment status. Part 2 is a list of symptoms and signs that can be assessed in a clinical interview and from data provided by informants and other sources, such as case notes. The first section of Part 2 is a checklist of 40 symptoms and signs (see Appendix B), common in depressive disorders and defined in the glossary accompanying the schedule. The ratings on these symptoms and signs are made in relation to (a) the time when the symptom or sign was present (two ratings are made, one for the month preceding the interview, and another for appearance of the symptom at any time during the current episode of illness); and (b) the intensity or degree of manifestation of the symptom (absent, mild, occasionally severe or continuously present). The checklist also includes open-ended items that allow the recording of rare or culture-specific symptoms. The second section of Part 2 consists of 18 items related to the past history of the patient – for example, number of past episodes, presence of precipitating factors, and presence of mental disorder in relatives. Part 3 contains items for the recording of the diagnosis, of the impression of the overall severity of the condition, and for the classification of the patient's diagnosis. In each case, the investigator is requested to make a diagnosis in terms that he would customarily use in his own practice. In addition he is requested to "trans-late" his diagnosis into a category of the ICD. Also in Part 3, the investigator is required to rate the severity of the condition, to specify the clinical syndrome in addition to the nosological diagnosis, and to indicate the five most important items (symptoms or history data) that he considered to be the reasons for selecting a particular diagnostic category.

It should be noted that no diagnostic "key" or "algorithm" has been originally developed for the WHO-SADD, since one of the purposes of the clinical study in which it was first employed was precisely the exploration of the reasons psychiatrists give for choosing one or another diagnostic label for a depressive state.

An excerpt from the accompanying glossary is given in Appendix C.

Reliability of WHO-SADD Assessment. To determine the reliability of the assessment of patients with the WHO-SADD, a series of rating exercises were carried out in the centers participating in the WHO study.

During an exercise the same patient was rated simultaneously by two or more psychiatrists, one of them filling in the schedule while conducting the interview and the other (or others) observing and making independent ratings. The observer(s) was (were) given an opportunity to ask clarifying questions at the end of the interview.

A total of 83 such rating exercises was performed in the five centers.

Three groups of items were distinguished for the assessment of reliability – sociodemographic items, symptoms and signs of the patient's present state, and past history items.

For purposes of analysis, some of the items were regrouped. Ratings on symptoms and signs were dichotomized into "present" and "absent" categories by taking ratings 0, "not applicable" and "uncertain", as negative, and ratings 1 and 2 as positive.

The data from all 83 reliability exercises were first analyzed together; subsequently values for individual centers were calculated.

Reliability was evaluated in terms of three coefficients:

1. Agreement ratio a, defined as the number of ratings for which the raters achieved agreement divided by the total number of ratings
2. The probability coefficient π, which represents the solution of

$$a = \pi^2 + (1-\pi)^2$$

where a is the agreement ratio
3. The φ coefficient for dichotomous variables

$$\varphi = \frac{\chi^2}{N}$$

where N is the total number of ratings.[4]

In case of complete agreement, a, π, and φ equal 1.0; the lowest possible value for π is 0.5, while a and φ may reach a value of 0. For easier comparison between π and φ, the latter coefficient may be transformed to $\varphi' = (\varphi+1)/2$, with a range of possible values for φ' of 0.5–1.0.

An overview of the average values of the reliability coefficients for the three main parts of the schedule, and for each of the five centers, is provided in Table 9.3. The levels of reliability in intracenter assessments were generally high. Agreement on sociodemographic characteristics was 0.98. The symptoms and signs, too, could be assessed with high reliability, and the average π-value was 0.96. The reliability of the psychiatric history items was slightly lower (0.91).

Of particular interest is the question concerning the reliability of individual items within each section of the instrument.

Sociodemographic variables can be assessed very reliably, and the coefficients for items such as age, sex, residence, and marital status are close to 1. Some difficulties have arisen with the item "highest level of education" ($\pi = 0.93$), because the rating instruction at the time of the original reliability assessments was not sufficiently precise (this has been corrected in the latest version of the schedule).

Table 9.3. Average reliability π of WHO-SADD by item groups

	Basle	Montreal	Nagasaki	Teheran	Tokyo	All centers combined
Sociodemographic	0.94	0.98	0.95	0.99	0.99	0.98
Symptoms and signs	0.93	0.96	0.97	0.99	0.93	0.96
Psychiatric history	0.98	0.90	0.90	0.99	0.95	0.91

---

[4] For a detailed discussion of the reliability measurements employed in the WHO study, see Annex 1 of the study report [13].

The WHO-SADD symptom profile consists of 39 psychiatric symptoms and signs and one item on physical disease, rated as present/absent during the last week (in the final version of the WHO-SADD this was changed to the last month) before the interview, and as present/absent at any time before this period. Analyses were first carried out separately to determine the reliability in assessing symptoms present during the last week and at any time during the episode. Then both ratings were combined so that a symptom was considered to be present when it was coded 1 or 2 in either of these time intervals. There was no change in the level of reliability when the ratings of "last week" and "any time in the episode" were combined.

The reliability profile, combining the reliability exercises of all centers, showed that the delusional items of the checklist (such as delusions of guilt, hypochondriasis, impoverishment, nihilism, and others) had π-values between 1.00 and 0.96, i.e., indicating higher reliabilities than any other symptom items (Table 9.4).

Delusions, however, were rated as present in only 0.6% of the patients. The high agreement ($\pi = 0.99$) of the psychiatrists on items concerning delusions was therefore agreement on the absence of these symptoms. On the basis of the data available, no definite conclusion can be drawn about the probability of "correctly" assessing the presence of a delusional symptom. At the other extreme, a frequent symptom like sadness was rated as present in more than 90% of the patients in the reliability exercise. The high π-value for this symptom, therefore, reflects mainly the reliability of agreement in rating the item as present. For most of the other symptoms and signs in the schedule there was sufficient variation in frequency to interpret π as the average probability in assessing the symptoms "correctly," both when symptoms were present and when they were absent.

It should be noted that a low φ'-value in this context does not necessarily mean low reliability, since the actual agreement between the raters was almost complete. The rarity of any item (delusional symptoms in this instance) tends to lower the value of reliability coefficients, like the φ'-value, which assesses agreement on both absence and presence of the item. This is not the case with the π-value, for which *separate* values can be computed for presence and absence of a given item.

The symptom reliability profile for all centers combined is shown in Fig. 9.1. The confidence intervals at the level of 95% are also shown. In this diagram reliability is expressed in terms of the probabilities π. The average of all the 39 π-values is 0.96, which corresponds to an average agreement ratio of 0.92. None of the symptoms has a π-value less than 0.90, and only ten symptoms were assessed with a reliability less than or equal to 0.94.

Table 9.4. Symptoms with very high reliability of assessment of absence or presence

Symptom	π	φ'
1. Sadness	0.99	0.92
21. Delusions of hypochondriasis	0.99[a]	0.81
22. Delusions of impoverishment	0.99[a]	0.81
23. Other delusions	0.99[a]	–
12. Loss of ability to concentrate	0.98	0.92
20. Delusions of guilt	0.96[a]	0.67

[a] Agreement on absence of the symptom.

The WHO Instruments for the Assessment of Depressive Disorders

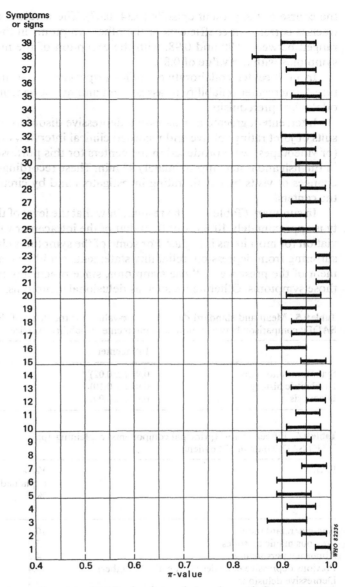

Fig. 9.1. Reliability: intracenter – all centers combined – for each (number-coded) symptom or sign. Reliability coefficients are indicated with lower and upper confidence limits (95%). Reproduced from [13] by permission of the World Health Organization

There was considerable variation of the level of reliability at which items describing the past history of the patient could be assessed. While the number of previous depressive episodes and the number of years since the first depressive episode could be assessed with high reliability (values 0.95–0.98), the corresponding values for manic episodes were rather low: 0.68–0.77. Similar difficulties arose when rating the course of the present episode (0.34-0.67). The π-values or the transformed intraclass correlation coefficients of the other symptoms in this part of the schedule ranged between 0.90 and 0.98, with the exception of the number of years free of symptoms with a π-value of 0.86.

In multicenter collaborative studies (especially those involving different cultures), intercenter reliability of assessment and measurements is an essential methodological prerequisite.

Intercenter agreement in assessing depressive disorders was examined using results of joint ratings of live and recorded clinical interviews with patients. Ten films (or videotapes) were produced in the centers for this purpose. The interviews were in English and lasted approximately 45 min. These recordings were rated during exchanges of visits by collaborating investigators and by circulating material among the centers.

In summary (Table 9.5), the results show that the level of the intercenter reliability is approximately 10% lower than that of the intracenter values. The standard deviation for most items is higher. For some of the symptoms characteristic of patients suffering from depression, reliability statements could be made only on the assessment of the presence of those symptoms, since practically no patient was without those symptoms. Other items, such as delusional symptoms, could be assessed only

Table 9.5. Mean and standard deviation of π-values for the items of three sections of the WHO-SADD: comparison between intra- and intercenter reliability exercise

	Intracenter	Intercenter
Symptoms and signs	0.96 (±0.02)	0.88 (±0.07)
Psychiatric history	0.91 (±0.10)	0.83 (±0.11)
Diagnosis	0.92 (±0.09)	0.82 (±0.17)

Table 9.6. Fifteen factors (principal components) explaining approximately 50% of the variance on WHO-SADD data in 573 patients

Factor	Variance explained %	Cumulative variance explained %
Anergia/retardation	10.1	10.1
Previous manic episodes	5.2	15.3
Abnormal personality	4.2	19.5
Previous depressive episodes (unspecified number)	3.4	22.9
Depressive delusions	3.2	26.1
Dejection	3.0	29.1
Marital status	2.7	31.8
Socioeconomic status	2.7	34.5
Sleep disturbance	2.5	37.0
Anxiety/agitation	2.2	39.2
Previous manic episodes (unspecified number)	2.2	41.4
Hypochondriasis	2.1	43.5
Other symptoms	1.9	45.4
Changed appetite and body weight	1.9	47.3
Employment: working hours	1.8	49.1

in terms of reliability for measuring their absence. Nevertheless, none of the items assessed was of insufficient reliability, and all π-values were significantly above 0.5.

Factor Analysis of WHO-SADD. The data on 573 patients with clinical diagnoses of nonorganic depressive illnesses were subjected to principal component analysis, in order to simplify comparisons between subgroups of patients and provide a more concise description of depressive symptomatology that can be rated on the WHO-SADD.

The first 15 factors obtained by principal component analysis[5] explained approximately 50% of the variance in the cross-cultural data (Table 9.6). Most of the factors turned out to be easily interpretable from a clinical point of view. For example, the first factor (anergia/retardation), which explained over 10% of the variance, was loaded by the following 12 items:

	Loading
Loss of interest	0.668
Psychomotor retardation	0.656
Slowness of thought	0.650
Indecisiveness	0.620
Lack of energy	0.609
Loss of ability to concentrate	0.603
Lack of contact	0.572
Joylessness	0.488
Changed perception of time	0.481
Disruption of social functioning	0.475
Decrease of libido	0.459
Sadness	0.415

The highest loadings are on items describing a syndrome of anergic retarded depression, with which other items of depressive symptomatology, such as joylessness, sadness, and decrease of libido, correlate, as could be clinically predicted.

Other examples are factor 5 (depressive delusions), loaded by the following five items:

	Loading
Delusions of impoverishment	0.774
Delusions of guilt	0.749
Hypochondriacal delusions	0.480
Ideas of impoverishment	0.464
Ideas of persecution and reference	0.420

and factor 6 (dejection):

	Loading
Hopelessness	0.641
Feelings of guilt and self-reproach	0.518
Ideas of insufficiency, inadequacy and worthlessness, lack of self-confidence	0.414
Sadness	0.406

---
[5] Only factor loadings equal to, or greater than 0.4 were considered in the analysis

The results of the principal component analysis were used to examine the relationship between clinical data, such as symptomatology and past history items, and the diagnostic classification of patients with depressive disorders. For this purpose, the different diagnostic rubrics applied to the patients in the research centers were assembled into two major categories, endogenous depressions and psychogenic depressions, in the following manner:

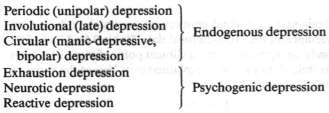

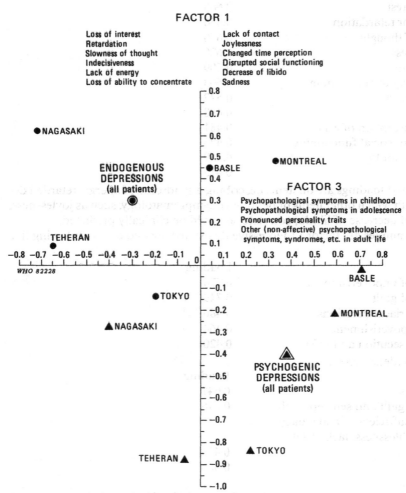

Fig. 9.2. Differences between endogenous and psychogenic depressive disorders in terms of two orthogonal factors ($P = 0.01$, MANOVA). Reproduced from [13] by permission of the World Health Organization

The results of multivariate analysis of variance (MANOVA) demonstrated that two orthogonal factors, factor 1 (anergia/retardation) and factor 3 (abnormal personality), distinguished best between the two diagnostic groups (Fig. 9.2). Patients with the diagnosis of endogenous depression had high scores on factor 1 and low scores on factor 3, while patients with the diagnosis of psychogenic depression showed the reverse pattern and had high scores on factor 3 and low scores on factor 1. The analysis also revealed interesting similarities and differences between the centers. For example, the similarity of both endogenous depressives and psychogenic depressives in Basle and Montreal is as striking as the magnitude of the differences between the patients assessed in Tokyo and in Nagasaki.

Discriminant function analysis demonstrated that endogenous and psychogenic depressive illnesses could be separated in terms of mean scores for factors 1 and 3, with misclassification rates ranging from 21.9% to 34.0% (average 28.3%) in the different centers.

The individual WHO-SADD items that discriminated best between the two types of depression varied somewhat from center to center, but they could all be related to the clinical stereotypes of the endogenous and psychogenic depressions which have been proposed by supporters of this classification. These discriminating items were used consistently in the centers, since the misclassification rates obtained with only five items were as low as 6.0%–9.8% in three centers, and 15.5% and 18.7% in the remaining two. In all centers combined, the items discriminating best between endogenous and psychogenic depression were: presence of continual psychological stress and history of psychopathological symptoms in childhood – characteristic of psychogenic depression; and psychomotor retardation, early awakening, and a history of past depressive episodes – characteristic of endogenous depression.

Relationship of WHO-SADD to Other Instruments for Assessment of Depression

As pointed out above, the WHO-SADD assessment produces three profiles describing a patient with a depressive disorder: a demographic profile, a symptomatological profile, and a past history profile. The formulation of a diagnosis is left to the clinical judgement of the rater, and there is no inbuilt diagnostic score or algorithm. However, attempts have been made to link WHO-SADD data to some of the widely used diagnostic scales that have found applications in many clinical trials of antidepressants. Thus, Bech et al. [1] have transformed the rating scales for 17 of the WHO-SADD items [selected for their correspondence to the 17-item version of the Hamilton Depression Scale (5)], and adapted them to the so-called Newcastle weighted scores for diagnostic differentiation between endogenous and nonendogenous depressions [3, 10, 11]

Similarly, Katschnig et al. [8] have demonstrated by applying discriminant function analysis to data on 77 patients who had dual assessments that WHO-SADD symptoms discriminate very well (91% correct classification) between patients identified as "cases" and as "noncases" by the General Health Questionnaire [4].

In a more recent study, Bech et al. [2] extended such work further and identified WHO-SADD item combinations which can lead to close approximations to the Research Diagnostic Criteria (RDC) and DSM (Diagnostic and Statistical Manual of Mental Disorders) -III diagnoses of major depression and melancholia. The two subscales derived from WHO-SADD, a 16-item severity (melancholia) scale and a 10-item endogenous/nonendogenous diagnostic scale, have been found to command satisfactory interrater reliability.

A comparison between the item contents of WHO-SADD and the SADS [14], which has been developed in conjunction with the RDC and applied in the NIMH (National Institute of Mental Health) Collaborative Program on the Psychobiology of Depression [9], is presented in Appendix D.[6]

The Follow-up Version of WHO-SADD

The FU-SADD has three principal parts (in addition to the introductory sections for the recording of patient identification data and general information about the interview).

The first main part is designed for the assessment of the patient's present mental state at the time of the follow-up. It is identical to the symptomatology section of WHO-SADD (which allows 40 symptoms to be rated) but contains some added special provisions for the recording of neurologic and physical signs and symptoms, such as memory loss, tremor, or disturbance of gait and equilibrium.

The second part is designed for recording information about the clinical course of the illness over the preceding 5 years (or 10 years in another modification of the FU-SADD). It includes a synopsis of episodes and intervals, with appropriate definitions, and a checklist for rating detailed descriptive features of each episode and each interval. The checklist for the individual episode contains items describing the clinical type of the episode (e.g., depressive, manic, initially depressive then manic, initially manic then depressive, mixed, circular, other), items dealing with various treatments, and provisions for writing down a brief narrative summary of the main features of the episode.

The third part of the schedule contains a checklist of important life events which may have occurred in the follow-up period and sections for detailed recording of information about changes in residence and housing, education, religion, occupation and employment, use of drugs and alcohol, social relationships and social functioning, self-care, and contacts with the law. For patients who have died prior to the follow-up date, any available data about the causes and circumstances of death are recorded in a special section.

With some modification the FU-SADD has been used for both 5-year and 10-year follow-up assessments of patients in different cultures, and its applicability has been found to be satisfactory.

---

[6] The comparative analysis of the contents of the two schedules has been carried out by the late Dr Robert W. Shapiro (unpublished data).

Training in the Use of WHO-SADD

A training procedure for psychiatrists, psychologists, and other researchers intending to use the instrument is now well established and has been tested repeatedly over the last few years. Originally, each field research center participating in the WHO study prepared several films or videotapes of interviews with depressive patients based on the WHO-SADD schedule. They were recorded in the local languages and used extensively in the training of raters; in addition, several of these recordings were used in intercenter training and reliability exercises. For the reliability exercises they were at first either dubbed in English or supplied with an English transcript. Dubbing was abandoned because of the difficulty of achieving correspondence between the patient's observable expression and psychomotor behavior and the dubbing reader's tone and inflexion of voice; only videotapes made originally in English were used as intercenter exercises. Later in the project audiotapes were added to the training tools.

In addition to films and tapes, each center prepared a number of detailed case histories, which were used for discussion during the meetings of collaborating investigators and for diagnostic reliability exercises.

Before data collection began, each investigator had completed at least ten assessments of patients with WHO-SADD. When new investigators joined the project they were fully trained by experienced users of the schedule and had to carry out at least ten interviews under supervision before beginning to assess patients independently.

At present, standard training in the use of WHO-SADD can be provided by several centers which have accumulated extensive experience with the instrument.[7]

Conclusion

The three interrelated instruments developed by an international network of collaborating investigators coordinated by WHO – the Screening Form, the WHO Schedule for Assessment of Depressive Disorders (WHO-SADD), and the follow-up version of SADD – represent a convenient and easy-to-use battery for the selection, clinical assessment, and follow-up reassessment of patients with "functional" depressive disorders. The instruments require brief training in their use, follow conventional clinical lines of inquiry into patients' history and symptoms, and are adaptable to different languages, cultural environments, interviewing styles, and diagnostic systems. They have been shown to be equally useful in clinical, psychopharmacological, and epidemiological research.

---

[7] Information about such training possibilities can be obtained on request from the WHO Division of Mental Health, Geneva.

Appendix A

Screening Form

Patient's surname (optional)_____

Patient's first name_____

Age_____ Sex_____
(in years)

Exclusion Categories
(ring)

1. Definite physical disease, toxic disorder or cerebral damage or disease
2. Mental retardation (IQ 70 or less)
3. Presence of one or more of the following symptoms:
   3.1. Thought withdrawal or intrusion, echo of thoughts
   3.2. Delusion of being controlled
   3.3. Elaborate delusional system of delusions other than guilt, hypochondriasis, impoverishment, nihilism
   3.4. Elaborate hallucinations with content other than depressive (e.g., not a voice calling the patient names, or saying "kill yourself" etc.)
4. Presence of severe language or hearing difficulties

Inclusion Categories

Presence of at least two of the following symptoms:
(ring as many as present)

1. Depressive mood
2. Suicidal thoughts
3. Hopelessness
4. Feeling of worthlessness
5. Hypochondriasis and/or anxiety
6. Feeling of diminution of ability
7. Self-reproach or guilt
8. Inability to feel or enjoy

This patient is (ring):

Excluded   Included
                                           if included
                                           WHO number_____

Appendix B WHO-SADD Symptom Checklist

Part 2. Symptoms, Signs and History

2.A Symptoms and signs

Coding instructions: 0 = Absent
1 = Present, mild
2 = Present, continuously or in severe form
9 = Interviewer not sure or information not sufficient

If no positive rating in rubric "last month", consider also rubric "any time in this episode". If rated positively under "last month" leave box "any time in this episode" empty.

Symptom number	Last month	Any time in this episode
1. Sadness, depressed mood	☐	☐
2. Joylessness, inability to enjoy	☐	☐
3. Hopelessness	☐	☐
4. Anxiety and/or tension	☐	☐
5. Aggression	☐	☐
6. Irritability	☐	☐
7. Lack of energy	☐	☐
8. Disruption of social functioning	☐	☐
9. Desire to be alone	☐	☐
10. Subjective experience of slowness and retardation of thought (Rate 9 if question understood by patient; objectively observed slowness should be rated in item 36.)	☐	☐
11. Indecisiveness	☐	☐
12. Lack of self-confidence	☐	☐
13. Loss of interest	☐	☐
14. Loss of ability to concentrate	☐	☐
15. Subjective experience of loss of memory	☐	☐
16. Early awakening	☐	☐
17. Inability to fall asleep	☐	☐
18. Fitful, restless sleep	☐	☐
19. Hypersomnia	☐	☐
20. Lack of appetite	☐	☐

21. Change of body weight ☐ ☐
22. Constipation ☐ ☐
23. Feelings of pressure ☐ ☐
24. Other somatic signs and symptoms (specify) ☐ ☐
25. Other psychological symptoms (specify) ☐ ☐
26. Decrease of libido ☐ ☐
27. Change of perception of time ☐ ☐
(If patient unable to understand question rate 9)
28. Suicidal ideas ☐ ☐

For the symptoms number 29–33 an additional code = 3 is to be used when the respective symptom is of delusional nature.

29. Feelings and/or ideas of guilt and self-reproach ☐ ☐
30. Ideas of insufficiency, inadequacy and worthlessness ☐ ☐
31. Hypochondriasis ☐ ☐
32. Ideas of impoverishment ☐ ☐
33. Ideas of reference and/or persecution ☐ ☐
34. Other delusions (specify) ☐ ☐
35. Disorders of perception: illusions or hallucinations ☐ ☐
(Use code = 3 if hallucinations)
36. Psychomotor retardation ☐ ☐
37. Psychomotor restlessness and agitation, diurnal fluctuation of mood: ☐ ☐
38. Worse in the morning than at any other time during the day ☐ ☐
39. Worse in the evening than at any other time during the day ☐ ☐
40. Physical disease or infirmity (specify) ☐ ☐

Appendix C   Excerpt from the WHO-SADD Glossary

14. Loss of ability to concentrate. Difficulty in focusing and sustaining attention. The interviewer's probing about this item should proceed so as to distinguish loss of the ability to concentrate from "Subjective experience of slowness and retardation of thought" (Item 10) and "Subjective experience of loss of memory" (Item 15). Do not rate positive if the patient stopped engaging in an activity because of loss of interest (e.g., not following a TV programme through).

Recommended probes:
- Can you concentrate on what you are doing as well as before?
- Can you concentrate on your daily tasks and activities?
- Is it more difficult for you to read a book or even a newspaper?
- Can you follow right through a television programme, or do you lose the thread of the action?
- Have you become more forgetful lately?

Examples of characteristic responses

Difficulty in collecting thoughts, "cannot concentrate on my newspaper", "cannot concentrate on what people are saying", "cannot concentrate on my favourite television programme". The patient may describe a feeling of "heaviness in the head", or of being unable to "think a matter through", and tends to avoid thinking about complicated matters.

Appendix D

Comparison of initial evaluation assessments in NIMH and WHO Collaborative Depression Studies: Psychopathology

	SADS	WHO-SADD
Time Frame	Week during current episode when each symptom was at its worst, and past week	Past month and any time during this episode
Ratings	6-point scale (not at all, slight, mild, moderate, severe, extreme)	3-point scale (absent, present mild, present continuously or severe)
	SADS	SADD
Psychosocial Factors	Additional schedules must be used to record such information	Marital status Hours per week of work Highest level of education Occupation Religion Socioeconomic status
Pattern of course	Longitudinal picture of episodes and intervals since first onset of affective disorder. Duration, type of onset for current episode.	Numbers of depressive and manic episodes, and numbers of intervals. Duration, type of onset for current episode.
Past history of psychiatric disorder other than affective disorder	Yes, specific disorders	Yes, nonspecific

Treatment prior to inclusion	Duration and dose ranges for antidepressants, lithium (serum levels), number of ECT. Yes or no for others.	Yes or no for all, past 2 weeks anytime this episode
Diagnosis	RDC – operational definitions keyed to SADS	ICD Basle classification other local classification

Symptoms assessed in both SADS and SADD

Depressed mood	Suicidal ideas
Hopelessness	Guilt
Irritability	Negative self-image
Lack of energy	Hypochondriasis
Psychomotor retardation	Ideas and delusions of reference
Agitation	Diurnal variation
Indecisiveness	Social withdrawal
Difficulty concentrating	
Early awakening	
Initial insomnia	
Hypersomnia	
Loss of appetite	
Weight change	

Symptoms assessed in SADD and not in SADS
Disruption of social functioning
Lack of self-confidence
Fitful, restless sleep
Constipation
Feeling of pressure
Change in perception of time
Ideas of impoverishment

Symptoms assessed in both, but handled differently
Joylessness, loss of interest
Decreased libido – part of loss of interest or pleasure item in SADS, handled separately in SADD
Anxiety – divided into psychic and somatic anxiety in SADS
Aggression – distinction made in SADS between aggression during mania and before or after mania
Delusions other than reference or impoverishment and hallucinations – specific types asked for in SADS

Symptoms assessed in SADS and not in SADD

Moderate insomnia	Bizarre behavior
Distinct quality of mood	Distractibility
Worrying	Self-pity
Panic attacks	Demandingness and dependency
Phobias	Incoherence
Obsessions or compulsions	Loosening of association

Manic symptoms, e.g. elevated mood,
increased energy, grandiosity
Poor judgement
Antisocial behavior

Poverty of content
Neologisms

References

1. Bech, P., Gram, L. F., Reisby, N., and Rafaelsen, O. J. 1980. The WHO Depression Scale: relationship to the Newcastle scales. Acta Psychiatr. Scand. 62: 140-153.
2. Bech, P., Gjerris, A., Andersen, J., and Rafaelsen, O. J. 1984. The WHO Schedule for Standardized Assessment of Depressive Disorders: item-combinations and inter-observer reliability. In press.
3. Carney, M. W. P., Roth, M., and Garside, R. F. 1965. The diagnosis of depressive illness and the prediction of ECT response. Br. J. Psychiatry 3: 659-674.
4. Goldberg, D. P. 1972. The Detection of Psychiatric Illness by Questionnaire. Oxford University Press, Oxford.
5. Hamilton, M. 1967. Development of a rating scale for primary depressive illness. Brit. J. Soc. Clin. Psychol. 6: 278-296.
6. Jablensky, A., Sartorius N., Gulbinat, W., and Ernberg, G. 1981. Characteristics of depressive patients contacting psychiatric services in four cultures. Acta Psychiatr. Scand. 63: 367-383.
7. Jablensky, A., Milenkov, K., and Temkov, I. 1982. Depressive disorders and depressive symptoms among patients making their first contact with a mental health service. In: T. Ban et al. (Eds.) Prevention and Treatment of Depression. University Park Press, Baltimore.
8. Katschnig, H., Berner, W., Haushofer, M., Barfuss, M., and Seelig, P. 1980. Psychiatric case identification in general practice: self-rating versus interview. Acta Psychiatr. Scand. 62 (suppl.): 285.
9. Katz, M. M. Secunda, S. K. Hirschfeld, R. M. A., and Koslow, S. H. 1979. NIMH Clinical Research Branch collaborative program on the psychobiology of depression. Arch. Gen. Psychiatry 36: 765-771.
10. Kerr, T. A. et al. 1972. The assessment and prediction of outcome in affective disorders. Br. J. Psychiatry 121: 167-174.
11. Roth, M. et al. 1972. Studies in the classification of depressive disorders. Br. J. Psychiatry 121: 147-161.
12. Sartorius, N. Jablensky, A., Gulbinat, W., and Ernberg, G. 1980. WHO Collaborative Study: assessment of depressive disorders. Psychol. Med. 10: 743-749.
13. Sartorius, N., Davidian, H., Ernberg, G., Fenton, F. R., Fujii, I., Gastpar, M., Gulbinat, W., Jablensky, A., Kielholz, P., Lehmann, H. E., Naraghi, N., Shimizu, M., Shinfuku, N., and Takahashi, R. 1983. Depressive Disorders in Different Cultures. World Health Organization, Geneva.
14. Spitzer, R. L. and Endicott, J. 1975. Schedule for Affective Disorders and Schizophrenia (SADS), 2nd Ed. New York State Psychiatric Institute, New York.
15. Takahashi R., Sakuma, A., Hara, T., Kazamatsuri, H., Hori, A., Saito, Y., Murasaki, M., Oguchi, T., Sakurai, Y., Yuzuriha, T., Takemura, M., Kurokawa, H., and Kurita, H. 1979. Comparison of efficacy of amoxapine and imipramine in a multi-clinic double-blind study using the WHO Schedule for Standard Assessment of Patients with Depressive Disorders. J. Int. Med. Res. 7: 7-18.
16. Wilson, J. M. and Jungner, G. 1968. Principles and Practice of Screening for Disease. (Public Health Papers Ser. No. 34). World Health Organization, Geneva.
17. Wing, J. K., Cooper, J. E., and Sartorius, N. 1973. Measurement and Classification of Psychiatric Symptoms. Cambridge University Press, Cambridge.

Chapter 10   AMDP-III in the Assessment of Depression

B. WOGGON

Introduction

In 1965 the Association for Methodology and Documentation in Psychiatry (AMP) was founded by several German-speaking psychiatrists from Germany, Switzerland, and Austria [3]. The AMP system was developed for the documentation of psychopathological and somatic symptoms which are characteristic of the description of psychiatric patients. In 1971 the first edition of the AMP manual was published [21], followed by the second edition in 1972 [22]. In 1979 the third, revised edition of the manual was published, and the name of the system was changed into AMDP [1]. One of the reasons for this change was the prevention of further confusion with cyclic AMP. Equally important was the wish to emphasize that the new version of the system represents the result of many years of methodological work [11] concerning the reliability of symptoms. Unreliable items were excluded or their description in the manual improved.

Description of the AMDP System

The AMDP system consists of five parts, each printed on a single sheet of paper: (1) anamnesis – demographic data, (2) anamnesis – life events, (3) anamnesis – historical data, (4) psychopathological symptoms, and (5) somatic signs.

This paper concentrates on parts 4 and 5. The 100 psychopathological symptoms (Table 10.1) and 40 somatic signs (Table 10.2) are clearly arranged into groups, a useful help for the rater.

Table 10.1. List of AMDP-III psychopathological symptoms [13]

Disorders of consciousness
 1. Lowered vigilance
 2. Clouded consciousness
 3. Narrowed consciousness
 4. Expanded consciousness

Disturbances of orientation
 5. Time
 6. Place
 7. Situation
 8. Self

Disorders of attention and memory
 9. Apperception
 10. Concentration
 11. Memorization
 12. Retention
 13. Confabulation
 14. Paramnesia

Table 10.1 (continued)

Formal disturbances of thinking
15. inhibited (experienced)
16. Retarded (observed)
17. Circumstantial
18. Restricted
19. Perseveration
20. Rumination
21. Pressured thinking
22. Flight of ideas
23. Tangential
24. Blocking
25. Incoherence
26. Neologisms

Fears, compulsions
27. Suspiciousness
28. Hypochondriasis
29. Phobias
30. Obsessive thoughts
31. Compulsive impulses
32. Compulsive actions

Delusions
33. Delusional mood
34. Delusional perception
35. Sudden delusional ideas
36. Delusional ideas
37. Systematized delusions
38. Delusional dynamics
39. Delusions of reference
40. Delusions of persecution
41. Delusions of jealousy
42. Delusions of guilt
43. Delusions of impoverishment
44. Hypochondriacal delusions
45. Delusions of grandeur
46. Other delusions

Disorders of perception
47. Illusions
48. Verbal hallucinations
49. Other auditory hallucinations
50. Visual hallucinations
51. Bodily hallucinations
52. Olfactory/gustatory hallucinations

Disorders of ego
53. Derealization
54. Depersonalization
55. Thought broadcasting
56. Thought withdrawal
57. Thought insertion
58. Other feelings of alien influence

Disorders of affect
59. Perplexity
60. Feeling of loss of feelings
61. Blunted affect
62. Loss of vitality
63. Depressed mood
64. Hopelessness
65. Anxiety
66. Euphoria
67. Dysphoria
68. Irritability
69. Inner restlessness
70. Complaining
71. Feelings of inadequacy
72. Exaggerated self-confidence
73. Feelings of guilt
74. Feelings of impoverishment
75. Ambivalence
76. Parathymia
77. Affective lability
78. Affective incontinence
79. Affective rigidity

Disturbances of drive and psychomotility
80. Lack of drive
81. Inhibition of drive
82. Increased drive
83. Motor restlessness
84. Parakinesis
85. Mannerisms
86. Histrionic
87. Mutism
88. Logorrhea

Circadian disturbances
89. Worse in a.m.
90. Worse in p.m.
91. Better in p.m.

Other disturbances
92. Reduced social contact
93. Excessive social contact
94. Aggressiveness
95. Suicidal tendencies
96. Self-mutilation
97. Lack of feeling of illness
98. Lack of insight
99. Refusal of treatment
100. Lack of self-care

Supplementary items
– Reliability of information

Table 10.2. List of AMDP-III somatic symptoms [13]

Sleep disturbances
101. Difficulty falling asleep
102. Interrupted sleep
103. Shortened sleep
104. Early awakening
105. Drowsiness

Appetite disturbances
106. Decreased appetite
107. Excessive appetite
108. Excessive thirst
109. Decreased libido

Gastrointestinal disturbances
110. Hypersalivation
111. Dry mouth
112. Nausea
113. Vomiting
114. Gastric discomfort
115. Constipation
116. Diarrhea

Cardiac-respiratory disturbances
117. Breathing difficulties
118. Dizziness
119. Palpitation
120. Cardiac pain

Other autonomic disturbances
121. Blurred vision
122. Increased sweating
123. Seborrhea
124. Micturition difficulties
125. Menstrual difficulties

General disturbances
126. Headache
127. Back pain
128. Heaviness in legs
129. Hot flashes
130. Chills
131. Conversion symptoms

Neurological disorders
132. Hypertonia
133. Hypotonia
134. Tremor
135. Dyskinesia (acute)
136. Hypokinesis
137. Akathisia
138. Ataxia
139. Nystagmus
140. Paresthesia

Supplementary items
- Laterality
- Convulsions

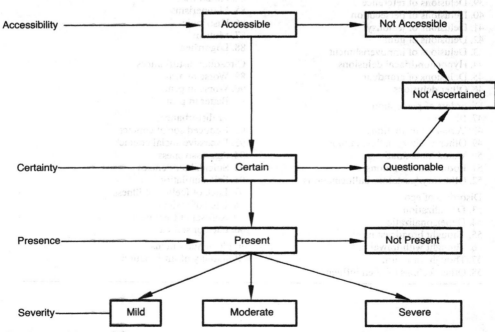

Fig. 10.1 Decision tree [13]

The rating of each symptom can be represented by four judgmental steps (Fig. 10.1): (1) A symptom is accessible and thus rateable when the necessary information is available. If a symptom is not rateable it should be documented as not ascertained. Example: A mute patient cannot give the necessary information for rating formal disorders of thinking. (2) If the rater is uncertain about the presence or absence of a symptom (reliability of information) he or she should rate the symptom as not ascertained. (3) Decision about presence or absence of a symptom. (4) If a symptom is present, its degree of severity should be estimated as mild, moderate, or severe. The judgment should be based on intensity and duration of a symptom. With fluctuating symptoms the highest intensity should be rated.

Every evaluation of psychopathological and somatic symptoms is based on a cross-section of a defined period, for example, 24 h. The rating of many symptoms combines subjective (reported by the patient) and objective (noticed by the doctor, nurses or family) information [24]. A trained rater needs on average 45 min for a complete AMDP interview [27].

Validity

If somebody wants to select a rating scale for a drug trial, sensitivity to change and reliability are very important criteria: But the most important point is the validity of the rating scale, especially the content validity. Content validity means in this context the extent to which a rating scale represents symptoms which are relevant in psychopharmacology for the measurement of change. The rating scale should reflect the most important changes of the symptomatology which can occur during treatment. Psychotropic drugs are not only able to induce a quantitative improvement or deterioration of a psychopathological picture but they may also cause qualitative changes. If we treat a depressed patient with an antidepressant drug the depressive symptomatology cannot only diminish gradually but a mixed state of manic and depressive symptoms may develop. A high dose of an anticholinergic tricyclic or tetracyclic antidepressant drug may induce a confusional state with disorientation of time and space. These two examples show the advantages of a rating scale with a broad spectrum of symptoms compared with a rating scale including only a narrow selection of psychopathological symptoms. The AMDP system has the broadest range of symptoms compared with other well-known rating scales, such as the Hamilton Rating Scale for Depression [14, 15], the Brief Psychiatric Rating Scale [19], the Inpatient Multidimensional Psychiatric Scale [17], and the Comprehensive Psychopathological Rating Scale [6]. Furthermore the AMDP system includes a sufficient number of somatic symptoms which may occur as signs of the illness or as side effects of the drug treatment [5].

Sensitivity to Change

The old version of the AMDP system (AMP system) has been used in a large number of drug trials, especially of antipsychotic and antidepressant drugs [2]. The results of these studies show the usability of the AMDP system for drug trials and its sensitivity to change.

In our own trials with antidepressant drugs we use both the AMDP system and the Hamilton Rating Scale for Depression. This gives us the possibility for international comparisons. Both rating scales show the same results concerning the improvement of typical depressive symptoms [5]. In addition the AMDP system gives a more detailed picture of qualitative changes, for example, switches into hypomania or mania, and of side effects.

Interrater Reliability

The interrater reliability of a rating scale is determined by a detailed description of each item and the training of the raters. Similar to other rating scales the interrater reliability of the AMDP symptoms varies in a relatively wide range [27]. The interrater reliability of syndromes is higher than the one of symptoms [9]. In a recent study the interrater reliability of AMP symptoms and AMDP symptoms was compared [16]. Based on a more precise description of AMDP items their interrater reliability is slightly better. Forty-three symptoms showed a good interrater reliability ($K \geq 0.6$; percent of agreement $\geq 80\%$) and 25 a moderate one ($K = 0.4-0.59$; percent of agreement, 70%-78%).

Besides the training it is very important to use the manual when documenting the symptoms on the AMDP sheets. Otherwise the probability of misunderstandings and mistakes is relatively high.

Subscales

Based on factor analyses five different sets of first-order factors of the AMP system have been used [7, 12, 18, 23, 24]. The similarities between these different syndrome solutions show that comparable syndromes can be identified in different patient samples [8]. In our own studies we used the syndrome solution of Baumann [7] for data analysis. Not unexpectedly the structure of these first-order factors proved to be not sample independent [4]. This was the reason for the construction of subscales based on second-order factors [28], which are not only sample independent but show a stable structure during 20 days of treatment [29] and are closely correlated to factors of the Hamilton Rating Scale for Depression, the Brief Psychiatric Rating Scale, and the Inpatient Multidimensional Psychiatric Rating Scale [26].

Table 10.3. Primary syndromes[a]

Syndrome	Symptoms (item numbers)
Paranoid hallucinating	33 34 35 36 37 38 39 40 48 51 54 56 58
Depressive	20 60 62 63 64 71 73 81 89 102 103 104 106
Psychoorganic	2 5 6 7 8 9 11 12 13 100
Manic	22 66 72 82 83 88 93
Hostile	27 67 68 94 97 98 99
Autonomic	28 112 117 118 119 120 122 126 129
Apathetic	15 16 17 18 61 79 80 92
Obsessive-compulsive	30 31 32
Neurological[b]	132 133 134 135 136 137 138 139 Convulsions

[a] Reprinted by permission from Pietzcker, A. et al.: The syndrome scales in the AMDP system. In: J. Angst, U. Baumann, D. Bobon, H. Helmchen, H. Hippius (eds.) Modern Problems of Pharmacopsychiatry. Copyright 1983, Karger, Basel.
[b] This is an "ad hoc" syndrome built on the basis of clinical consideration not by factor analysis

Table 10.4. Second-order syndromes[a]

Syndrome	Symptoms (item numbers)
Psychotic syndrome	33 34 35 36 37 38 39 40 48 51 54 56 58 97 98
Depressive syndrome	15 16 20 60 62 63 64 71 73 80 81 89 92 102 106 18
Psychoorganic syndrome	2 5 6 7 8 9 11 12 13 100

[a] Reprinted by permission of Pietzcker, A. et al.: The syndrome scales in the AMDP system. In: J. Angst, U. Baumann, D. Bobon, H. Helmchen, H. Hippius (eds.) Modern Problems of Pharmacopsychiatry. Copyright 1983, Karger, Basel.

For the new AMDP system first-order and second-order scales have been constructed based on the data of 2313 patients from the Psychiatric University Hospitals of Munich and Berlin. The statistical details have already been published [20]. Table 10.3 shows the nine first-order factors. Eight of them are based on factor analysis and one on clinical considerations. Table 10.4 shows the symptoms which are included in the three second-order syndromes, giving comprehensive pictures of psychotic, depressive, and psychoorganic symptomatology.

Summary

The AMDP system is a psychopathological rating scale with a broad spectrum of symptoms, valid for the assessment of depression, mania, schizophrenia, psychoorganic psychosis, neurosis, and side effects of psychotropic drugs. It is not recommended to use the subscales selectively for the rating of patients. Items of the subscales are selected from the total items used for data analysis. The AMDP system is not only used in German-speaking countries but has been adapted for use in the following languages: Croatian, Danish, Dutch, English, French, Greek, Italian, Japanese, Portuguese, Russian, and Spanish. Its use in many drug trials shows its usability for this purpose and the results demonstrate its sensitivity to change.

References

1. AMDP, Arbeitsgemeinschaft für Methodik und Dokumentation in der Psychiatrie. 1979. Das AMDP-System. 3rd Ed., Springer, Berlin Heidelberg New York.
2. AMDP. 1983. Empirische Studien zur Psychopathologie - Testmanual zum AMDP-System. Springer, Berlin Heidelberg New York.
3. Angst, J., and Woggon, B. 1983. The validity of the AMP system for its use in clinical psychopharmacology. In: J. Angst, U. Baumann, D. Bobon, H. Helmchen, and H. Hippius (eds.), AMDP-System in Pharmacopsychiatry. Modern Problems of Pharmacopsychiatry no. 20. Karger, Basel.
4. Angst, J., Battegay, R., Bente, D., Berner, P., Brören, W., Curnu, F., Dick, P., Engelmeier, M.-P., Heimann, H., Heinrich, K., Helmchen, H., Hippius, H., Pöldinger, W., Schmidlin, P., Schmitt, W., and Weis, P. 1969. Das Dokumentations-System der Arbeitsgemeinschaft für Methodik und Dokumentation in der Psychiatrie. Arzneimittelforsch. 19: 339-405.
5. Angst, J., Dittrich, A., and Woggon, B. 1979. Reproduzierbarkeit der Faktorenstruktur des AMP-Systems. International Pharmacopsychiatry 14: 319-324.
6. Åsberg, M., Montgomery, S. A., Perris, C., Schalling, D., and Sedvall, G. 1978. A comprehensive psychopathological rating scale. Acta Psychiatr. Scand. (suppl.) 271: 5-27.
7. Baumann, U. 1974. Diagnostische Differenzierungsfähigkeit von Psychopathologie-Skalen. Arch. Psychiatr. Nervenkr. 219: 89-103.
8. Baumann, U., and Woggon, B. 1979. Interrater-Reliabilität bei Diagnosen, AMP-Syndromen und AMP-Symptomen. Arch. Psychiatr. Nervenkr. 227: 3-15.
9. Baumann, U., Pietzcker, A., and Woggon, B. 1983. Syndromes and scales in the AMP-System. In: J. Angst, U. Baumann, D. Bobon, H. Helmchen, and H. Hippius (eds.), AMDP-System in Pharmacopsychiatry. Modern Problems of Pharmacopsychiatry, no. 20. Karger, Basel.
10. Bobon, D. 1983. Foreign adaptations of the AMDP system. In: J. Angst, U. Baumann, D. Bobon, H. Helmchen, and H. Hippius (eds.), AMDP-System in Pharmacopsychiatry. Modern Problems of Pharmacopsychiatry, no. 20. Karger, Basel.
11. Fähndrich, E., and Helmchen, H. 1983. From AMP to AMDP. In: J. Angst, U. Baumann, D. Bobon, H. Helmchen, and H. Hippius (eds.), AMDP-System in Pharmacopsychiatry. Modern Problems of Pharmacopsychiatry, no. 20. Karger, Basel.
12. Gebhardt, R., Pietzcker, A., Freudenthal, K., and Langer, C. 1981. Die Bildung von Syndromen im AMP-System. Arch. Psychiatr. Nervenkr. 231: 93-109.
13. Guy, W., and Ban, T. A. 1982. The AMDP-System. Manual for the Assessment and Documentation of Psychopathology. Springer, Berlin Heidelberg New York.
14. Hamilton, M. 1960. A rating scale for depression. J. Neurol. Neurosurg. Psychiatry 23: 56-62.
15. Hamilton, M. 1967. Development of a rating scale for primary depressive illness. Br. J. Soc. Clin. Psychol. 6: 278-296.
16. Kuny, S., Luckner, N. von, Bänninger, R., Baur, P., Eichenberger, G., and Woggon, B. 1983. Interrater reliability of AMDP and AMP symptoms. In: J. Angst, U. Baumann, D. Bobon, H. Helmchen, and H. Hippius (eds.), AMDP-System in Pharmacopsychiatry. Modern Problems of Pharmacopsychiatry, no. 20, Karger, Basel.
17. Lorr, M., Klett, C. J., McNair, D. M., and Lasky, J. J. 1963. Inpatient Multidimensional Psychiatric Scale (IMPS). Consulting Psychologists Press, Palo Alto.
18. Mombour, W., Gammel, G., Zerssen, D. von, and Heyse, M. 1973. Die Objektivierung psychiatrischer Syndrome durch multifaktorielle Analyse des psychopathologischen Befundes. Nervenarzt 44: 352-358.
19. Overall, J. E., and Gorham, D. R. 1962. The brief psychiatric rating scale. Psychol. Rep. 10: 799-812.
20. Pietzcker, A., Gebhardt, R., Strauss, A., Stöckel, M., Langer, C., and Freudenthal, K. 1983. The syndrome scales in the AMDP system. In: J. Angst, U. Baumann, D. Bobon, H. Helmchen, and H. Hippius (eds.), AMDP-System in Pharmacopsychiatry. Modern Problems of Pharmacopsychiatry, no. 20. Karger, Basel.
21. Scharfetter, C. 1971. Das AMP-System. Manual zur Dokumentation psychiatrischer Befunde. Springer, Berlin Heidelberg New York.

22. Scharfetter, C. 1972. Das AMP-System. Manual. 2nd Ed. Springer, Berlin Heidelberg New York.
23. Sulz-Blume, B., Sulz, K.D., Cranach, M. von. 1979. Zur Stabilität der Faktorenstruktur der AMDP-Skala. Arch. Psychiatr. Nervenkr. 227: 353-366.
24. Wegscheider, R. 1977. Empirische Diagnostik aufgrund klinischer Schätzskalen. Unpublished doctoral dissertation, University of Munich.
25. Woggon, B. 1979. Einstufung von AMP-Symptomen bezüglich Fremd- und Selbstbeurteilung. International Pharmacopsychiatry 14: 158-169.
26. Woggon, B. 1979. Untersuchung zur Validität der übergeordneten AMP-Skalen durch Vergleich mit der Hamilton-Depressions-Skala, BPRS und IMPS. International Pharmacopsychiatry 14: 338-349.
27. Woggon, B., and Dittrich, A. 1979. Konstruktion übergeordneter AMP-Skalen: "manisch-depressives" und "schizophrenes" Syndrom. International Pharmacopsychiatry 14: 325-337.
28. Woggon, B., Baumann, U., and Angst, J. 1978. Interrater-Reliabilität von AMP-Symptomen. Arch. Psychiatr. Nervenkr. 225: 73-85.
29. Woggon, B., Dittrich, A., Luckner, N. von, and Keller, W. 1980. Untersuchung zur Stabilität der faktoriellen Struktur des AMP-Systems im Behandlungsverlauf. International Pharmacopsychiatry 15: 350-364.

Chapter 11 Rating of Depression with a Subscale of the CPRS[1]

C. PERRIS

The CPRS [1] is a Comprehensive Psychopathological Rating Scale that has been developed by a working group with the Swedish Medical Research Council. It is currently used in the Scandinavian countries and is available in many languages.[2] The different national editions are not just a translation of the original Swedish scale, but they have been worked out by bilingual psychiatrists familiar not only with ratings but also with the idiomatic use of psychiatric terminology in the different countries. Such an approach to the translation of CPRS has largely contributed to making it easily communicable and highly reliable among psychiatrists with different linguistic backgrounds.

In 1971, when the work of constructing the CPRS began, it appeared that the market was saturated with easily accessible and accurate rating instruments and that the development of a new scale would be a superfluous task. However, a thorough study of the rating tools available at that time soon showed that, despite the great number of excellent rating scales on the market, very few had been constructed explicitly for the measurement of change in psychopathology, and that even fewer were comprehensive enough to cover a wide range of psychiatric disorders.

In this chapter, emphasis is given to that part of the CPRS used in the rating of affective disorders, and principally of depression. However, it seems appropriate to introduce very briefly the principles on which the construction of the CPRS was based, to enable the reader to see the differences from other similar instruments now available.

The Principles on Which the CPRS Is Based

Psychiatric rating instruments are usually constructed for a very specific purpose, for example, to assess habitual personality characteristics of the subject, to help in the diagnostic process and the following classification of a disorder, to facilitate the monitoring of psychopathological changes in the course of a treatment, or to describe the patient's behavior in the ward. Unfortunately, it is ignored too often that scales constructed for one purpose cannot be used for another.

---

[1] Supported in part by a grant from the Swedish Medical Research Council (grant no. 21X-5244)
[2] The CPRS is available in the following languages: American and British English, Czechoslovakian, Danish, French, German, Hungarian, Italian, Japanese, Norwegian, Polish, Portuguese, Russian, Serbo-Croatian, Spanish and Swedish.

In selecting the items to be included in the CPRS the general principle was followed that they had to be considered particularly relevant for psychiatric illness, liable to change with time-limited treatment, and capable of being elicited in the course of a psychiatric interview. As a consequence, variables of a pronounced trait character were excluded. Also avoided were variables likely to be heavily influenced by sociocultural differences in order to increase generalizability in the use of the scale or variables – such as intelligence – that are usually measured rather than rated.

The constructors have also avoided, as far as possible, using items that have become too closely identified with particular psychiatric syndromes (e.g., depression, anxiety, paranoia), and preferred a more elementary denomination of symptoms and signs. Another important general principle that has inspired the construction of the CPRS has been that of keeping separate items referring to the subjective report or complaint of the patient (symptoms) from those referring to the rater's observation (signs). We believe that such a distinction, rarely taken into account in other instruments, is more likely to increase the accuracy of the rating than using a more or less haphazard weighting between symptoms and signs as it very likely occurs when no distinction between symptoms and signs is made.

It is widely recognized that many of the commonly used psychiatric terms are ambiguous and rated unreliably. For that reason, an explicit description of each item is provided, with a specific warning for keeping separate variables that could be confounded.

It is also a common experience that a similarity between some items and the theoretical prejudices of the rater might be an important source of error in ratings. In fact, it is difficult for a less sophisticated rater to avoid an inference that a patient with depressively colored delusions also has a depressed mood, is worried, and has considerable inner tension. In order to avoid these inferences, items likely to be confused are supplemented with the warning "distinguish from ...". Obviously, the warning does not imply that the other items are not present, but that a careful separate scrutiny of each of them has to be made.

A thorough attempt has been made to formulate the descriptions of the items in everyday language rather than in technical terms in order to make the scale easily understandable by mental health workers with different levels of training. This point is of particular interest for the use of the scale in countries where a shortage of highly trained manpower has stimulated the training of other professional categories as raters. "Anxiety," as an example, is a term too broad and vague to apply to the specific psychopathological symptoms associated with it. To avoid problems with its interpretation it has been replaced by "worrying" and "inner tension." Furthermore, in line with a separation of anxiety into two components "psychic" and "somatic" [15] the variable "muscular tension" has been included.

Scoring Rules

Far too often, scales aimed at the quantification of psychopathology are scored in vaguely defined steps as "slight," "moderate," and "severe," which allow for a wide range of interpretations. At the other extreme are those instruments where the ambition to obtain a meticulous operational definition of each step has been pushed beyond the limits of any practical utility. It also happens that rating instruments comprising several subscales do not use a consistent scoring system for all the items taken into account. In order to try to avoid these shortcomings, the scale steps 0, 1, 2, and 3 of all variables of the CPRS have been operationally defined according to the general rule described below. In addition, we suggest the use of (undefined) half-steps, at the discretion of the rater, to increase the sensitivity of the scale.

The rule followed in the definition of the steps was:
3 Should be a description of an extreme degree of pathology.
2 Should be a description of subjective experiences or behavior that would always be considered clearly pathological in the circumstances.
1 A description that could apply to a pathological deviation from the individual's own norm, but might equally be considered at the borders of a normal variant in some people.
0 Absence of the particular symptom.

In the rating of items referring to variables for which wide individual variations in the normal population as well as between different age groups do occur, e. g., sexual interest and sleep, patients are explicitly asked to compare their present state with their own habitual functioning, which is then taken to be the norm.

An example of an item is as follows:

Fatigability

Representing the experience of tiring more easily than usual. When lassitude is extreme, this item is difficult to evaluate. If impossible do not rate. Distinguish from lassitude.
0 Ordinary staying power. Not easily fatigued.
1 Tires easily but does not have to take a break more often than usual.
2 Easily wearied. Frequently forced to pause and rest.
3 Exhaustion interrupts almost all activities or even makes them impossible.

Use of the Scale

The scale can be used by all trained mental health workers, the essential requirement for a rater being his/her training and experience in interviewing psychiatric patients. It is recommended that the rater should become familiar with the scale in training sessions before using it for evaluation in a research project. As will be mentioned below, a satisfactory level of interrater reliability can be achieved in a few training sessions also by naive raters.

Obviously, the scale could be used as a questionnaire during an interview and the ratings could be based on specific answers. Such a procedure would probably enhance reliability, but much information could be lost. We suggest that an interview technique that is as close as possible to the clinical psychiatric interview should be used. When such an interview is completed it is opportune to check what information is available for the rating of every item.

In carrying out the rating interview the span of time that the rating is supposed to cover must be decided. The choice of such a span may vary from covering the last few days to the very moment of the interview and depends on the purpose of the rating. In practice, when rating patients in the course of, for example, a treatment trial, it would be convenient to refer to the last 2-3 days before the rating. Whatever span of time has been preferred, it must be observed that the same principle is applied through the whole trial. The CPRS can be used in its whole, or preferably as a pool of items from which those relevant for a study to be carried out can be selected. Such a selection to be used for the assessment of depression will be described in more detail below.

Reliability and Validity of the CPRS

Versions of the CPRS, both in Swedish and in other languages, have been in use for some years. During this time a series of studies of interrater reliability have been carried out [9]. These have included both trained and untrained doctors as well as other professionals and have been undertaken both in Sweden and abroad. In some training sessions, videotaped interviews have been used both to train neophytes and to assess reliability [11]. They have proved that the CPRS is easy to communicate and its use easy to learn. Table 11.1 shows some of the principal results of the reliability studies. It is evident that a very satisfactory level of agreement can be reached both among doctors and research workers belonging to other professional groups.

However, it should be kept in mind that a high reliability obtained in training sessions, when all the participants are highly motivated to do their best, might not necessarily reflect what will in fact occur in the course of an investigation lasting for months. Table 11.2 illustrates just this situation. It can be seen that the reliability coefficients show some fluctuations, but that most of them remain at an acceptable level. Such fluctuations are usually, in part, due to a possible decrease in motivation by the raters the longer the study lasts, and in part to a more general difficulty in reaching a high degree of agreement when rating intermediate levels of psychopathology. For this reason, training sessions should always comprise patients with a wide range of psychopathology. Furthermore, some control of the interrater reliability should occur at appropriate intervals during the course of a study in order to maintain a high level of motivation.

Table 11.1. CPRS: Interrater reliability

	Two Swedish psychiatrists	Four Italian psychiatrists
Reported symptoms		
Sadness	0.97	0.92
Elation	0.93	0.89
Worrying over trifles	0.83	0.97
Inner tension	0.94	0.93
Hostile feelings	0.88	0.94
Inability to feel	0.68	0.90
Pessimistic thoughts	0.94	0.89
Suicidal thoughts	0.96	_[a]
Hypochondriasis	0.81	0.64
Compulsive thoughts	0.83	0.93
Indecision	0.97	0.77
Inertia	0.88	0.73
Fatigability	0.92	0.95
Depersonalization	0.92	0.83
Derealization	0.89	0.81
Ideas of persecution	0.77	0.81
Illusions and hallucinations	0.82	0.90
Observed signs		
Incongruity of affect	0.83	0.89
Incoherent speech	0.77	0.87
Withdrawal	0.77	0.93
Perseveration	0.69	0.97
Slowness of movement	0.76	0.71
Hallucinatory behavior	0.69	0.71
Agitation	0.63	0.86
Apparent sadness	0.80	0.23
Mannerisms and postures	0.80	0.68
Hostility	0.63	0.91
Pressure of speech	0.62	0.83
Reduced speech	0.76	0.92
Overactivity	0.47	0.89

[a] The item was rated 0 or was not included in the subscale

Table 11.2. Interrater reliability for some items of the CPRS during the course of a trial.[a] (From Gullberg 1976, unpublished)

Item	Ratings and relative coefficients		
	0 w	2 w	4 w
Hallucinations	0.84	0.91	0.69
Depersonalization	0.89	0.78	0.50
Withdrawal	0.82	0.79	0.60
Perseveration	0.66	0.73	0.85
Ideas of reference and persecution	0.77	0.92	0.97

[a] Two Swedish psychiatrists

Table 11.3. CPRS: changes in total score of subscale for depression comprising 21 items

	Total score before treatment $\overline{X} \pm SD$	Total score after treatment $\overline{X} \pm SD$	P
Patients who improved ($n=18$)	46.9 ± 8.8	17.9 ± 5.2	<0.01
Patients who did not improve ($n=12$)	46.6 ± 10.5	45.6 ± 10.1	NS
P	NS	<0.001	

Table 11.4. Differentiation between psychotic and nonpsychotic depressed patients. Adapted from [3a]

	Psychotic ($n=20$)	Nonpsychotic ($n=20$)	Mann-Whitney U	P
Cronholm and Ottosson Rating Scale for Depression (CORSD) Total score	14.9 ± 0.9	12.1 ± 1.0	130	NS
CPRS: 13-item subscale for depression Total score	17.3 ± 0.7	11.8 ± 0.9	56	<0.001

Although reliability may give some information about validity, other ways of assessing validity have to be used. So, for example, validity can be assessed by examining the ability of the scale to discriminate between patients belonging to different diagnostic categories or, when the aim is to detect changes, to differentiate on the basis of a clinical judgment between patients who are ill and patients who have recovered. When objective measures are available, the validity of a rating may be determined by ascertaining the degree of agreement between the results obtained with the objective measurement and those obtained with the rating scale. Also comparisons with results obtained by using both the CPRS and other well-established scales for measuring psychopathology in the same subjects can give information about the concurrent validity [1]. In Tables 11.3 and 11.4 are given a few examples which may give some information about the validity of the CPRS. Additional examples will be given later on in this chapter.

The Derivation of a Subscale for Depression and Its Applications

It has been mentioned earlier in this chapter that the CPRS can be used as a pool of items from which to extract those relevant for the rating of a well-defined disorder. Although the whole scale can be used easily especially if one wants to map the possible occurrence of less common symptoms in a given syndrome, it is preferable to make a choice of relevant items to avoid the noise of superfluous items.

Groups of items from the CPRS have been repeatedly used for the rating of depressive syndromes.

An Early Attempt in Umeå

In Umeå an arbitrarily derived subscale for depression comprised the following 21 items:

Sadness	Failing memory
Inner tension	Reduced appetite
Hostile feelings	Reduced sleep
Inability to feel	Reduced sexual interest
Pessimistic thoughts	Autonomic disturbances
Suicidal thoughts	Aches and pains
Hypochondriasis	Apparent sadness
Worrying over trifles	Reduced speech
Indecision	Slowness of movements
Lassitude	Agitation
Concentration difficulties	

The subscale has been used for some time, both in studies of depressed patients [5, 10, 14] and as a measure to investigate possible differences in psychopathology in transcultural studies [12]. When using the 21-item subscale no significant differences emerged between male and female patients nor were significant correlations between its total score and age found (Table 11.5).

A principal component factor analysis with Varimax rotation carried out on this subscale [10] yielded two principal factors – the first of them corresponding to the core of the depressive syndrome and the second to a component of retardation. Also these two factors did not show any significant difference among the sexes, nor

Table 11.5. CPRS: depression subscale (21 items)

Patients	Mean score	SD	Spearman rank correlation coefficients	
			Age	Zung scale
Male $(n=48)$	24.7	9.4	0.10	0.30*
Female $(n=75)$	22.6	8.3	−0.02	0.67***
t (d.f. = 121)		1.31 NS		

* $P<0.05$; *** $P<0.001$

Table 11.6. CPRS: depression subscale (21 items): principal component factors. Difference between sexes and correlation with age

		Factor score			Correlation with age (r_s)
		Mean	SD		
Factor I	M $(n=48)$	9.6	3.9	M+F $(n=123)$	0.01
	F $(n=75)$	9.1	4.0		
Factor II	M $(n=48)$	5.1	2.7	M+F $(n=123)$	0.10
	F $(n=75)$	4.4	2.5		

any significant correlation with age (Table 11.6). However, when analyzing correlations between single symptoms or signs and age, the results showed the occurrence of a few significant relationships (Table 11.7).

The patients in the study mentioned so far had also completed Zung's Self-Rating Scale for Depression [16]. As can be seen in Table 11.8 small, but statistically significant, correlations were found between the two scales with the exception of the part of the CPRS concerning observed signs.

The 21-item subscale proved capable of differentiating between psychotic and nonpsychotic depressed patients as classified by means of the Multiaspect Classification Model (MACM) developed in Umeå (Table 11.9) [4, 8].

In a transcultural study of age-, sex- and diagnosis-matched Italian and Swedish depressed patients consecutively admitted to an Italian and a Swedish department of psychiatry [12], no statistically significant difference in the total score of this subscale was found. However, a few statistically significant differences between the two series emerged concerning single items. Thus, Italian patients received a higher score on the variables "sadness," "reduced appetite," "pessimistic thoughts," "hypochondriasis," "apparent sadness," "reduced speech," and "slowness of movement," whereas Swedish patients on average scored higher on the variable "inability to feel."

Table 11.7. Significant correlations between CPRS variables and age (r_s)

CPRS variable	Male ($n=48$)	Female ($n=75$)	M+F ($n=123$)
Inner tension	0.23*		0.17*
Hostile feelings	−0.31**		
Worrying over trifles			0.19**
Compulsive thoughts	−0.26*		
Phobias		−0.20*	−0.15*
Rituals		−0.19*	−0.19**
Indecision	0.27*		
Concentration difficulties		−0.25**	
Failing memory	0.27*		0.16*
Aches and pain	0.25*		
Labile emotional response		0.22*	

* $P<0.05$; ** $P<0.01$

Table 11.8. Correlation coefficients within the variables of the whole CPRS and between them and the Zung scale (r_s)

	CPRS Reported symptoms	CPRS Observed signs	Zung Scale
CPRS			
Total score	0.94***	0.72***	0.48***
Subtotal reported symptoms		0.52***	0.52***
Subtotal observed signs			0.23
Factor I			0.48***
Factor II			0.26**

** $P<0.01$; *** $P<0.001$

Table 11.9. Differences in age and rating scores between psychotic and nonpsychotic patients according to the MACM

Present status	Age	CPRS (whole)			CPRS depression subscale (21 items)			Zung
		Total score	Reported symptoms	Observed signs	Total	Factor I	Factor II	
Psychotic (n=20)	48.1±10.9	44.6±11.6	33.7±10.4	11.0±3.0	27.2±7.1	10.5±3.8	6.5±1.8	53.7±4.2
Nonpsychotic (n=103)	43.9±14.5	31.7±11.0	24.4±8.6	7.2±3.8	22.2±7.2	9.0±3.8	4.2±2.5	52.1±9.5
t (d.f.=121)	0.99	3.87	3.46	3.36	2.37	1.38	3.21	0.49
P		<0.001	<0.001	<0.001	<0.02		<0.01	

The 21-item subscale has been used in our Department, also in the monitoring of psychopathological changes in the course of (unpublished) clinical trials. On these occasions, the scale proved to be capable of differentiating those patients who had clinically substantially improved from those who did not benefit from the therapy.

A Depression Subscale Sensitive to Change Derived by Montgomery and Åsberg

Montgomery and Åsberg [7] have presented their own subscale of the CPRS to be used in depression derived from a study of 54 English and 52 Swedish patients. The subscale, eventually comprising only ten items, was obtained after a primary selection of the most commonly occurring symptoms in primary depressive illness in the combined sample. As a secondary selection those items were eventually retained (ten) which showed the largest changes with treatment and the highest correlation to overall change. Also this subscale proved to have a high reliability, with coefficients ranging from 0.89 to 0.97 with different rater pairs. Moreover, its capacity to differentiate between responders and nonresponders to antidepressant treatment proved to be better than with the Hamilton Rating Scale [3], indicating a greater sensitivity to change. This last conclusion is hardly surprising because of the principle used in selecting the items in the subscale and because the Hamilton Scale was not originally constructed to monitor changes in relation to treatment. A shortcoming of the subscale proposed by Montgomery and Åsberg consists of the very limited number of items it contains. Since only those items which showed the largest changes with certain well-limited treatments were included, it is possible that symptoms or signs still clinically relevant, but not influenced by the tried treatments, will not be identified, thus limiting an accurate identification of the therapeutic profile of new treatments.

A More Recent Subscale for Depression Derived in Umeå

During a comprehensive investigation of depressed patients that has been going on at the Department of Psychiatry of Umeå University since 1976, patients who have consecutively attended the Department as either out- or inpatients have been consistently rated with the whole CPRS as well as with a battery of other scales. From an analysis of 209 patients who participated in the study, a new subscale for depression was derived as follows. The frequency distribution of the scores on each item of the CPRS was analyzed in the whole group. From this analysis, those items on which at least 70% of the patients received a score of one or more were chosen to represent the subscale for depression.

The resultant scale consisted of 28 items, of which 20 refer to reported symptoms (items No. 1, 3-9, 11, 13-19, 21, 23-25 in the original version - Åsberg et al. [1]) and eight refer to observed signs (items No. 41, 44, 46, 49, 54, 60, 61, 63) (see Appendix A). On this subscale a series of further analyses was carried out. The internal consistency of the whole subscale proved to be satisfactory (Cronbach alpha = 0.86).

A test-retest of 61 patients rated when first in contact with psychiatric care and later on when recovered from the depressive illness showed highly significant differences ($P<0.001$) in the total score as well as in the single items but for those referring to hypochondriasis and aches and pains for which no statistically significant difference emerged. However, it should be mentioned that the patients in this part of the study had very low initial scores on these two variables (Table 11.10).

Several of the items of the 28-item subscale were capable of significantly differentiating among patients classified according to the Newcastle Index and divided in quartiles according to their score. These items were: pessimistic thoughts, worrying over trifles, indecision, lassitude, failing memory, reduced sleep, and muscular tension. Also, significant differences in the expected direction occurred when patients were divided into unipolars ($n=61$), bipolars ($n=22$), neurotic-reactive ($n=68$),

Table 11.10. CPRS ratings at admission and at discharge in 61 patients

	At admission $\bar{X}$	SD	At discharge $\bar{X}$	SD	Wilcoxon's test	P
1. Sadness	1.5	0.8	0.6	0.6	−6.2	***
3. Inner tension	1.3	0.9	0.6	0.7	−5.4	***
4. Hostile feelings	0.5	0.7	0.2	0.4	−3.5	***
5. Inability to feel	1.4	0.9	0.6	0.6	−5.7	***
6. Pessimistic thoughts	1.2	0.8	0.5	0.6	−5.2	***
7. Suicidal thoughts	0.7	0.8	0.2	0.5	−4.1	***
8. Hypochondriasis	0.3	0.6	0.2	0.5	−1.0	NS
9. Worrying over trifles	1.2	0.9	0.7	0.7	−5.0	***
11. Phobias	0.6	0.9	0.2	0.5	−3.0	**
13. Indecision	1.1	0.9	0.4	0.6	−5.5	***
14. Lassitude	1.4	0.9	0.5	0.7	−5.6	***
15. Fatigability	1.3	1.0	0.5	0.7	−5.2	***
16. Concentration difficulties	1.3	0.9	0.6	0.7	−5.4	***
17. Failing memory	0.9	0.8	0.4	0.6	−4.3	***
18. Reduced appetite	0.7	0.8	0.3	0.6	−4.0	***
19. Reduced sleep	1.2	1.0	0.5	0.7	−4.8	***
21. Reduced sexual interest	1.2	1.2	0.7	0.9	−3.2	***
23. Autonomic disturbances	1.3	0.7	0.8	0.7	−4.2	***
24. Aches and pains	0.7	0.8	0.6	0.8	−1.2	NS
25. Muscular tension	1.1	1.0	0.7	0.9	−3.7	***
41. Apparent sadness	1.5	0.8	0.6	0.6	−5.8	***
44. Labile emotional responses	0.4	0.6	0.3	0.5	−2.2	*
46. Autonomic disturbances	0.8	0.7	0.5	0.6	−3.3	***
49. Withdrawal	0.4	0.6	0.3	0.4	−3.2	***
54. Reduced speech	0.4	0.6	0.2	0.4	−2.3	*
60. Slowness of movement	0.8	0.8	0.3	0.5	−3.2	***
61. Agitation	0.5	0.7	0.3	0.6	−2.9	**
63. Muscular tension	1.1	0.8	0.7	0.7	−3.6	***

* $P<0.05$; ** $P<0.01$; *** $P<0.001$

and those suffering from an unspecified affective disorder – depressive type ($n=57$) (Table 11.11). One hundred and sixty of the patients in the study had also completed the Zung Self-Rating Scale for Depression. The results of the correlation between the two scales are presented in Table 11.12.

As in the case of the 21-item subscale mentioned earlier in this paper the correlation coefficients are, as expected, higher for the reported (and for the whole scale) than for the observed variables.

On this 28-item subscale a new principal component factor analysis with Varimax rotation has been carried out. Four factors emerged explaining about 44% of the variance. These factors are presented in Table 11.13 together with an analysis of

Table 11.11. CPRS ratings in diagnostic subgroups

	Unipolar $\overline{X}$	SD	Bipolar $\overline{X}$	SD	Unspecified depression (UNS) $\overline{X}$	SD	Reactive-neurotic depression (RND) $\overline{X}$	SD	P
1. Sadness	1.6	0.8	1.2	1.0	1.5	1.0	1.5	0.7	
3. Inner tension	1.6	0.8	1.0	0.9	1.4	0.9	1.2	0.8	*
4. Hostile feelings	0.4	0.6	0.5	0.7	0.5	0.7	0.6	0.8	
5. Inability to feel	1.5	0.9	1.0	1.0	1.3	1.0	1.4	0.8	
6. Pessimistic thoughts	1.3	0.7	1.0	0.9	1.3	1.0	1.0	0.8	I
7. Suicidal thoughts	0.7	0.8	0.7	0.8	0.6	0.8	0.7	0.8	
8. Hypochondriasis	0.3	0.7	0.4	0.7	0.3	0.6	0.2	0.6	
9. Worrying over trifles	1.4	0.9	1.2	0.9	1.3	0.9	1.0	0.8	*
11. Phobias	0.5	0.8	0.6	0.9	0.6	0.9	0.7	0.9	
13. Indecision	1.3	0.9	1.2	0.8	1.3	1.0	0.8	0.8	***
14. Lassitude	1.5	0.8	1.2	0.8	1.6	1.0	1.2	0.8	*
15. Fatigability	1.5	0.9	1.2	0.8	1.4	1.1	1.2	0.9	I
16. Concentration difficulties	1.3	0.9	1.3	0.8	1.3	1.0	1.3	0.8	
17. Failing memory	1.1	0.9	1.1	0.9	1.0	0.8	0.6	0.7	***
18. Reduced appetite	0.7	0.8	0.3	0.7	0.8	0.9	0.6	0.8	I
19. Reduced sleep	1.2	1.1	0.8	1.1	1.1	1.1	1.2	1.0	
21. Reduced sexual interest	1.2	1.2	1.3	1.2	1.3	1.3	1.0	1.1	
23. Autonomic disturbances	1.2	0.7	1.4	0.8	1.3	0.7	1.4	0.7	
24. Aches and pains	0.7	0.7	0.6	0.8	0.7	0.9	0.8	0.7	
25. Muscular tension	1.2	1.0	0.7	0.9	1.0	1.0	1.4	0.9	**
41. Apparent sadness	1.6	0.8	1.4	0.8	1.6	1.0	1.4	0.7	
44. Labile emotional responses	0.5	0.7	0.1	0.5	0.2	0.4	0.4	0.6	*
46. Autonomic disturbances	0.9	0.6	0.8	0.9	0.8	0.8	0.9	0.6	
49. Withdrawal	0.4	0.5	0.5	0.7	0.7	0.6	0.3	0.5	***
54. Reduced speech	0.4	0.6	0.6	0.7	0.5	0.8	0.3	0.4	
60. Slowness of movement	0.8	0.8	1.0	0.8	0.8	0.9	0.6	0.8	
61. Agitation	0.5	0.7	0.3	0.6	0.5	0.7	0.6	0.6	
63. Muscular tension	1.2	0.8	1.0	0.9	1.1	0.9	1.1	0.7	

I $P<0.10>0.05$;   * $P<0.05$;   ** $P<0.01$;   *** $P<0.001$

Table 11.12. Correlations with the Zung scale (Spearman rank correlation coefficient (r_s))

CPRS variables	
Reported	0.65***
Observed	0.35***
Total	0.64***

*** $P<0.001$

Table 11.13. Factor analysis of CPRS depression subscale

		Loading	% of variance
Factor I	3. Inner tension	0.53	24.9
	9. Worrying over trifles	0.64	
	13. Indecision	0.76	
	14. Lassitude	0.61	
	15. Fatigability	0.67	
	16. Concentration difficulties	0.64	
	17. Failing memory	0.61	
	23. Autonomic disturbances	0.43	
Factor II	1. Sadness	0.56	7.6
	4. Hostile feelings	0.31	
	5. Inability to feel	0.50	
	6. Pessimistic thoughts	0.45	
	7. Suicidal thoughts	0.44	
	18. Reduced appetite	0.54	
	19. Reduced sleep	0.51	
	25. Muscular tension	0.57	
	46. Autonomic disturbances	0.42	
	61. Agitation	0.42	
	63. Muscular tension	0.64	
Factor III	41. Apparent sadness	0.54	6.0
	49. Withdrawal	0.55	
	54. Reduced speech	0.76	
	60. Slowness of movement	0.76	
Factor IV	8. Hypochondriasis	0.57	5.2
	11. Phobias	0.50	
	24. Aches and pains	0.34	
	44. Labile emotional responses	−0.62	
Factor I to factor IV			43.7

their internal consistency. With the exception of factor 4, comprising one negative loading, the Cronbach alpha [2] seems to be satisfactory.

An analysis of possible differences between the sexes showed that female patients ($n=130$) scored lower on the variable "indecision" ($P<0.02$) and higher on the variables "aches and pains" ($P<0.002$) and "reported" ($P<0.03$) and "observed muscular tension" ($P<0.05$) than male patients, independently of age. Several variables showed slight, but significant, correlation with age, the correlation coefficients being, however, no higher than 0.30 ("reduced sexual interest" in male patients).

Thus, the 28-item subscale mentioned above is a feasible and reliable instrument for the assessment of the severity of a depressive syndrome and for the monitoring of possible changes in psychopathology in the course of a treatment.

The Problem of the Rating of Manic Symptoms

Patients undergoing antidepressive treatment, and specifically bipolar patients in a depressive phase, may undergo a switch to mania in the course of, e.g., a clinical trial. On such an occasion, the research worker might want to be able to record the degree of manic symptom shown by the patient.

Also for this purpose the CPRS is a particularly suitable tool. In fact, variables referring specifically to manic symptoms can be taken from the pool and easily added to the subscale for depression when appropriate. The variables, which should be included for the purpose mentioned above, are as follows: "elated mood," "increased sexual interest," and "disrupted thoughts" among the reported symptoms, and "elated mood," "distractability," "pressure of speech," "flight of ideas," "incoherent speech," "overactivity," and "agitation" among the observed signs.

Recently, we have added [13] a few items to the original 65 contained in the CPRS. Two of them refer particularly to manic manifestations, namely "increased energy" among the reported variables and "disinhibition" among the observed variables. The format of these items is the same as the others in the CPRS, and their reliability is as high as the other items (coefficients ranged from 0.90 to 0.95 in different training sessions). These items are given in extenso in Appendix B.

A factor analytical study of the German version of the CPRS has been carried out recently by Maurer et al. [6]. Those authors were able to identify a subscale for manic syndromes comprising items 2, 4, 32, 42, 43, 53, 54, 55, 59, and 60 from the original pool of 65 items.

Conclusions

The CPRS – a comprehensive scale for the rating of psychopathology, and in particular its 28-item subscale described in this chapter – has proved to be a highly reliable and easily communicable instrument for the rating of depressive syndromes. The 28 items in the subscale specifically recommended for the rating of depression have proved to be valid for differentiating between sick and recovered patients, and also for demonstrating clinical differences among diagnostic subgroups. The subscale is largely independent of age and sex, and correlates well with self-rating instruments for depression. The variables in the subscale are sensitive to change; thus the scale is particularly suitable in the monitoring of psychopathological changes in the course of antidepressive treatment. The possibility of adding further variables for the rating of manic symptoms allows recording of manic symptoms due to treatment. Unskilled raters can achieve a high level of reliability with only a few training sessions, and videotaped interviews can be used for such a purpose. The application of the subscale in practice does not require more than about 20 min.

Appendix A List of the 28 Items Selected as a Subscale for Depression[3]

The numeration of the items is the same as in the full CPRS

Reported
1. Sadness
3. Inner tension
4. Hostile feelings
5. Inability to feel
6. Pessimistic thoughts
7. Suicidal thoughts
8. Hypochondriasis
9. Worrying over trifles
11. Phobias
13. Indecision
14. Lassitude
15. Fatigability
16. Concentration difficulties
17. Failing memory
18. Reduced appetite
19. Reduced sleep
21. Reduced sexual interest
23. Autonomic disturbances
24. Aches and pains
25. Muscular tension

Observed
41. Apparent sadness
44. Labile emotional responses
46. Autonomic disturbances
49. Withdrawal
54. Reduced speech
60. Slowness of movement
61. Agitation
63. Muscular tension

---

[3] The description of the variables and the steps of the ratings can be found in Åsberg et al. [1]

Appendix B   Added Items

Depression

Reported

Negative Self-evaluation

Representing ideas of self-depreciation and feelings of worthlessness which may incapacitate social functioning.
   Rate according to extension, intensity, degree of incapacity, and degree of further elaboration.
   Distinguish from pessimistic thoughts (6).

0 Occasional feelings of inferiority may occur in the circumstances.
1 Predominant feelings of inferiority and worthlessness but areas in which he/she does not feel inferior or worthless are also acknowledged.
2 Pervasive feelings of worthlessness, also on occasions when he/she should feel at ease. Recurrent themes of self-depreciation during the interview.
3 Unrelenting and painful feelings of worthlessness that seriously hamper social functioning, and may lead to secondary delusional elaborations.

Social Withdrawal

Representing the report of active behavior aimed at avoiding interaction with other people.
   Distinguish from inability to feel (5), lassitude (14), and (observed) withdrawal (49).

0 No active efforts at avoiding people. The degree of interaction is dependent upon the circumstances.
1 Prefers to be alone, but can occasionally accept meeting friends and acquaintances.
2 Active efforts to avoid meetings or interaction with people outside the household. Has stopped paying or receiving calls from friends.
3 Complete social isolation, also from relatives. Prefers to spend a large part of the day in bed to avoid social contacts.

Mania

Reported

Increased Energy

Representing the experience of being able to carry out much more than usual, or much more than other people in similar circumstances can do without becoming tired.

Distinguish from elation (2) and ideas of grandeur (32). Fatigability is scored zero when this item is positive.

0 Normal alternation of periods of energetic behavior and tiredness.
1 More energetic than usual. It is easy to think of new enterprises. It feels much easier than usual to engage in work and other activities.
2 Predominant feeling of increased energy. Contemporaneous start of different activities. Reduced need for rest and/or sleep.
3 Intensively increased level of activity. Feelings of being able to cope with any amount of work without becoming tired. Several unrelated activities are started at the same time. "Never tired."

Observed

Disinhibition

Representing a clear deviance from shared behavioral standards that is manifest during the interview, and is expressed in speech, gestures, or postures.

0 No manifest deviance from expected social behavior.
1 Overfamiliar in his/her relation to the interviewer. Free and uninhibited talk on sensitive personal matters.
2 Dwells freely upon sexual information. Verbal sexual hints to the interviewer. Uses swearwords or produces noisy alimentary release.
3 Completely disinhibited in relation to the interviewer. Makes open sexual advances. Exhibitionism.

References

1. Åsberg, M., Perris, C., Schalling, D., and Sedvall, G. (eds.). 1978. The CPRS - Development and applications of a psychiatric rating scale. Acta Psychiatr. Scand. (suppl. 271).
2. Cronbach, L.J. 1951. Coefficient alpha and the internal structure of tests. Psychometrika 16: 297-334.
3. Hamilton, M. 1960. A rating scale for depression. J. Neurol. Neurosurg. Psychiatry 23: 56-62.
3a. Knorring, von, L., and Strandman, E. 1982. A comparison between Cronholm-Ottosson De-

pression Rating Scale and variables concerned with depressive symptomatology in the comprehensive Psychopathological Rating Scale – CPRS. Acta Psychiatr. Scand. (suppl. 271): 45–51.
4. Knorring, von, L., Perris, C., Jacobsson, L., and Rosenberg, B. 1980. Multi-Aspects Classification of Mental Disorders (MACM). Neuropsychobiology 6: 101–108.
5. Knorring, von, L., Perris, C., Eiseman, M., Eriksson, U., and Perris, H. 1983. Pain as a symptom in depressive disorders. I. Relationship to diagnostic subgroups and depressive symptomatology. Pain 15: 19–26.
6. Maurer, M., Kuny, S., Dittrich, A., and Woggon, B. 1982. Skalenkonstruktion der deutschsprachigen Version der Comprehensive Psychopathological Rating Scale (CPRS). Int. Pharmacopsychiat. 17: 338–353.
7. Montgomery, S., and Åsberg, M. 1979. A new depression scale designed to be sensitive to change. Br. J. Psychiatry 134: 382–389.
8. Ottosson, J-O., and Perris, C. 1973. Multidimensional classification of mental disorders. Psychol. Med. 3: 238–243.
9. Perris, C. 1979. Reliability and validity studies of the Comprehensive Psychopathological Rating Scale (CPRS). Prog. Neuropsychopharmacol. 3: 413–421.
10. Perris, C., and Eisemann, M. 1980. Some biological correlates of clinical symptomatology and of personality characteristics in depressed patients. In: K. Achté, V. Aalberg, and J. Lönnqvist (eds.), Psychopathology of Depression. Psychiatria Fennica, Suppl., pp. 27–39.
11. Perris, C., Eriksson, U., Jacobsson, L., Lindström, H., and Perris, H. 1979. Interprofessional communicability and reliability of the Comprehensive Psychopathological Rating Scale (CPRS) as assessed by video-taped interviews. Acta Psychiatr. Scand. 60: 144–148.
12. Perris, C., Eisemann, M., Eriksson, U., Perris, H., Kemali, D., Amati, A., DelVecchio, M., and Vacca, L. 1981. Transcultural aspects of depressive symptomatology. Psychiatria Clin. (Basel) 14: 69–80.
13. Perris, C., Eisemann, M., Knorring, von, L., and Perris, H. 1984. Presentation of a subscale for the rating of depression and some additional items to the Comprehensive Psychopathological Rating Scale. Acta Psychiatr. Scand. 70: 261–274.
14. Perris, H., Eisemann, M., Eriksson, U., Knorring, von, L., and Perris, C. 1983. Attempts to validate a classification of unipolar depression based on family data. Neuropsychobiology 9: 103–107.
15. Schalling, D., Cronholm, B., Åsberg, M., and Espmark, S. 1973. Rations of psychic and somatic anxiety indicants. Acta Psychiatr. Scand. 49: 353–368.
16. Zung, W. W. K. 1965. A self-rating depression scale. Arch. Gen. Psychiatry 12: 63–70.

Chapter 12 A Self-Report Inventory on Depressive Symptomatology (QD2) and Its Abridged Form (QD2A)

P. PICHOT

There are numerous self-report inventories for the assessment of depressive symptomatology. The advantages and drawbacks of such questionnaires have often been discussed. From the theoretical viewpoint, their chief disadvantage is that they reflect only the symptoms felt, which represent merely a part of the information the physician requires to reach a diagnosis, and from the practical viewpoint, that they are suitable for use only by patients with sufficient insight and an adequate vocabulary. On the other hand, technically their use is easy and they do not call, unlike the Observer's Rating Scales, for the participation of a competent psychiatrist; thus, when they are short, they provide a practical means of epidemiological screening. The two inventories devised in recent years at the Clinique des Maladies mentales et de l'Encéphale, Paris, are intended for the assessment of depressive symptomatology [5, 6]. The first (QD2), which comprises 52 items, is applicable in the field of research. It provides a quantitative assessment of the intensity of the depression and, if the subscales isolated by factor analysis are employed, of the principle symptomatic dimensions of the syndrome. The second (QD2A), which was derived from the first by item analysis, consists of 13 items chosen in such a way that they constitute the best possible combination of items for the detection of people with depression in the general population, among patients with organic disease, or among psychiatric patients.

Construction of Questionnaire QD1

Item Bank. The initial bank of 151 items was built up on the basis of the depression questionnaires most in use, namely:

- The Hopkins Symptoms Check List [2] with 58 items
- The Beck-Pichot Scale [4] with 13 items
- Scale D of the Minnesota Multiphasic Personality Inventory (MMPI) [3] with 60 items
- The Zung Depression Scale [8] with 20 items

The way in which the items are presented varies from one inventory to another. For example, Scale D of the MMPI consists of statements calling for the answer "true" or "false"; the Beck Scale includes four statements for each item corresponding to degrees of intensity of the symptom, from which the subject must select the one which corresponds to his present condition; and the Zung Scale comprises four degrees of response per item.

Analysis of Item Content. With a view to an analysis of their content, the 151 items were submitted to five experts. The following principles were adopted:

The number of content categories to be established by the experts was in principle unlimited (up to 151 if they considered that all the items were specific).
An "items excluded" category was established, to which were relegated items whose content seemed to the experts to be unconnected with depression.
Each expert had to start with the longest questionnaire and use it to frame categories as discriminating as possible, then take a second questionnaire and distribute the items among the categories previously created or, if necessary, create new ones. One and the same item could belong to two categories if its contents were heterogeneous or its wording ambiguous.

In this way, five classifications of category content of the 151 items were obtained.

A preliminary examination consigned 17 items to the "items excluded" category. These were essentially items from Scale D of the MMPI, of the type "I sometimes tease animals."

The five classifications of the remaining 134 items were then analyzed. Correspondences between classifications were sought and the nuclei of these categories defined, starting for this pupose from a cross-table of categories, questionnaires, and experts. Certain categories proved to be homogeneous, since the same items had been grouped together by the five experts, while agreement regarding others was less complete. In such cases a discussion took place in order to arrive at a consensus. Finally, 78 categories were defined, 54 agreed on by all five experts and 24 agreed on by three or four of them.

Certain categories which dealt at too great a length with some aspect of the symptomatology (for example, somatic symptoms) were eliminated, as well as those whose content was ambiguous. On the other hand, new categories were created to strengthen certain aspects which seemed to be lacking or inadequately represented in the four inventories analyzed (for example, guilt feelings or ideas of suicide).

The end result was 52 categories, whose content was worded in the form of statements calling for a "true" of "false" answer. The wording is simple and avoids negative phrasing (of the type "I cannot ..."), a frequent source of error in such questionnaires. To eliminate the effect of response attitudes as far as possible, 34 statements were worded in such a way that a depressed subject would tend to answer "true", and 18 were worded in the contrary manner, calling for the answer "false" from a depressed person. The 52 items constitute inventory QD1.

Factor Analysis of the Results. Inventory QD1 was applied to a sample of 204 subjects in a clinically depressive state. The results were subjected to principal component analysis, and Varimax rotation was carried out on the first four components. While, according to the content of the items, two of the factors could be interpreted as "anxiety" and "guilt feelings," the other two could not be interpreted. It became apparent that one of the factors grouped together exclusively items worded in a way that did not indicate depression (items to which the depressed subject was more likely to answer "false") while the other grouped together exclusively items worded in a way that did indicate depression. It was thus found that items very close in meaning were allocated, according to their wording, to one or the other factor; for example, the pairs:

44. I have no difficulty in doing things I was accustomed to do (factor I)
36. I must force myself to do anything at all (factor IV)

or

39. I am able to reach a decision as easily as usual (factor I)
2. I have to ask others what I should do (factor IV)

It thus seems that the two factors which comprise the elements most characteristic of depression are formal factors reflecting a response attitude.

Similar findings have been made in a neighboring field. In 1970 Spielberger et al. [7] compiled a State-Trait Anxiety Inventory, or STAI, consisting of items referring, according to their wording, either to a stable personality disposition (Anxiety-Trait) or to a present emotional state (Anxiety-State). To avoid the role played by response attitudes, each of the subscales included an approximately equal number of items, a positive response which corresponded to the presence of anxiety (Anxiety +), and of items where the presence of anxiety was indicated by a negative response (Anxiety −). The STAI is one of the most widely used anxiety inventories, and has given rise to numerous experimental studies. In 1980, Spielberger et al. [7] reported the results of a factor analysis and observed that they had obtained not two orthogonal factors (Anxiety-State, Anxiety-Trait) as the construction of the inventory postulated, but four, corresponding to Anxiety-State +, Anxiety-State −, Anxiety-Trait +, and Anxiety-Trait −. In other words, in the factor structure the form of the item (+ or −) played just as important a role as did the psychological content (Trait or State). Bernstein and Eveland in 1982 [1] discussed the problem thoroughly from the statistical viewpoint and concluded, in particular, that "the most deplorable characteristic (of the STAI) was that the differences between the positive and negative items were approximately as large as the differences between the State and Trait items..."

It follows from these results that in inventories whose aim is to detect pathologic characteristics all the items should be worded as uniformly as possible. If this is not done the "form of the item" variance masks the "content of the item" variance, making delimitation of the subjacent psychopathological dimensions impossible.

In view of the results obtained, it was decided to reword the 18 items which, in QD1, were drafted in such a way that they called for the answer "false" from depressed persons. The content remained the same, but in the new version the question always called for the answer "true" from the depressed person. For example:

44. (QD1) I have no difficulty in doing things I was accustomed to do
has become
44. (QD2) I have difficulty in doing things I was accustomed to do.

The QD2 Inventory

Factor Analysis. Inventory QD2 (see Appendix A) was applied to 150 subjects in a clinically depressive state.

A principal component analysis was done. All the items show positive saturation in the first principal component, corresponding to 23.8% of the total variance. This component can therefore be regarded as a general factor of depression. The

A Self-Report Inventory on Depressive Symptomatology (QD2)

Table 12.1. The most and the least saturated items in the first principal component

40. I feel sad at present	0.695
19. I am disappointed and disgusted with myself	0.694
39. I am unable to reach a decision as easily as usual	0.687
20. When I have the slightest thing to do I feel blocked or prevented	0.665
44. I have difficulty in doing things I was accustomed to do	0.662
10. I perspire more than usual	0.172
35. At present I am more constipated than usual	0.172
7. I am less interested than usual in sex	0.143
28. My weight has changed	0.138
33. At present I am unable to stay still	0.119

Table 12.2. Varimax rotations – three and four-factor solutions

Items	I	I'	III	III'	II	IV'	II'
44	79	78					
36	71	70					
50	68	67					
1	66	66					
12	65	65					
34	61	60					
22	59	57					
4	54	53					
52	52	52					
20	52	51			43	47	
39	50	48			43	40	
16	44	43					
47	44	44					
9	43						45
24			65	63			
5			64	62			
27			59	60			
15			52	51			
45			52	54			
14			50	57	48	47	
10			47	51			
46			43	43			
23					71	68	
38					71	69	
19					69	67	
32					64	66	
29					63	65	
51					63	63	
40					62	68	
8					58	58	
3					56	52	
21	43		42		56	63	
42					55	48	46
25					48	40	43
6					43		
13					43		42
49					43		
37							58
11							52

most saturated items concern mood and general drive, while the less saturated items concern anxiety symptoms (10, 33) and somatic symptoms (35, 7, 28) (Table 12.1).

In order to determine the number of principal components to submit to Varimax rotation, i.e., those that can be regarded as significant, the Romeder simulation method was used. The latter suggested that only three components should be retained. Nevertheless, we felt it useful also to carry out a rotation of the first four components for comparative purposes (Table 12.2).

Both solutions can be interpreted, the four-factor one introducing a new dimension, prime II. However, since the latter was less well defined than the first three, it seemed preferable to adopt the three-factor solution.

From the psychopathological viewpoint, factor I/I prime defines the feeling of loss of general drive, of "élan vital," and corresponds very precisely to what German authors term *"Antriebsverlust."*

Items with a saturation of 0.60 or more in the two solutions are:

44. I have difficulty in doing things I was accustomed to do
36. I must force myself to do anything at all
50. I work less easily than before
 1. I now find it difficult to get going
12. I have no energy
34. I do things less quickly than usual

Factor III/III' is an anxiety factor, relating to the somatic manifestations of anxiety. The items with a saturation of 0.60 or more in one or both solutions are:

24. I have the feeling that my heart is beating harder than usual or is racing
 5. I feel that there is a lump in my throat
27. I feel very tense at present

Factor II/IV' is a depressive mood/pessimism factor.

The items with a saturation of 0.60 or more in both solutions are:

23. I've had enough of life and wish it were ended
38. I feel it would be better if I were dead
19. I am disappointed and disgusted with myself
32. I feel blue
29. I have no hope for the future
51. At present my life seems empty
40. I feel sad at present

Homogeneity. Homogeneity was studied by calculating the contingency coefficient for each item. All the coefficients are significant at a level above 0.01, except for two that are significant at the 0.05 level.

Reliability. The reliability coefficient, employing the split-half method with the Spearman-Brown correction, is $r=0.93$. Identical values were found for groups of normal subjects, somatic patients, and nondepressed psychiatric patients to whom the inventory was applied.

Concurrent Validity. The QD2 was applied to a group of 81 depressed subjects at the same time as the Zung inventory. The correlation between the results was 0.85.

Empirical Validity (Discriminatory Power). We applied the questionnaire to four groups: 157 depressed subjects, 89 normal subjects, 90 subjects hospitalized for so-

Table 12.3. Mean values of the QD2 scores of the four groups of subjects and significance of the differences

Subjects	N	M	Standard deviation	t 1 Depressed	2 Normal	3 Somatic
1 Depressed	157	32.22	11.07			
2 Normal	89	9.57	7.67	18.28		
3 Somatic	90	18.64	11.61	9.00	6.17	
4 Mental	145	24.34	12.10	5.88	11.45	3.55

Table 12.4. Mean value of the QD2 in three subgroups of depressed subjects defined by clinical intensity of symptoms and significance of the differences

Intensity of depression	N	M	Standard deviation	t 1 Serious	2 Moderate
1 Serious	33	37,09	10,83		
2 Moderate	77	32,22	9,95	2,24**	
3 Slight	40	28,42	11,98	3,25***	1,72*

* 0.10, ** 0.05, *** 0.01

matic illness, and 145 subjects who had psychiatric disturbances, but who, after examination, were regarded as free from depressive symptoms. The subjects hospitalized for somatic illness had not undergone psychiatric examination, and it is probable that depressive symptoms coexisted in some of them (Table 12.3).

The differences between the mean values were all significant above the 0.01 level.

Empirical Validity (Correlation with Intensity of Depression). The intensity of depression in the group of depressed subjects had been estimated by the clinicians on a three-point scale (slight, moderate, serious; Table 12.4).

The QD2 scale scores for the three subgroups show a significant difference. The correlation between the score and the clinical degree of depression (triserial *r*) is 0.30.

Conclusions. The QD2 inventory provides a tool whose homogeneity, reliability, and validity are very satisfactory. It makes possible an assessment of three dimensions of the syndrome (feeling of loss of general drive, depressed mood, and anxiety) by adding the scores for the items corresponding to those dimensions.

The QD2A Inventory

Depressed patients often answer the inventory questions hesitantly and slowly, so that when the number of items exceeds 50 it becomes difficult to obtain satisfactory replies, even by encouraging the patient. Although the presentation of the items has deliberately been made simple, even an inventory like the QD2 takes at least 30 min to apply in the case of a subject suffering from relatively deep depression with retardation, despite the presence of a psychologist who encourages the patient to reply. This is acceptable in experimental work where the aim is to obtain a precise estimate of the intensity of the depression and of the components of the syndrome, but not when the purpose is to employ an inventory for large-scale screening so as to detect the presence of a probable depressive state in a population of subjects regarded as normal, of somatic patients, or of psychiatric patients. The aim is then solely to reach a probable diagnosis of depression, not to assess the symptomatic dimensions. Under these conditions, an inventory should be devised comprising items with the best possible discriminatory value and whose number is governed by two contradictory objectives: rapid application and acceptable reliability. The abridged QD2A scale was constructed along these lines by making an empirical selection of 13 items from the QD2 scale.

Principles of the Item Analysis Resulting in the QD2A Inventory. The QD2A inventory was required to satisfy the following conditions:

(1) Best possible discrimination between normal subjects and subjects clinically considered to be depressed
(2) Correlation with the clinically estimated intensity of the depression
(3) Best possible discrimination between subjects not depressed but suffering from a somatic condition, and subjects clinically considered to be depressed
(4) Best possible discrimination between subjects manifesting mental disturbances without a depressive component and subjects clinically considered to be depressed

In practice, a scale constructed on the basis of criteria (1) and (2) can be used for epidemiology of the general population, a scale constructed on the basis of criteria (2) and (3) for detecting depressed subjects among patients suffering from a somatic complaint, and a scale constructed on the basis of (2) and (4) for rapid detection of depressed subjects in a psychiatric milieu.

In theory, analyses of items based on each of the criteria result in different abridged scales. But for obvious practical reasons, if empirical study were to show this to be possible it would be preferable to construct a single abridged scale, provided that its discriminatory value were satisfactory from the different viewpoints considered.

Steps in Item Analysis. The initial analysis covered a sample of 157 depressed patients and a sample of 89 subjects regarded as normal (students and medical personnel). The chi square between the frequencies of answers to the items was calculated for each item and the items were classified in decreasing order of chi-square values.

A second analysis covered the sample of 157 depressed patients and a random sample of 90 patients hospitalized in the somatic medicine services of the Hôpital de Luxembourg. These patients had not undergone psychiatric examination, so that it is probable that a certain proportion of them were suffering from a depressive state, apart from their physical affection. The only consequence this fact can have is to lower the discriminatory level, but it cannot influence the classification of the items from this viewpoint. The items were arranged in decreasing order of the chi-square values calculated.

A Self-Report Inventory on Depressive Symptomatology (QD2)

Table 12.5. Correlation between the classification of the items in relation to their discriminatory value according to the four criteria

	1	2	3	4
1. Rank discrimination depressed/normal	–			
2. Rank correlation with intensity	0.29	–		
3. Rank discrimination depressed/somatic subjects	0.61	0.64	–	
4. Rank discrimination depressed/psychiatric subjects	0.67	0.40	0.47	–

A third analysis covered the sample of 157 depressed patients and a group of 145 mental cases who were outpatients of or hospitalized in the Clinique des Maladies mentales, Paris. After a thorough clinical examination, none of these patients had been considered to suffer from a primary depressive syndrome or a depressive syndrome in addition to their other psychiatric symptoms. The items were arranged in decreasing order of the chi-square values calculated.

A fourth analysis consisted in correlating biserial $r(r^{bis})$, the answer to each item with the clinically estimated intensity of the depression in the sample of 157 depressed subjects, and in arranging the items in accordance with the decreasing values of the correlation coefficients.

Choice of the 13 Items in QD2A. The four item analyses result in different classifications. In order to compare them, the rank correlations (ρ) between the four classifications were calculated (Table 12.5). The coefficients vary between 0.29 and 0.67, with a mean of 0.51.

In these circumstances it seemed acceptable to combine the four item analyses so as to obtain a single list of 13 items – inventory QD2A. The technique, chosen arbitrarily, consisted in calculating the sum of the ranks of each item in the four analyses and retaining those items having the lowest totals (Table 12.6).

Homogeneity. The contingency coefficient Φ was calculated for each item. All the coefficients are significant at a 0.01 level.

Reliability. The reliability coefficient calculated by the split-half method with the Spearman-Brown correction is 0.84 for the group of depressed patients.

Concurrent Validity. The correlation in the group of depression cases, for the QD2 scale with 52 items, is 0.91. With the Zung inventory the correlation is 0.65 for a sample of 81 depression cases. It should be noted that this value is distinctly lower than that obtained on correlating the QD2 and the Zung Inventory for the same sample (0.85). The significance of this fact will be considered later on.

Empirical Validity: Discriminatory Power. Comparison of the means reveals t values that are all significant at the 0.01 threshold. As compared with the depression cases, the t values reflect the decrease in quality of discrimination when normal subjects ($t = 19.30$), somatic patients ($t = 11.36$) and mental patients ($t = 6.98$) are considered, although the lowest of the three values still remains highly significant (Table 12.7).

Table 12.6. Sum of ranks obtained for each item in accordance with the four-item analysis criteria

Item	Sum of ranks	Ranks Depressed/ normal	Depressed/ somatic	Depressed/ psychiatric	Intensity	Item	Sum of ranks	Ranks Depressed/ normal	Depressed/ somatic	Depressed/ psychiatric	Intensity
51	23,5	6	1	5	11,5	48	98	43	33	19	3
6	36	14	8	13	1	49	99	18	28	36	17
12	38	8	16	12	2	25	103	30	15	30	28
20	39	2	4	9	24	23	105	36	18	45	6
19	42	10	3	25	4	4	114	44	23	42	5
36	47	9	13	3	22	14	121	48	43	21	9
44	51,5	1	18,5	6	26	42	123,5	42	29	38	14,5
40	52	21	14	7	10	46	128	37	36	28	27
37	56	16	2	15	23	17	135	27	42	20	46
16	58	5	11	8	34	7	138	24	39	32	43
11	59,5	13	19	16	11,5	5	139	38	27	37	37
29	68	23	21	11	13	35	152	28	35	47	42
21	69,5	3	31	10	25,5	43	153	39	24	39	51
9	70	29	5	29	7	2	155	40	32	51	32
32	71	20	19	1	31	47	159	22	37	52	48
13	72	25	7	24	16	27	164	47	45	31	41
34	72,5	11	41	2	18,5	41	165	49	40	26	40
39	74	12	10	22	30	24	168	34	44	40	50
8	75,5	17	6	27	25,5	10	169	33	50	34	52
3	77	15	9	33	20	26	175	45	38	48	44
1	77,5	32	7	14	14,5	33	175	52	48	46	29
31	83	7	22	18	36	18	176	46	49	43	38
50	88	19	30	4	35	15	179	35	46	49	49
22	89	26	25	17	21	28	180	41	50	50	39
38	92	31	12	41	8	45	184	50	52	35	47
52	94	4	34	23	33	30	187	51	47	44	45

A Self-Report Inventory on Depressive Symptomatology (QD2)

Table 12.7. Mean values of QD2A scores of the four groups of subjects and significance of the differences

	N	M	Standard deviation	t 1 Depressed	2 Normal	3 Somatic
1 Depressed	157	9.54	3.56			
2 Normal	89	2.15	2.42	19.30		
3 Somatic	90	4.20	3.55	11.36	4.53	
4 Mental	145	6.44	4.12	6.98	10.05	4.43

Table 12.8. Mean QD2A values in three subgroups of depressed subjects defined by clinical intensity of symptoms and significance of differences

	N	M	Standard deviation	t 1 Serious	2 Moderate
Intensity of depression					
1 Serious	33	11.09	3.36		
2 Moderate	84	9.70	3.35	2.06*	
3 Slight	40	7.95	3.71	3.84**	2.53*

* 0.05;   ** 0.01

Empirical Validity: Ccorrelation with Intensity of Depression. The differences between serious and moderate depression, and between moderate and slight depressions, are all significant at the 0.05 level, and between serious and slight depression at the 0.01 level (Table 12.8).

Choice of a Cutting Score. Since the aim of the inventory is to detect depressions, the proportion of false-positives and of false-negatives in relation to the discriminatory threshold adopted must be determined, in order to choose an optimal threshold.

In practice, the choice of the threshold from which the total QD2A score is considered to indicate the presence of a depression will depend on the user's decision. The lower the threshold selected, the fewer false-negatives there will be (depressed subjects not recognized as such), and the higher the number of false-positives (nondepressed subjects regarded as depressed).

If, for example, the threshold 3/4 is taken (regarding as depressed all subjects with a score of 4 or above) then only 9% of depressed subjects will "escape," but 22% of normal subjects will be considered as depressed as well as 54% of somatic patients and 70% of psychiatric patients. Conversely, if 10/11 is taken as the threshold, this will allow 48% of depressed persons to "escape," but on the other hand only 6% of somatic patients, 24% of psychiatric patients, and no normal subjects will be regarded as depressed. If the aim is a special application of the inventory so as to leave practically no depressed subjects undetected, then the lower threshold (3/4) will be selected, but this will be at the expense of a large proportion of false-positives. The converse situation arises if a high threshold is adopted, for example, 10/11 (Table 12.9).

Table 12.9. Discriminatory value of QD2A – Percentage of true- and false-positives in the different groups

	Threshold							
	3/4	4/5	5/6	6/7	7/8	8/9	9/10	10/11
False-negatives Percentage of depressed persons considered to be nondepressed	8.92	12.10	17.20	19.11	22.29	27.39	34.39	48.41
False-positives Percentage of normal subjects considered to be depressed	22.47	15.73	11.23	4.49	4.49	4.49	1.16	0.00
Percentage of somatic patients considered to be depressed	54.44	43.33	31.11	23.33	17.78	13.33	10.00	5.56
Percentage of mental patients considered to be depressed	70.34	60.69	55.17	50.34	42.76	33.79	28.28	24.14

Table 12.10. Percentage of subjects wrongly classified in accordance with threshold (the optimal solutions have been underlined)

Threshold	Depressed + normal subjects	Depressed + somatic patients	Depressed + mental patients
3/4	15.70	31.68	39.63
4/5	13.92	27.72	36.40
5/6	14.22	24.16	36.19
6/7	<u>11.80</u>	21.22	34.73
7/8	13.39	20.04	32.53
8/9	15.94	<u>20.36</u>	30.39
9/10	17.76	22.20	<u>31.34</u>
10/11	24.21	26.99	36.28

The optimal solution may be calculated by estimating the percentage of false-diagnoses (false-positives + false-negatives) in relation to the total number of subjects. It should be mentioned, however, that the result is based on a series of assumptions. A precise calculation would require Bayes' formulae to be borne in mind, which take into consideration the a priori probability of the appearance of a depressed subject in the population examined – a probability which, in fact, is not known. This being so, it is customary to assign an arbitrary value of ½ to that probability, i.e. to consider that the group examined includes an equal number of depressed and nondepressed subjects. Table 12.10 gives the results of this calculation. The percentages given correspond to the false diagnoses (false-positives and false-negatives) for the different thresholds in three populations of subjects: depressed and normal subjects in equal numbers; depressed and somatic patients in equal numbers; and depressed and nondepressed mental patients in equal numbers.

A Self-Report Inventory on Depressive Symptomatology (QD2)

Table 12.11. Detection of depressed subjects by psychiatric clinical examination and by inventory QD2A among 112 patients attending because of somatic illness

	Considered by the QD2A as	
	Normal	Depressed
Clinically depressed	3	28
Clinically nondepressed	73	8

On adopting the cutting score 6/7, a figure of 4.49% false-positives and 19.11% false-negatives is obtained.

Cross-Validation of Discriminatory Power. The results reported concern groups that have been used for item analysis. In these circumstances, it is usual for the values obtained to be over-evaluated, and it is necessary to confirm them by cross-validation, in which the same inventory is applied with the same cutting score to a fresh sample. In three outpatient departments of a general hospital (rheumatology, gastric and diabetic diseases, cardiology), 112 consecutive patients were clinically examined by a psychiatrist who, after examining them thoroughly, indicated whether the subject suffered from a clinically significant depressive syndrome, independently of the complaint for which he was attending the outpatient department. The subjects also completed the QD2A without the psychiatrist knowing the result.

The psychiatrist considered that 26.7% of the subjects suffered from a depression, while 32% of them had a score of 7 or over in inventory QD2A (Table 12.11). Comparison between the QD2A results (cutting score 6/7) and the clinical criteria shows that the inventory produced 9.8% false-positives and 9.6% false-negatives, or a total diagnostic error of 9.8% (11 wrong diagnoses out of 112). These results are slightly better than those obtained with the groups used for item analysis.

Conclusions. Inventory QD2A thus seems to be a screening tool with satisfactory validity. It should be stressed that the 13 items of which it consists were chosen empirically in relation to the aim pursued (their discriminatory value). It can be seen that none of the 13 items belongs to the anxiety factor. Anxiety is one of the important dimensions of depressive symptomatology, but it is not a diagnostic criterion. This particular technique for selecting the items probably explains why the correlation with Zung's inventory, which was 0.85 for the 52-item QD2, is only 0.65 for the 13-item QD2A. Both Zung's inventory and the QD2 concern in principle all aspects of depressive symptomatology, whereas the QD2A deals only with those which have a discriminatory value for the diagnosis of depression.

Appendix A

Inventory QD2

		I	1. I now find it difficult to get going
			2. I have to ask others what I should do
		II	3. I have been less successful in life than most people
		I	4. At present I am neglecting myself
		III	5. I feel that there is a lump in my throat
X		II	6. I have difficulty in shaking off the evil thoughts that pass through my head
			7. I am less interested than usual in sex
		II	8. I feel useless
		I	9. I am now obliged to check and re-check whatever I am doing
		III	10. I perspire more than usual
X			11. My memory does not seem to be as good as it used to be
X		I	12. I have no energy
		II	13. I feel guilty
		II, III	14. At the moment, I feel particularly nervous
		III	15. I have a feeling of heaviness in the arms and legs
X		I	16. I have less pleasure now in doing things that please or interest me than previously
			17. I seem more tired than usual without any reason
			18. At present my appetite is not so good as it used to be
X		II	19. I am disappointed and disgusted with myself
X	I, II		20. When I have the slightest thing to do I feel blocked or prevented
X	I, II		21. At present I feel less happy than most people
		I	22. At present I find it difficult to concentrate my attention on any work or occupation
		II	23. I've had enough of life and wish it were ended
		III	24. I have the impression that my heart is beating harder than usual or is racing
		II	25. I feel myself to be less capable or intelligent than most other people
			26. At present I often want to be alone
		III	27. I feel very tense at present
			28. My weight has changed
X		II	29. I have no hope for the future
			30. I have pains in the small of my back
			31. I now avoid certain activities, places or things for they frighten me
		II	32. I feel blue
			33. At present I am unable to stay still
		I	34. I do things less quickly than usual
			35. At present I am more constipated than usual
X		I	36. I must force myself to do anything at all
X			37. My mind is not as clear as usual

A Self-Report Inventory on Depressive Symptomatology (QD2)

        II 38. I feel it would be better if I were dead
  I, II 39. I am unable to reach a decision as easily as usual
X   II 40. I feel sad at present
           41. I do not sleep as well as usual
    II 42. I reproach myself for things
        43. I have the feeling that other people do not understand me
X   I 44. I have difficulty in doing things I was accustomed to do
    III 45. I'm more irritable than usual
    III 46. At present it takes little to make me cry
    I 47. I worry about my health
        48. At present things worry and torment me
    II 49. I am full of a feeling of fear
    I 50. I work less easily than before
X   II 51. At present my life seems empty
    I 52. I feel I am in a state of general weakness

The inventory can be presented in the usual way, on a sheet. However, if possible, it is advisable to type each statement on a card, and to submit the statements to the subject in any order. Two cards marked true and false are placed in front of the subject and he is asked to put each statement opposite the card corresponding to what he is feeling at that time. If necessary, the subject is encouraged by stressing the fact that it is essential for the 52 statements to be classified. It is also possible to read out each statement to the subject, but no comment should be made, and in particular, the text should never be paraphrased. The answers obtained should be entered on an answer sheet. The total depression score is the number of "true" answers; that for the "feeling of loss of general drive" factor is the number of "true" answers to the 15 saturated items in factor I (preceded by I); that for the "anxiety" factor is the number of "true" answers to the 8 saturated items in factor III (preceded by III); while that for the "depressive mood" factor is the number of "true" answers to the 18 saturated items in factor II (preceded by II).

The 13 items which constitute inventory QD2A are preceded by "X".

References

1. Bernstein, I. H., and Eveland, D. C. 1982. State vs. trait anxiety: a case study in confirmatory factor analysis. Personality and Individual Differences 3: 361–372.
2. Derogatis, L. E., Lipman, R. S., Rickels, K., Uhlenhuth, E. H., and Covi, L. 1974. The Hopkins Symptom Checklist (HSCL). A measure of primary symptom dimensions. In: P. Pichot (ed.) Psychological Measurements in Psychopharmacology. Mod. Probl. Pharmacopsychiatry, Vol. 7. Karger, Basel.
3. Hathaway, S. R., McKinley, J. C. 1942–47. Minnesota Multiphasic Personality Inventory, revised edition. Psychological Corporation, New York.
4. Pichot, P., Piret, J., Clyde, D. J. 1966. Analyse de la symptomatologie dépressive subjective. Revue de Psychologie appliquée 16: 105–115.
5. Pichot, P., Boyer, P., Pull, C. B., Rein, W., Simon, M., and Thibault, A. 1985. Un questionnaire

d'auto-évaluation de la symptomatologie dépressive, le Questionnaire QD2. I. Construction, structure factorielle et propriétés métrologiques. Revue de Psychologie appliquée 34: 229–250.
6. Pichot, P., Boyer, P., Pull, C. B., Rein, W., Simon, M., and Thibault, A. 1985. Un questionnaire d'auto-évaluation de la symptomatologie dépressive, le Questionnaire QD2. II. Forme abrégée QD2A. Revue de Psychologie appliquée 34: 323–340.
7. Spielberger, C. S., Vagg, P. R., Barker, L. R., Duham, G. W., and Westbury, L. G. 1980. The factor structure of the State-Trait Anxiety Inventory. In: I. G. Sarason, and C. D. Spielberger (eds.) Stress and Anxiety, Vol. 7. Hemisphere, Washington, DC.
8. Zung, W. W. K. 1965. A self-rating depression scale. Arch. gen. Psychiatry 13: 508–515.

Chapter 13   Applications of the Beck Depression Inventory

R. A. STEER, A. T. BECK, and B. GARRISON

Introduction

Twenty-one years have passed since the Beck Depression Inventory (BDI) was first described by Beck et al. [16]. Over the years, two important reviews about the psychometric properties of the BDI have been written by Beck and Beamesderfer [15] and Mayer [123]. The former review stressed aspects of reliability and validity, whereas the latter review also compared the BDI with other self-report measures of depression.

The present review does not focus upon the psychometric properties of the BDI or with its comparisons to other instruments; instead, it describes how the BDI has been employed over the past 21 years. Reliability and validity considerations are discussed briefly where appropriate, but the emphasis is upon the broad spectrum of psychosocial and medical problems to which the BDI has been addressed.

The review must be highly selective because the records of the Center for Cognitive Therapy, which has acted as a clearinghouse for the dissemination of the BDI, indicate that it has been used in over 500 reported studies. One of the most impressive features about this body of research about the BDI is the worldwide trend for its routine inclusion within psychological test batteries as a touchstone against which to compare assessments derived from other measures.

Since the current review is addressed to an audience of international readers, the authors have also decided to restrict their review to articles published in scientific journals which are available to the worldwide scientific community. Such a decision is, however, unfortunate since a number of important studies about the BDI have involved doctoral and masters theses, not to mention unpublished papers written for health care agencies and academic institutions.

All of the references describing studies of depression in the present chapter have employed the BDI as a measurement instrument for assessing the intensity of depression. However, to avoid the constant repetition of mentioning the BDI, the words "depression" or "depressed" are frequently used by themselves to represent "depression as measured by the BDI" or "depressed according to the BDI."

By way of a brief overview, the present review also describes how the BDI has grown from its original use as a brief psychiatric screening instrument to its employment as a powerful assessment tool. The BDI is sensitive to changes associated with psychopharmacological trials, varying psychotherapeutic techniques, and a variety of medical problems. It has been translated into a variety of languages, which will be listed later, and modified to extend its applicability from adults to children. Although specifically developed to assess depression in psychiatric patients, the BDI is also appropriate for detecting depression in normal adults.

Brief Description of BDI

The BDI was derived from clinical observations about the attitudes and symptoms displayed by depressed psychiatric patients [16]. The observations were systematically reduced to 21 symptoms and attitudes which could be rated from 0 to 3 in terms of intensity. Importantly, the items were chosen to assess the intensity of depression and were not selected to reflect any developmental theory of depression. The symptoms and attitudes were (1) mood, (2) pessimism, (3) sense of failure, (4) lack of satisfaction, (5) guilt feelings, (6) sense of punishment, (7) self-dislike, (8) self-accusation, (9) suicidal wishes, (10) crying, (11) irritability, (12) social withdrawal, (13) indecisiveness, (14) distortion of body image, (15) work inhibition, (16) sleep disturbance, (17) fatigability, (18) loss of appetite, (19) weight loss, (20) somatic preoccupation, and (21) loss of libido. Although it was initially designed to be administered by trained interviewers, the BDI is most often used as a self-administered scale.

The BDI's first psychometric studies were based upon 606 patients routinely admitted to the psychiatric outpatient and inpatient services of a large metropolitan hospital serving lower socioeconomic classes [13]. The odd-even internal reliability coefficient was 0.86 for this sample, and the BDI total scores correlated 0.65 with clinicians' ratings of depression. Many of the studies included in this review have further evaluated the concurrent, construct, and discriminant validities of the BDI within different clinical and normal samples; the magnitudes of internal reliability coefficients and associations with clinical ratings reported therein were found to mirror those reported in this initial 1961 study.

Although Beck and Beamesderfer [15] contended that cutoff scores on the BDI should be based upon the purposes for which decisions about the intensity of depression are to be made, their broad guidelines will be followed throughout this review when describing mild, moderate, and severe levels of depression. Mild (low) scores are less than 4; moderate (medium) is between 14 and 20; and severe is 21 and above. Unless otherwise indicated, the use of "mild," "moderate," and "severe" levels of depression throughout the remainder of this chapter will refer to the aforementioned ranges.

Psychiatric Appraisals

Clinical Ratings

Over the past 21 years, the BDI's psychometric properties have been reportedly investigated within different samples of psychiatric patients. May et al. [122] confirmed Beck et al.'s [16] report that the BDI was significantly related to clinical ratings of depression ($r = 0.65$). Further corroborations for the high level of agreement between the BDI and clinical ratings were reported by Salkind [155], Williams et al. [184], Beck et al. [17], Bech et al. [12], Davies et al. [59], and Bailey and Coppen [6]. The magnitude of the correlations between clinical ratings and the BDI ranged between 0.60 and 0.90, and the sample sizes varied widely.

Discriminant Validity

The BDI's relationships with psychiatric ratings scales and psychological tests have also been extensively studied and have generally yielded correlations which ranged between 0.50 and 0.80 [123]. The substantial correlations (i.e., r's > 0.50) of the BDI with other psychometric instruments [12, 59, 86, 160] have caused some researchers [123, 126] to question its ability to distinguish between depression and other types of psychiatric syndromes. However, the BDI has discriminated between psychiatric patients displaying different types of depression [59] and has been shown previously by Schnurr et al. [160] to differentiate among psychiatric diagnoses, such as schizophrenia and psychotic depression. Nevertheless, the BDI is associated with measures of anxiety [27, 119, 160].

Langevin and Stancer [109] have suggested that the BDI displays weak construct methodology and may simply reflect social desirability; the Pearson product-moment correlation between Edwards' Social Desirability Scale and the BDI was -0.83. Low self-esteem is crucial to the diagnosis of depression, however, and would be expected theoretically [13] to be related to social desirability.

Stability

The test-retest stability of the BDI appears to be quite high and in the 0.70s [139]; however, the psychological set which the respondent is asked to hold while taking the instrument is crucial. If the respondent is asked to describe himself or herself for just today, then the BDI is evaluating state depression which would not be expected to display much stability. On the other hand, if the patient describes himself or herself for at least the past week, then the BDI is assumed to be measuring trait depression; the stability coefficients would be higher.

Factor Analytic Studies

A number of researchers have employed the BDI to ascertain whether or not there are distinct components of depression. The BDI has been factor analyzed for hospitalized psychiatric patients [57, 142, 179], attempted suicides [14], alcoholics [78, 168, 170], drug addicts [163], and mildly depressed samples [20, 81]. Distinctions have arisen in the compositions of the reported components or factors, but the differences appear relatively small compared with diverse clinical samples and factor-analytic methodologies that have been employed. Some studies, such as Beck and Lester's [14], have employed principal components analyses in which orthogonal factors were extracted. Steer et al. [170] have questioned the principal components approach since the BDI is composed of items displaying high item-total correlations and intercorrelations; principal factor techniques employing oblique rotations were recommended.

Tanaka and Huba [174] reported having used hierarchical confirmatory factor analyses with previously published BDI intercorrelation matrices and found that the BDI represents three correlated primary factors – negative attitudes/suicide, physiological, and performance difficulty. These three factors, in turn, described one second-order general factor representing overall depression. It is important to note that across the various factor-analytic studies which have been reported for the BDI, the major dimension is a cognitive self-evaluative one.

Psychosocial Correlates

With the acceptance of the BDI as a valid measure of depression, it has now been used to help establish the construct validity of newly developed instruments. Lubin [119] used the BDI to validate a variety of adjective checklists which he had developed to assess depression, and Spitzer et al. [167] also employed the BDI in assessing the construct validity of the Mental Status Schedule. Bloom and Brady [27] have reported that the BDI was positively correlated with the depression scale in the Multiple Adjective Checklist.

Biological Correlates

Another important area in which the BDI has been used involves studying its relationship with physiological changes attributed to depression. Brooksbank and Coppen [33] described BDI scores as positively related to elevated corticosteroid plasma levels in reactive and mixed depression; Bursten and Rass [39] also indicated that BDI scores were positively associated with elevated corticosteroid levels in depressed patients. The occurrence of monoamine precursors [43], increased indoleamines [52], derangement in the normal synthesis of adrenal cortical hormones [97], elevated blood sugar levels [93], and 17-OHCS excretion [171] have also been found to be positively correlated to depression as measured by the BDI.

Electrophysiological Correlates

The BDI has been reported by Rimon et al. [149] to be related to residual muscle activity in unselected depressive patients, and Wiet [183] has reported that more frequent non-Gaussian cumulated amplitude distributions in the right control hemisphere of college students, as reflected by EEGs, were positively related to BDI total scores. Furthermore, Carney et al. [42] have indicated that changes in BDI scores were related to initial zygomatic-facial-electromyography indices.

Sleep Disturbance

Some of the earliest work exploring the relationships between the BDI and biological processes involved monitoring depression in sleep studies. Widmann, Prange, and Cochrane [182] found that increased sleep was related to lower levels of depression. Other types of sleep research were described by Hauri and Hawkins [91], Claghorn et al. [47], and Mendels and Hawkins [127]. All of these studies revealed that the BDI was sensitive to levels of depression which were related to changes in sleep patterns and behavior.

Cross-cultural Applications

The cross-cultural applications of the BDI are many, and the BDI has been translated into a number of different languages. For example, a critical review of the Spanish edition of the BDI was presented by Lopez, Chamorro, and Serrano [118], and Barcia and Galiana [8] have also described its use with alcoholism and suicide problems in Spain. Lopez and Chamorro [117] have indicated that there were no sex differences or age-related differences for Spanish samples, and the Spanish BDI mean levels of intensity were comparable to the psychiatric samples originally reported by Beck et al. [16]. Recently, Comas-Diaz [50] has also indicated that the Spanish BDI was successful in detecting changes in depression related to behavior therapy interventions employed with Puerto Rican women.

There is a German translation of the BDI [72, 92, 120], and the Polish BDI detected changes in depression related to antidepressant therapy [23].

An Indian version of the BDI has been reported by Ajamany and Nandi [2]. Bech et al. [11, 12] have used the BDI in Denmark in a variety of medical studies, and Delay et al. [60] have reported that the BDI has been quite successful in discriminating between different psychiatric diagnoses within French samples. There is a Finnish BDI [177], and the Japanese version has been reported by Shinfuku [164]. Furthermore, Tarighati [175] has indicated that the BDI was successful in measuring levels of depression in Iranian heroin addicts.

The levels of intensity and the factor structures of the BDI for different nationalities vary. Metcalfe and Goldman [129] reported that the intensity of depression was lower in British psychiatric samples than in American ones. However, for Spanish samples, the levels of intensity appear to be comparable [117] to United States samples. Probably the most comprehensive racial comparisons have been reported by Marsella et al. [121] with Hawaiian college students, and there is an indication that Oriental women have higher intensities of depression than Oriental men; and Caucasian men appear to describe the lowest level of depression. However, these samples were based upon college students and more detailed cross-national studies should be conducted with clinical populations.

Normal Populations

Students

The BDI over the past 10 years has increasingly been employed to screen for depressive symptomatology in student populations. For example, Baumgart and Oliver [9] in studying 275 students have reported that the BDI indicated no sex ratio and gender differences when it was administered anonymously. Bosse et al. [30] in assessing the retrospective descriptions of 158 sophomores found that 41% had described moderate to severe depression in their preceding freshman year; whereas, Bumberry et al. [35] had indicated that the BDI scores of 56 university students correlated 0.77 with psychiatric ratings of depression; this level is comparable to such relationships with psychiatric patients.

Beck et al. [17] had developed a 13-item version of the full BDI which had been shown to display extremely high ($r = 0.91$) correlations with the full BDI, and this instrument has also been employed successfully in screening college students. The abbreviated BDI has also suggested that perhaps 28% of elementary and high school students ($N = 21$) may be diagnosed as depressed [41] and 60% had depressive symptoms.

Similar rates of depression to those described above were described by Hammen [88]. Interestingly, clinically assessed depression was eventually observed in approximately 50% of the college students who had been identified by the BDI as moderately depressed, and Hammen and Padesky [89] found that several BDI items differentiated between 972 men and 1300 women. The men cried less, felt more social withdrawal, and described themselves more as failures than women; whereas, the women were more indecisive and expressed more self-dislike than the men.

Oliver and Burkham [139] indicated that the 3-week test-retest stability of the BDI was high, 0.78 in college students, and 17% (BDI > 10) were depressed. Importantly, 69% of the 17% who were initially depressed were still depressed 3 weeks later. There was no difference in level of depression with respect to sex, but the BDI was inversely related to grade level.

Sacco [153] has cautioned that special care is required for the use of the BDI in college populations, especially with those volunteering for experiments. The BDI should not be used as a screening criterion after the students have been identified for a particular study to avoid contamination with outcome criteria.

Psychosocial Correlates

The types of correlational studies described for psychiatric patients have also been reported for college students. Little and McPhail [115] found that the BDI was significantly correlated with the Aiken Visual Analog Test, and Prociuk et al. [145] reported that the BDI was significantly related to hopelessness in college students. The Depression Adjective Checklist [46], Luscher Color Test [48], Minnesota Multiphasic Personality Inventory (MMPI-D) Scale [36], and Moos Ward Environment Scale [148] are a few of the different types of scales that have also been shown to be related to depression as measured by the BDI in normal populations.

Etiology of Depression

The BDI has been used in a number of studies which attempted to ascertain not only the etiology of depression, but also its cognitive-behavioral deficits. Loeb et al. [116] studied the relationship between BDI scores and feedback for task performance in depressed persons and found that favorable feedback regarding performance improved a patient's outlook about the future, level of aspiration, and productivity.

A number of researchers testing hypotheses derived from the learned helplessness model of depression [130] have also studied the relationships between performance and depression. In general, these studies have used the BDI as a screening instrument [62, 90, 136, 154, 156]. The findings are often conflicting, and the disparity may be related to the differences in the screening criteria set for the BDI cutoff scores. For example, the majority of the college samples have employed BDI scores for indicating depression as > 10; whereas other studies have set BDI levels as > 15. In contrast to results reported by Loeb et al. [116], the studies with cutoff scores at 10 seem to indicate that depressed patients react more adversely to negative feedback than to positive feedback about their performance.

Another issue related to helplessness which has been tested with hospitalized patients has involved locus of control [69]. Depressed patients were found to describe less control over their lives than nondepressed individuals.

The role of cognitive deficits in differentiating between types of depressed persons as measured by the BDI has been widely studied. Braff and Beck [31] reported that schizophrenic patients demonstrated more cognitive deficits than depressed patients who, in turn, demonstrated more deficits than normals. Hammen [87] stated that undergraduates displayed different patterns of depression when subjected to varying levels of life stress, and Frost, Graf, and Becker [76] found that depressed persons made more self-devaluations about themselves than nondepressed persons. Furthermore, Roth et al. [150] have indicated that depressed persons overestimated negative and underestimated positive behaviors, whereas Baker and Jessup [7] have suggested that verbal processes may be more characteristic of depressed people than visual imagery. Krantz and Hammen [108] have studied cognitive biases in depression.

Interpersonal problem solving in depression has also been studied rather extensively with the BDI, and Gotlib and Asarnow [79] have indicated that depression varies inversely with interpersonal problem solving. Derry and Kuiper [63] have reported that schematic processing and self-reference differ in depressed people, and Dobson and Dobson [64] have also found that there are different types of problem-solving strategies employed by depressed and nondepressed individuals.

The BDI has also been used to study psychoanalytic formulations about the etiology of depression. Gottschalk et al. [82] investigated the relationship between depression and hostility, and Forrest and Hokanson [74] have indicated that depressed persons have a higher precedence for self-punitive behavior. In 98 female college students, Schwarz et al. [162] found that fathers who consistently expressed their feelings about their children had children with lower levels of depression than those who inconsistently expressed their feelings. The consistent expression of positive feelings toward the children by their parents was associated with less vulnerability to adult depression as measured by the BDI.

Therapeutic Response

As previously mentioned, the BDI has frequently been employed with patients to estimate their responses to treatment; the BDI is used in a pre- and posttest design, and decreases in mean depression scores are considered to represent positive response to treatment. Perhaps, the most frequent use of the BDI has been in comparative trials of psychotropic medications. The BDI was shown to be sensitive to tricyclic medications [19, 32, 38, 53, 113], and decreases in depression associated with lithium carbonate have also been mentioned by Mendels et al. [128].

Green and Stafduhar [85] measured changes in depression using the BDI with respect to electroconvulsive therapy (ECT), and other researchers have also reported that changes in depression associated with ECT can be assessed by the BDI [32, 54, 56, 73, 180].

Inpatient treatment produces quite remarkable changes in BDI scores. For example, Metcalfe and Goldman [129] reported admission BDI scores of 26.18 (SD = 8.75) and discharge scores of 7.15 (SD = 6.23) for 14 men and 23 women given inpatient treatment. Philip [141], in studying patients who did not respond to treatment, has indicated that the higher BDI scores were associated with lack of improvement, and Taylor and Marshall [176] have indicated that the BDI is sensitive to subtle changes in mildly depressed patients. Johnson and Heather [99], Blackburn and Bishop [25], and Bigman and Crocker [22] have all found that the BDI can detect changes in levels of depression related to treatment.

Cognitive-behavioral approaches to the treatment of depression have also been shown to produce decreases in depression using the BDI. Rush et al. [152], in studying 41 unipolar depressives were able to detect significant decreases in depression through the use of cognitive-behavior therapy as opposed to imipramine, and these decreases in depression were reported by Kovacs [107] as being more sustained with cognitive-behavior therapy than with psychopharmacotherapy alone. Another cognitive therapy comparison with psychopharmacology was performed by Blackburn et al. [26], and Antonuccio et al. [4] have indicated that the BDI is sensitive to the treatment of depression in group therapy. Jarvinen and Gold [98] reported that the BDI was able to detect a decrease of levels of depression in college students, related to the use of imagery therapy.

The BDI was employed in comparison of short-term therapy, relaxation therapy, behavior therapy, and drug therapy by McLean and Hakstian [125] and had been used to assess the efficacy of smoking reduction techniques by Graff et al. [84]. However, the BDI has not always been capable of detecting changes in depression associated with treatment [103].

The assessment of marriage difficulties and sexual problems has also been investigated with the BDI. Coleman and Miller [49] indicated that depression was related to marital maladjustment, and Watson and Bamber [178] in a small study of general practice patients reported that marriage and sexual dysfunctioning were related to depression. Winokur et al. [185] have described depression as important in family planning and emotional distress, and Ellis et al. [68] have studied the prevalence of depression in rape victims.

In the evaluation of the relationship between suicidal behavior and depression, Silver et al. [165] revealed that 80% of suicide attempters were depressed, and Lester and Beck [112] found that depression was particularly high in suicide attempters who were also alcoholics or drug abusers.

In summary, the BDI has been successful in detecting changes in depression associated with a wide variety of different treatments in psychiatry. Surprisingly, the magnitude of changes appears to be substantial. The mean pretest scores for the studies presented above were over 20, whereas the mean posttest scores were below 10. Beck and Beamesderfer's [15] cutoff ranges for the BDI would, therefore, suggest that the typical patient had moved from severe depression to nondepression after treatment. Such a finding argues that future psychotherapeutic interventions for depression should be able to support at least a 10-point drop in pre- and posttest BDI scores to be comparable with existing therapies.

Substance Abuse

The role of depression in alcoholism has been studied by Beck et al. [18], O'Leary et al. [138], and Donovan and O'Leary [65, 66], who have all concluded that alcoholics display moderate to severe levels of depression as measured by the BDI. Zielinski [187] has reported that about 42% of alcoholics may be clinically depressed. However, Steer, McElroy, and Beck [170] have found mild levels of depression in outpatient alcoholics of lower socio-economic status.

DeLeon [61] described depression as prevalent in drug addicts admitted to a therapeutic community. Dorus and Senay [67] also challenged the supposedly high prevalence of depression in methadone patients, and Steer et al. [169] found mild levels of depression in newly admitted methadone patients.

Within a Vietnam veteran population, composed mostly of drug abusers and medical patients, Nace et al. [134] found that in 202 veterans who had returned home for an average of 28 months, 33% were depressed according to the BDI.

Rounsaville et al. [151] concluded that the short version of the BDI was more sensitive to specific types of depression in the screening of drug patients than the Hamilton Psychiatric Rating Scale for Depression, the Raskin, or the SCL-90; and Reynolds and Gould [147] have indicated that the correlation between the long and the short forms of the BDI for 163 methadone patients was 0.93.

Finally, turning to another type of addiction, Creden et al. [55] has indicated that high caffeine consumers are more depressed as assessed by the BDI than low caffeine consumers.

Health Care

Another exciting area into which the BDI has moved has been in the assessment of depression accompanying different types of medical problems. Parens et al. [140] found that high BDI depression scores were related to a number of reported illnesses.

Moffic and Paykel [131] found that 24% of the new admissions to a medical ward were depressed, and 5% more became depressed during their 1st week in the hospital. However, medical patients were less depressed than psychiatric patients.

Armstrong et al. [5] reported that the BDI was related to medical distress as measured by the Cornell Medical Index, and Kaplan et al. [100] also found that it was associated with a series of problems as described by the Health Behaviors Questionnaire; smokers had higher mean BDI scores than nonsmokers, drug users had higher mean BDI scores than non-users, and under- and overweight persons had higher mean BDI scores than those who believed that their weights were comparable to others.

In assessing depression in 526 medical outpatients, Nielsen and Williams [137] indicated that 12.2% had mild depressions, 5.5% had moderate depressions, and 0.6% had severe depressions. Importantly, the physicians failed to diagnose the depression in 50% of the patients whom the BDI had suggested were depressed.

Beyond associations with physical complaints and health behavior, the BDI has been employed with persons suffering from a variety of known diseases. For example, Graff [83] and Fischer [71] used the BDI in assessing depression among the obese and those undergoing therapeutic fasting. Bech and Hey [10] also employed the BDI with obese patients who were undergoing bypass surgery, and Schuffel et al. [159] and Schwab et al. [161] applied it in patients with abdominal complaints. Piper et al. [143] studied depression in duodenal ulcer patients and found that duodenal ulcer patients were more depressed than matched controls.

The assessment of depression in cancer patients has been reported by Leiber et al. [111], Plumb and Holland [144], Bluhm et al. [28], and Blumberg and Loudon [29]. The latter researchers, for example, reported that 25% of their cancer patients were depressed. However, all four sets of researchers have maintained that it is difficult to discriminate between the somatic depressive symptoms usually described by cancer patients and the prevalence of true depression; the nonsomatic symptoms, such as self-esteem, may be better indicators of depression in cancer patients than the somatic ones.

Khatami and Rush [104] and Mohamed et al. [132] have studied the role of depression in chronic pain patients. Again, it appears that depressed patients with pain may represent distinctive types of depressive illness.

To mention just a few of the other illnesses in which the BDI has been used, it has been employed with chronic prostatitis [102], hemodialysis [148], asthma [177], parkinsonism [51, 124], hypothyroidism [96], epilepsy [146], and skin disease (psoriasis) [70]. With respect to medical problems, the somatic complaints measured by the BDI must be carefully weighed before concluding that a medical patient is indeed depressed.

In the past few years, there has been increased interest in women's health care and its relationship to depression. Herzberg et al. [94] studied 261 women's reactions to oral contraceptives and their levels of depression as measured by the BDI. The BDI scores of women receiving first or repeated abortions [75], pregnant women [114], women who had experienced mastectomies [133], and menopausal women [157, 158] have also been reported in the literature.

In summary, the BDI appears to be quite successful in measuring depressive symptomatology associated with medical problems. Perhaps, the BDI's success in assessing depression in medical patients is attributable to what Mayer [123] considered to be one of its major deficits – that BDI stresses cognitive symptoms rather than affective and somatic ones. However, this emphasis upon the cognitive aspects of depression allows it to assess depression regardless of medical or other problems that accompany the diseases from which the patients are suffering.

Children and Adolescents

The BDI was originally developed for adult psychiatric patients and, as has already been described above, has also been successfully used with normal adults. In the latter half of the 1970s, its use was extended to children and adolescents. Kovacs and Beck [106] presented a review of depression in adolescence and childhood and have described a modified form of the BDI that was appropriate with younger age groups. However, the adult versions of both the long and the short BDI may be appropriate without modification for assessing depression in children. Albert and Beck [3] indicated that in 31 seventh graders and 32 eighth graders, 35% had significant levels of depression, and depression was more prevalent in early adolescence than adulthood. Delinquents also demonstrated high levels of depression (23%) as measured by the BDI [45]. Strober et al. [172] assessed 78 adolescent patients and found that the coefficient alpha was 0.79. Again, the correlation between clinical ratings and the BDI scores was high ($r = 0.76$).

Furthermore, Butensky et al. [40] have used the BDI in a project to assess coronary behavior proneness in children and teenagers; Sullivan [173] studied the relationship between depression and diabetes in 105 adolescent girls; and Ackerman et al. [1] have evaluated depression and peptic ulcer development in older children and adolescents.

Depression in childhood has also been investigated by Lefkowitz and Tesiny

[110] and found to correlate with popularity among 452 boys and 492 girls whose mean age was 10.24 years (SD = 0.78). Importantly, Whiting [181] has indicated that the BDI has been able to assess depression in adolescents which was not related to either their mothers' or fathers' level of depression.

However, as Kovacs and Beck [106] indicated, some researchers prefer to use the modified form of the BDI called the Child Depression Inventory (CDI) in assessing depression in children [101]. Kovacs [105] modified the original CDI form and extended it to 27 multiple items; this modification has been reported for 875 Canadian children to have a Cronbach coefficient alpha, an estimate of internal consistency, of 0.86, and it has a 1-month test-retest reliability of 0.72. Other researchers using the childhood form of the BDI are Brumback and Station [34] and Carlson and Cantwell [41].

The types of depressive symptoms measured by the CDI are comparable to those that are used in assessing adult depression. In fact, Cytryn et al. [58] have indicated that childhood depression, as assessed by Kovacs' modified CDI, conforms to Diagnostic and Statistical Manual (DSM-III) criteria. Childhood and adult depressive disorders appear to be very similar not only with respect to intensity, but also to symptom profile.

Depression in Older Adults

An extensive literature employing the BDI to measure depression in the elderly has not yet developed. May et al. [122] were among the first to study the problems of depression in the elderly using the BDI, and Zemore and Eames [186] compared 48 elderly persons living in homes for the aged, 31 living in the community waiting to be admitted to the homes for the elderly, and 424 younger adults. These latter researchers found that the levels of depression were comparable in the two elderly groups, but somatic symptoms were more prevalent in the elderly groups than in the younger group. Elderly persons may not be more depressed than younger groups if the somatic symptoms concurrent with the aging process are discounted.

Simpson et al. [166] have studied depression and social involvement in residential homes for the elderly. In studying 36 depressed persons over 61 years of age, Hussian and Lawrence [95] have indicated that problem-solving training may be important in reducing depression among the elderly, and Gallagher et al. [77] found that the BDI may be more internally consistent in older adults than it is with younger ones. They reported a Cronbach coefficient alpha of 0.91 with their sample of older persons.

Summary

Over the past 21 years, the BDI has grown from assessing depression in psychiatric samples to screening for depression in normal adults. It is now used to measure depression in children and older adults. The BDI continues to display a high degree of stability and internal consistency across various clinical populations and discriminates among the intensities of depression displayed by different diagnostic samples. It has also been shown to be sensitive to detecting changes in depression produced by different therapies. The BDI has now become an established instrument and is used to support the concurrent validity and construct validity of other instruments.

References

1. Ackerman, S., Manaker, S., and Cohen, M. 1981. Recent separation and the onset of peptic ulcer disease in older children and adolescents. Psychosom. Med. 43: 305-310.
2. Ajmany, S., and Nandi, D. N. 1973. Adaptation of A. T. Beck et al.'s An inventory for measuring depression. Indian Journal of Psychiatry 15: 386-390.
3. Albert, N., and Beck, A. T. 1975. Incidence of depression in early adolescence: A preliminary study. Journal of Youth and Adolescence 4: 301-307.
4. Antonuccio, D. O., Lewinsohn, P. M., and Steinmetz, J. L. 1982. Identification of therapist differences in a group treatment for depression. J. Consult. Clin. Psychol. 50: 433-435.
5. Armstrong, H. E., Goldenberg, E., and Stewart, D. 1980. Correlations between Beck Depression scores and physical complaints. Psychol. Rep. 46: 740-742.
6. Bailey, J., and Coppen, A. 1976. A comparison between the Hamilton Rating Scale and the Beck Inventory in the measurement of depression. Br. J. Psychiatry 128: 486-489.
7. Baker, L. L., and Jessup, B. A. 1980. The psychophysiology of affective verbal and visual information processing in dysphoria. Cognitive Therapy and Research 4: 135-148.
8. Barcia, S. D., and Galiana, C. M. 1976. Alcoholism and attempted suicide. Actas Luso Esp. Neurol. Psiquiatr. 4: 267-290.
9. Baumgart, E. P., and Oliver, J. M. 1981. Sex ratio and gender differences in depression in an unselected adult population. J. Clin. Psychol. 37: 570-574.
10. Bech, P., and Hey, H. 1979. Depression or asthenia related to metabolic disturbances in obese patients after intestinal bypass surgery. Acta Psychiatr. Scand. 59: 462-470.
11. Bech, P., Dein, E., Jacobsen, O., Vitger, J., and Bolwig, T. G. 1972. The depressive state syndrome. Quantitative evaluation: Correlation between clinical evaluation, objective rating scale (Hamilton) and self-rating scale (Beck's Depression Inventory). Nordisk Psvkiatrisk Tidsskrift 26: 358.
12. Bech, P., Gram, L. F., Dein, E., Jacobsen, O., Vitger, J., and Bolwig, T. G. 1975. Correlation between clinical assessment, Beck's self-rating scale and Hamilton's objective rating scale. Acta Psychiatr. Scand. 51: 161-170.
13. Beck, A. T. 1972. Depression: Causes and Treatment. University of Pennsylvania Press, Philadelphia.
14. Beck, A. T., and Lester, A. T. 1973. Components of depression in attempted suicides. J. Psychol. 85: 257-260.
15. Beck, A. T., and Beamesderfer, A. 1974. Assessment of depression: The depression inventory. In: P. Pichot (ed.), Psychological Measurements in Psychopharmacology, Modern Problems in Pharmacopsychiatry, pp. 151-169, Vol. 7. Karger, Basel.
16. Beck, A. T., Ward, C. H., Mendelson, M., Mock, J., and Erbaugh, J. 1961. An inventory for measuring depression. Arch. Gen. Psychiatry 4: 561-571.

17. Beck, A.T., Rial, W.Y., and Rickels, K. 1974. Short form of depression inventory: Cross validation. Psychol. Rep. 34: 1184-1186.
18. Beck, A.T., Weissman, A., and Kovacs, M. 1976. Alcoholism, hopelessness and suicidal behavior. J. Stud. Alcohol 37: 66-77.
19. Bellak, L., and Rosenberg, S. 1966. Effects of anti-depressant drugs on psychodynamics. Psychosomatic Medicine 7: 106-114.
20. Berndt, D.J. 1979. Taking items out of context: Dimensional shifts with the short form of the Beck Depression Inventory. Psychol. Rep. 45: 569-570.
21. Bierman, K.L. 1981. Relationship between stability of cognition and stability of depressive mood. Psychol. Rep. 48: 295-298.
22. Bigman, A., and Crocker, D. 1982. Effects of pleasant-activities manipulation on depression. J. Consult. Clin. Psychol. 50: 436-438.
23. Bilikiewicz, A., and Landowski, J. 1976. Evaluation of antidepressive action of maprotyline. Psychiatr. Pol. 10: 367-374.
24. Biro, M., Bozic, N., and Grmusa, M. 1974. MMPI and Beck scale for diagnosing depression. Anal. Zav. Mental. Zdrav. 6: 99-104.
25. Blackburn, I.M., and Bishop, S. 1981. Is there an alternative to drugs in the treatment of depressed ambulatory patients? Behavioral Psychotherapy 9: 96-104.
26. Blackburn, I.M., Bishop, S., Glen, A.I.M., Whalley, L.J., and Christie, W. 1981. The efficacy of cognitive therapy in depression: A treatment trial using cognitive therapy and pharmacotherapy, each alone and in combination. Br. J. Psychiatry 139: 181-189.
27. Bloom, P.M., and Brady, J.P. 1968. An ipsative validation of the multiple affect adjective check list. J. Clin. Psychol. 24: 45-46.
28. Bluhm, H.P., Glover, D., and Sanford, M.E. 1979. The at-home multidisciplinary rehabilitation team: A new trend in cancer rehabilitation. Rehabilitation Counseling Bulletin June: 419-423.
29. Blumberg, B.S., and London, W.T. 1980. Hepatitis B virus and primary hepato-cellular carcinoma: Relationship of "icrons" to cancer. Viruses in Naturally Occurring Cancers 7: 150-155.
30. Bosse, J.J., Croghan, L.M., Greenstein, M.B., Katz, N.W., Oliver, J.M., Powell, D.A., and Smith, W.R. 1975. Frequency of depression in the freshman year as measured in a random sample by a retrospective version of the BDI. J. Consult. Clin. Psychol. 43: 746-747.
31. Braff, D.L., and Beck, A.T. 1974. Thinking disorder in depression. Arch. Gen. Psychiatry 31: 456-459.
32. Broadhurst, A.D. 1970. L-Tryptophan vs. ECT (letter). Lancet 1: 1392-1392.
33. Brooksbank, B.W.L., and Coppen, A. 1967. Plasma 11-hydroxycorticosteroid in affective disorder. Br. J. Psychiatry 113: 395-404.
34. Brumback, R., and Station, D. 1980. Neuropsychological study of children during and after remission of endogenous depressive episodes. Percept. Mot. Skills 50: 1163-1167.
35. Bumberry, W., Oliver, J.M., and McClure, J.N. 1978. Validation of the Beck Depression Inventory in a university population using psychiatric estimate as the criterion. J. Consult. Clin. Psychol. 46: 150-155.
36. Burkhart, B.R., Gynther, M.D., and Fromuth, M.D. 1980. The relative predictive validity of subtle vs. obvious items on the MMPI depression scale. J. Clin. Psychol. 36: 748-751.
37. Burrows, G.D., Davies, B., and Scroggins, B.A. 1972. Plasma concentration of nontriptyline and clinical response in depressive illness. Lancet 2: 619-623.
38. Burrows, G.D., Foenander, G., Davies, B., and Scoggins, B.A. 1976. Rating scales as predictors of response to tricyclic antidepressants. Aust. N.Z. J. Psychiatry 10: 53-56.
39. Bursten, B., and Rass, J.J. 1965. Preoperative psychological state and corticosteroid levels of surgical patients. Psychosom. Med. 27: 309-316.
40. Butensky, A., Faralli, V., Hubner, D., and Waldron, J. 1976. Elements of the coronary prone behavior pattern in children and teenagers. J. Psychosom. Res. 20: 439-444.
41. Carlson, G.A., and Cantwell, D.P. 1980. A survey of depressive symptoms, syndrome and disorder in a child psychiatric population. J. Child. Psychol. Psychiatry 21: 10-25.
42. Carney, R.M., Hong, B.A., O'Connell, M.F., and Amado, H. 1981. Facial electromyography as a predictor of treatment outcome in depression. Br. J. Psychiatry 138: 485-489.
43. Carroll, B.J. 1971. Monoamine precursors in the treatment of depression. Clin. Pharmacol. Ther. 12: 743-761.

44. Carroll, B.J., Feinberg, M., Smouse, P.E., Rawson, S.G., and Greden, J.F. 1981. The Carroll rating scale for depression. I. Development, reliability and validation. Br. J. Psychiatry 138: 194-200.
45. Chiles, J.A., Miller, M.L., and Cox, G.B. 1980. Depression in an adolescent delinquent population. Arch. Gen. Psychiatry 37: 1179-1184.
46. Christenfeld, R., Lubin, B., and Satin, M. 1978. Concurrent validity of the Depression Adjective Checklist in a normal population. Am. J. Psychiatry 135: 582-583.
47. Claghorn, J.L., Mathew, R.J., Weinman, M.L., and Hruska, N. 1981. Daytime drowsiness and other sleep related symptoms such as attention and concentration difficulties, blurred vision and daytime sleepiness in depression. J. Clin. Psychiatry 42: 342-343.
48. Cohen, E., and Hunter, I. 1978. Severity of depression differentiated by a color selection test. Am. J. Psychiatry 135: 611-612.
49. Coleman, R.E., and Miller, A.G. 1975. The relationship between depression and marital maladjustment in a clinic population: A multitrait-multimethod study. J. Consult. Clin. Psychol. 43: 647-651.
50. Comas-Diaz, L. 1981. Effects of cognitive and behavioral group treatment on the depressive symptomatology of Puerto Rican women. J. Consult. Clin. Psychol. 49: 627-632.
51. Coppen, A., and Metcalfe, M. 1972. Levodopa and L-trytophan therapy in Parkinsonism. Lancet 1: 654-658.
52. Coppen, A., Prange, A.T., Whybrow, P.C., and Noguora, R. 1972. Abnormalities of indoleamines in affective disorders. Arch. Gen. Psychiatry 26: 474-478.
53. Coppen, A., Whybrow, P.C., Noguera, R., Maggs, R., and Prange, A.J. 1972. The comparative antidepressant value of L-trytophan and imipramine with and without attempted potentiation by liethrenine. Arch. Gen. Psychiatry 26: 234-241.
54. Costello, C.G., Belton, G.P., Abra, J.C., and Dunn, B.E. 1970. The amnesic and therapeutic effects of bilateral and unilateral ECT. Br. J. Psychiatry 116: 69-78.
55. Creden, J.F., Fontaine, P., Lubetsky, M., and Chamberlain, K. 1978. Anxiety and depression associated with caffeinism among psychiatric inpatients. Am. J. Psychiatry 135: 963-966.
56. Cronin, D., Bedley, P., Potts, L., Mather, M.D., Gardner, R.K., and Tobin, J.D. 1970. Unilateral and bilateral ECT: A study of memory disturbance and relief from depression. J. Neurol. Neurosurg. Psychiatry 33: 705-713.
57. Cropley, A.J., and Weckowicz, T.E. 1966. The dimensionality of clinical depression. Australian Journal of Psychology 18: 18-25.
58. Cytryn, L., McKnew, D.H., Jr., and Bunney, W.E., Jr. 1980. Diagnosis of depression in children: A reassessment. Am. J. Psychiatry 137: 22-25.
59. Davies, B., Burrows, G., and Poynton, C. 1975. A comparative study of fair depression rating scales. Aust. N.Z. J. Psychiatry 9: 21-24.
60. Delay, J., Pichot, P., Mirouze, R., and Peyrouzet, J.M. 1963. La nosologie des états dépressifs. Rapports entre l'étiologie et la sémiologie. 1. Position du problème. Encéphale 52: 481-496.
61. DeLeon, G. 1974. Phoenix House: Psychopathological signs among male and female drug-free residents. Addictive Diseases 1: 135-151.
62. DeMonbrean, B.G., and Craighead, E. 1977. Distortion of perception and recalled positive and neutral feedback in depression. Cognitive Therapy and Research 1: 311-329.
63. Derry, P.A., and Kuiper, N.A. 1981. Schematic processing and self-reference in clinical depression. J. Abnorm. Psychol. 90: 286-297.
64. Dobson, D.J., and Dobson, K.S. 1981. Problem-solving strategies in depressed and non-depressed college students. Cognitive Therapy and Research 5: 237-249.
65. Donovan, D.M., and O'Leary, M.R. 1976. Relationship between distortions in self-perception of depression and psychopathology. J. Clin. Psychol. 32: 16-19.
66. Donovan, D.M., and O'Leary, M.R. 1979. Depression, hypomania, and the expectation of future success among alcoholics. Cognitive Therapy and Research 3: 141-154.
67. Dorus, W., and Senay, E.C. 1980. Depression, demographic dimensions, and drug abuse. Am. J. Psychiatry 137: 699-704.
68. Ellis, E.M., Atkeson, B.M., and Calhoun, K.S. 1981. An assessment of long-term reaction to rape. J. Abnorm. Psychol. 90: 263-266.
69. Evans, R.G., and Dinning, W.D. 1978. Reductions in experienced control and depression in psychiatric inpatients: A test of the learned helplessness model. J. Clin. Psychol. 34: 609-613.

70. Fava, G. A., Perini, G. I., Santonastaso, P., and Fornasa, C. V. 1980. Life events and psychiatric distress in dermatological disease, psoriasis, chronic urticaria, and fungal infections. Br. J. Med. Psychiatry 53: 277-282.
71. Fischer, N. 1967. Obesity, affect, and therapeutic starvation. Arch. Gen. Psychiatry 17: 227-233.
72. Flegel, H. 1967. Probleme der Versuchsanordnung bei der klinischen Prüfung von Thymoleptika, Activ. Nerv. Super (Praha) 6: 383-385.
73. Fleminger, J. J., Horne, D. J., Hair, N. P. V., and Hott, P. N. 1970. Differential effects of unilateral and bilateral ECT. Am. J. Psychiat. 127: 430-436.
74. Forrest, M. S., and Hokanson, J. E. 1975. Depression and autonomic arousal reduction accompanying self-punitive behavior. J. Abnorm. Psychol. 84: 346-357.
75. Freeman, E. et al. 1979. Emotional distress patterns among women having first or repeat abortions. Obstet. Gynecol. 55: 630-636.
76. Frost, R. O., Graf, M., and Becker, J. 1979. Self-devaluation and depressed mood. J. Consult. Clin. Psychol. 47: 958-962.
77. Gallagher, D., Nies, G., and Thompson, L. W. 1982. Reliability of the Beck Depression Inventory with older adults. J. Consult. Clin. Psychol. 50: 152-153.
78. Gibson, S., and Becker, J. 1973. Alcoholism and depression: The factor structure of alcoholics' responses to depression inventories. Quarterly Journal of Studies on Alcohol 34: 400-408.
79. Gotlib, I. H., and Asarnow, R. F. 1979. Interpersonal and impersonal problem-solving skills in mildly and clinically depressed university students. J. Consult. Clin. Psychol. 47: 86-95.
80. Golin, S., and Terrell, F. 1977. Motivational and associative aspects of mild depression in skill and chance tests. J. Abnorm. Psychol. 86: 389-401.
81. Golin, S., and Hartz, M. A. 1979. A factor analysis of the Beck Depression Inventory in a mildly depressed population. J. Clin. Psychol. 35: 323-325.
82. Gottschalk, L. A., Gleser, G. C., and Springer, K. J. 1963. Three hostility scales applicable to verbal samples. Arch. Gen. Psychiatry 9: 254-279.
83. Graff, H. 1965. Overweight and emotions in the obesity clinic. Psychosom. Med. 6: 89-94.
84. Graff, H., Hammett, V. B. B., Bash, N., Fackler, W., Yanovski, A., and Goldman, A. 1966. Results of four antismoking therapy methods. Penn. Med. J. 69: 39-43.
85. Green, W. J., and Stafduhar, P. P. 1966. The effect of ECT on the sleep dream cycle in a psychotic depression. J. Nerv. Ment. Dis. 143: 123-134.
86. Grosscup, S. J., and Lewinsohn, P. M. 1980. Unpleasant and pleasant events, and mood. J. Clin. Psychol. 36: 252-259.
87. Hammen, C. L. 1978. Depression, distortion and life stress in college students. Cognitive Therapy and Research 2: 189-192.
88. Hammen, C. L. 1980. Depression in college students: Beyond the Beck Depression Inventory. J. Consult. Clin. Psychol. 48: 126-128.
89. Hammen, C. L., and Padesky, C. A. 1977. Sex differences in the expression of depressive responses on the BDI. J. Abnorm. Psychol. 36: 609-614.
90. Harvey, D. M. 1981. Depression and attributional style: Interpretations of important personal events. J. Abnorm. Psychol. 90: 134-142.
91. Hauri, P., and Hawkins, D. R. 1972. Sleep of depressed patients in remission. Psychophysiology 9: 136.
92. Heimann, Von H., Hursch, L., Eisert, H. G., and Huber, H. 1969. Klinische und experimentelle Objektivierung von Stimmungsveränderungen. Arzneimittelforsch. 19: 467-469.
93. Herzberg, B., Coppen, A., and Marks, V. 1968. Glucose tolerance in depression. Br. J. Psychiatry 114: 627-630.
94. Herzberg, B. N., Johnson, A. L., and Brown, S. 1970. Depressive symptoms and oral contraceptives. Br. Med. J. 5728: 142-145.
95. Hussian, R. A., and Lawrence, P. S. 1981. Social reinforcement of activity and problem-solving training in the treatment of depressed institutionalized elderly patients. Cognitive Therapy and Research 5: 57-69.
96. Jain, V. K. 1971. Affective disturbance in hypothyroidism. Br. J. Psychiatry 119: 279-280.
97. Jakobson, T., Stenback, A., Strandstrom, L., and Rimon, R. 1966. The excretion of urinary 11-deoxy- and 11-oxy-17-hydroxycorticosteroid in depressive patients during basal conditions and during the administration of methopyrapone. J. Psychosom. Res. 9: 363-374.

98. Jarvinen, P.J., and Gold, S.R. 1981. Imagery as an aid in reducing depression. J. Clin. Psychol. 37: 523-529.
99. Johnson, D.A.W., and Heather, B.B. 1974. The sensitivity of the Beck Depression Inventory to changes to symptomatology. Br. J. Psychiatry 125: 184-185.
100. Kaplan, S.L., Nissbaum, M., Skomorowsky, P., Shanker, I.R., and Ramsey, P. 1980. Health habits and depression in adolescence. Journal of Youth and Adolescence 9: 299-304.
101. Kazdin, A.E. 1981. Assessment techniques for childhood depression: a critical appraisal. J. Am. Acad. Child Psychiatry 20: 358-375.
102. Keltikansas, J., Jarvinen, H., and Lehtonen, T. 1981. Psychic disturbances in patients with chronic prostatitis. Ann. Clin. Res. 13: 45-59.
103. Kilpatrick, T.B., and Roth, S. 1978. An attempt to reverse performance deficits associated with depression and experimentally induced helplessness. J. Abnorm. Psychol. 87: 141-154.
104. Khatami, M., and Rush, A.J. 1978. A pilot study of the treatment of outpatients with chronic pain: Symptom control, stimulus control and social system intervention. Pain 5: 164-172.
105. Kovacs, M. 1981. Rating scales to assess depression in school-aged children. Acta Paedopsychiatrica (Basel) 46: 305-315.
106. Kovacs, M., and Beck, A.T. 1977. An empirical-clinical approach toward a definition of childhood depression. In: J.G. Schuterbrandt and A. Raskin (eds.), Depression in Childhood: Diagnosis, Treatment, and Conceptual Models. Raven Press, New York.
107. Kovacs, M., Rush, A.J., Beck, A.T., and Hollon, S.D. 1981. Depressed outpatients treated with cognitive therapy or pharmacotherapy: A one-year follow-up. Arch. Gen. Psychiatry 38: 33-39.
108. Krantz, S., and Hammen, C.L. 1979. Assessment of cognitive bias in depression. J. Abnorm. Psychiatry 88: 611-619.
109. Langevin, R., and Stancer, H. 1979. Evidence that depression rating scales primarily measure a social undesirability response set. Acta Psychiatr. Scand. 59: 70-79.
110. Lefkowitz, M.M., and Tesiny, E.P. 1980. Assessment of childhood depression. J. Consult. Clin. Psychol. 48: 43-40.
111. Leiber, L., Plumb, M.M., Gerstenzang, M.L., and Holland, J. 1976. The communication of affection between cancer patients and their spouses. Psychosom. Med. 38: 379-389.
112. Lester, D., and Beck, A.T. 1975. Attempted suicide in alcoholics and drug addicts. J. Stud. Alcohol 36: 162-164.
113. Lipsedge, M.S., and Rees, W.L. 1971. A double-blind comparison of doxepin and amitriptyline for the treatment of depression with anxiety. Psychopharmacologia 19: 153-162.
114. Lips, H.M. 1982. Somatic and emotional aspects of the normal pregnancy experience: The first 5 months. Am. J. Obstet. Gynecol. 142: 524-529.
115. Little, J.C., and McPhail, N.I. 1973. Measures of depressive mood at monthly intervals. Br. J. Psychiatry 122: 447-452.
116. Loeb, A., Beck, A.T., and Diggory, J. 1971. Differential effects of success and failure on depressed and non-depressed patients. J. Nerv. Ment. Dis. 152: 106-114.
117. Lopez, V.C., and Chamorro, T.E. 1976. Influencia de la edad, sexo y estado civil en el inventario de Beck. Actas Luso Esp. Neurol. Psiquiatr. 4: 105-140.
118. Lopez, V.C., Chamorro, T.E., and Serrano, E.U. 1976. Critical review of the Spanish adaptation of the Beck Questionnaire. Revista de Psicología General y Aplicada 31: 469-497.
119. Lubin, B. 1966. Fourteen brief depression adjective checklists. Arch. Gen. Psychiatry 15: 205-208.
120. Lukesch, H. 1974. Test criteria of the depression inventory of A.T. Beck. Psychologische Praxis (Basel) 18: 60-78.
121. Marsella, A.J., Sanborn, K.O., Kamooka, V., Shizuru, L., and Brennan, J. 1975. Cross-validation of self-report measures of depression among normal populations of Japanese, Chinese, and Caucasian ancestry. J. Clin. Psychol. 31: 281-287.
122. May, A.E., Urquhart, A., and Tarran, J. 1969. Self-evaluation of depression in various diagnostic and therapeutic groups. Arch. Gen. Psychiatry 21: 191-194.
123. Mayer, J.M. 1977. Assessment of depression. In: P.M. Reynolds (ed.), Advances in Psychological Assessment, pp. 358-425, Vol. 4. Jossig-Boss, San Francisco.
124. Mayeux, R., Stern, Y., Rosen, J., and Leventhal, J. 1981. Depression, intellectual impairment, and Parkinson's disease. Neurology 31: 645-650.

125. McLean, P. D., and Hakstian, A. R. 1979. Clinical depression: Comparative efficacy of outpatient treatments. J. Consult. Clin. Psychol. 47: 818–836.
126. Meites, K., Lovallo, W., and Pishkin, V. 1980. A comparison of four scales for anxiety, depression, and neuroticism. J. Clin. Psychol. 36: 427–432.
127. Mendels, J., and Hawkins, D. R. 1971. Sleep and depression. IV. Longitudinal studies. J. Nerv. Ment. Dis. 153: 251–272.
128. Mendels, J., Secunda, S. K., and Dyson, W. L. 1972. A controlled study of the antidepressant effects of lithium carbonate. Arch. Gen. Psychiatry 26: 154–157.
129. Metcalfe, M., and Goldman, E. 1965. Validation of an inventory for measuring depression. Br. J. Psychiatry 111: 240–242.
130. Miller, W. R., and Seligman, M. E. P. 1975. Depression and learned helplessness in men. J. Abnorm. Psychol. 84: 228–238.
131. Moffic, H. A., and Paykel, E. S. 1975. Depression in medical inpatients. Br. J. Psychiatry 126: 346–353.
132. Mohamed, S. N., Weisz, G. M., and Waring, E. M. 1978. The relationship of chronic pain to depression, marital adjustment and family dynamics. Pain 5: 285–292.
133. Morris, T. 1979. Psychological adjustment to mastectomy. Cancer Treat. Rev. 6: 41–61.
134. Nace, E. P., Meyers, A. L., O'Brien, C. P., Ream, N., and Mintz, J. 1977. Depression in veterans two years after Vietnam. Am. J. Psychiatry 134: 167–170.
135. Nelson, R. E., and Craighead, W. E. 1977. Selective recall of positive and negative feedback, self-control behaviors, and depression. J. Abnorm. Psychol. 86: 379–388.
136. Nelson, R. E., and Craighead, W. E. 1981. Tests of a self-control model of depression. Behavior Therapy 12: 123–129.
137. Nielson, A. C., and Williams, T. A. 1980. Depression in ambulatory medical patients. Arch. Gen. Psychiatry 37: 999–1004.
138. O'Leary, M. R., Donovan, D., Cysewski, B., and Chaney, E. F. 1977. Perceived locus of control, experienced control and depression: A trait model of depression. J. Clin. Psychol. 33: 164–167.
139. Oliver, J. M., and Burkham, R. 1979. Depression in university students: Duration, relation to calendar time, prevalence, and demographic correlates. J. Abnorm. Psychol. 88: 667–670.
140. Parens, H., McConville, B. J., and Kaplan, S. M. 1966. The prediction of frequency of illness from the response to separation: A preliminary study and replication attempt. Psychosom. Med. 28: 162–176.
141. Philip, A. E. 1971. Psychometric changes associated with response to drug treatment. Brit. J. Soc. Clin. Psychol. 10: 138–143.
142. Pichot, R., and Lemperiere, T. 1964. Analyse factorielle d'un questionnaire d'auto-évaluation des symptomes dépressifs. Revue de Psychologie Appliquée 14: 15–29.
143. Piper, D. W., Ariotti, D., Greis, M., and Brown, R. 1980. Chronic duodenal ulcer and depression. Scand. J. Gastroenterol. 15: 201–203.
144. Plumb, M. M., and Holland, J. 1977. Comparative studies of psychological function in patients with advanced cancer-1. Self-reported depressive symptoms. Psychom. Med. 39: 264–276.
145. Prociuk, T. J., Breen, L. J., and Lussier, R. J. 1976. Hopelessness, internal-external locus of control, and depression. J. Clin. Psychol. 32: 299–300.
146. Reynolds, E. H. 1970. Water, electrolytes and epilepsy. J. Neurol. Sci. 11: 327–358.
147. Reynolds, W. M., and Gould, J. W. 1981. A psychometric investigation of the standard and short form Beck Depression Inventory. J. Consult. Clin. Psychol. 49: 306–307.
148. Rhodes, L. M. 1981. Social climate perception and depression of patients and staff in a chronic hemodialysis unit. J. Nerv. Ment. Dis. 169: 169–175.
149. Rimon, R., Stenback, A., and Huhman, E. 1966. Electromyographic findings in depressive patients. J. Psychosom. Res. 10: 159–170.
150. Roth, D., Rehm, L. P., and Rozensky, R. H. 1980. Self-reward, self-punishment, and depression. Psychol. Rep. 47: 3–7.
151. Rounsaville, B. J., Weissman, M. M., Rosenberger, P. H., Wilber, C. H., and Kleber, H. D. 1979. Detecting depressive disorders in drug abusers: A comparison of screening instruments. J. Affect. Disord. 1: 255–257.
152. Rush, A. J., Beck, A. T., Kovacs, A. T., and Hollon, S. 1977. Comparative efficacy of cognitive therapy and pharmacotherapy in the treatment of depressed outpatients. Cognitive Therapy and Research 1: 17–37.

153. Sacco, W. P. 1981. Invalid use of the Beck Depression Inventory to identify depressed college-student subjects: A methodological comment. Cognitive Therapy and Research 5: 143-147.
154. Sacco, W. P., and Hokanson, J. E. 1978. Performance satisfaction of depressives under high and low success conditions. J. Clin. Psychol. 34: 907-909.
155. Salkind, M. R. 1969. Beck Depression Inventory in a general practice. J. R. Coll. Gen. Pract. 18: 267-271.
156. Saulnier, K., and Perlman, D. 1981. Inmates' attributions: Their antecedents and effects on coping. Criminal Justice Behavior 8: 159-172.
157. Schneider, M., and Brotherton, P. 1979. Physiological, psychological and situational stresses in depression during the climacteric. Maturitas 1: 153-158.
158. Schneider, M. A., Brotherton, P. L., and Hailes, J. 1977. Effect of exogenous oestrogens on depression in menopausal women. Med. J. Aust. 2: 162-163.
159. Schuffel, W., Schaumburg, C., Schenecke, O., and Wolfert, W. 1973. Functional abdominal complaints as a neurotic symptom. Psychother. Psychosom. 21: 235-240.
160. Schnurr, R., Hoaken, P. C., and Jarrett, F. J. 1976. Comparison of depression inventories in a clinical population. Can. Psychiatr. Assoc. J. 21: 473-476.
161. Schwab, J. J., Brown, J. M., and Holzer, C. E. 1968. Depression in medical inpatients with gastrointestinal diseases. Am. J. Gastroenterol. 49: 146-152.
162. Schwarz, J., Conrad, R., and Zuroff, D. C. 1979. Family structure and depression in female college students: Effects of parental conflict, decision-making power, and inconsistency of love. J. Abnorm. Psychol. 88: 398-406.
163. Shaw, B. F., Steer, R. A., Beck, A. T., and Schut, J. 1979. The structure of depression in heroin addicts. Br. J. Addict. 74: 295-303.
164. Shinfuku, N. 1973. Diagnosis of manic-depressive illness with special emphasis on the basic problems of diagnosis of depressive illness. Japanese Journal of Clinical Psychiatry 2: 5-12.
165. Silver, M. A., Bohnert, M., Beck, A. T., and Marcus, D. 1971. Relation of depression of attempted suicide and seriousness of intent. Arch. Gen. Psychiatry, 25: 573-575.
166. Simpson, S., Woods, R., and Britton, P. 1981. Depression and engagement in a residential home for the elderly. Behav. Res. Ther. 19: 435-438.
167. Spitzer, R. L., Fleiss, J. L., Endicott, J., and Cohen, J. 1967. Mental status schedule: Properties of factor analytically derived scales. Arch. Gen. Psychiatry 16: 479-493.
168. Steer, R. A., Shaw, B. F., Beck, A. T., and Fine, E. W. 1977. Structure of depression in black alcoholic men. Psychol. Rep. 41: 1235-1241.
169. Steer, R. A., Emery, G. C., and Beck, A. T. 1980. Correlates of self-reported and clinically assessed depression in male heroin addicts. J. Clin. Psychol. 36: 798-800.
170. Steer, R. A., McElroy, M., and Beck, A. T. 1982. Structure of depression in alcoholic men: A partial replication. Psychol. Rep. 50: 723-728.
171. Stenback, A., Jakobson, T., and Rimon, R. 1966. Depression and anxiety ratings in relation to the excretion of urinary total 17-OHCS in depressive subjects. J. Psychosom. Res. 9: 355-362.
172. Strober, M., Green, J., and Carlson, G. 1981. Utility of the Beck Depression Inventory with psychiatrically hospitalized adolescents. J. Consult. Clin. Psychol. 49: 482-483.
173. Sullivan, B. J. 1979. Adjustment in diabetic adolescent girls: II. Adjustment, self-esteem, and depression in diabetic adolescent girls. Psychosom. Med. 41: 127-138.
174. Tanaka, J. S., and Huba, G. J. 1982. Hierarchical confirmatory factor analysis establishing a general depression factor. Paper presented at the 1982 Annual Meeting of the Western Psychological Association, Sacramento, CA, April, 1982.
175. Tarighati, S. 1980. An exploratory study on depression in Iranian addicts. Int. J. Soc. Psychiatry 26: 196-199.
176. Taylor, F. G., and Marshall, W. L. 1977. Experimental analysis of a cognitive-behavioral therapy for depression. Cognitive Therapy and Research 1: 59-72.
177. Teiramaa, E. 1977. Psychosocial factors in the onset and course of asthma: A clinical study of 100 patients. Acta Universitatis Ouluonsis D-14: 135.
178. Watson, J. P., and Bamber, R. W. 1980. Some relationships between sex, marriage, and mood. J. Int. Med. Res. 8: 14-19.
179. Weckowicz, T. E., Muir, W., and Cropley, A. J. 1967. A factor analysis of the Beck inventory of depression. J. Consult. Psychol. 31: 193-198.

180. West, E. D. 1981. Electric convulsion therapy in depression: A double-blind controlled trial. Br. Med. J. 282: 355–357.
181. Whiting, S. 1981. The problem of depression in adolescence. Adolescence 16: 67–89.
182. Widmann, D. E., Prange, A. J., and Cochrane, C. M. 1967. Sleep as a sign and as a symptom in depressive illness. Diseases of the Nervous System 28: 314.
183. Wiet, S. G. 1981. Some quantitative hemispheric EEG measures reflecting the affective profile of students differing in university academic success. Biol. Psychol. 12: 25–42.
184. Williams, J. G., Barlow, D. H., and Agras, W. S. 1972. Behavioral measurement of severe depression. Arch. Gen. Psychiatry 27: 330–333.
185. Winokur, A., Rickels, K., Garcia, C., Huggins, G., and Guthrie, M. 1979. Emotional distress in family planning service patients. Advances in Planned Parenthood 14: 17–23.
186. Zemore, R., and Eames, N. 1979. Psychic and somatic symptoms of depression among young adults. Institutionalized aged and noninstitutionalized aged. J. Gerontol. 34: 716–722.
187. Zielinski, J. J. 1978. Situational determinants of assertive behavior in depressed alcoholics. J. Behav. Exp. Psychiatry 9: 103–107.

Chapter 14 The Hamilton Rating Scale for Depression

M. HAMILTON

Introduction

This observer-rating scale was designed in 1957 and a preliminary report published 3 years later [5]. Soon after, the introduction of many antidepressant drugs led to increasing interest in its use. A slightly modified form was published in a definitive paper [6]. The National Institute of Mental Health (United States) adopted a modified version (with three extra items) for use in its Early Clinical Drug Evaluation Programme, but subsequently reverted to the standard form. This promoted the use of the scale so that, in spite of its deficiencies and limitations, it has been described as the standard scale against which others are evaluated. It has been used all over the world and has been translated into nearly all the European languages; there is even a Korean translation [12].

The primary interest here is in the use of this scale, but an understanding of its characteristics and the basis of its construction will make its application much easier for the clinician. The scale was designed for a specific purpose: to measure the severity of illness in patients already diagnosed as suffering from a depressive illness. Although such a scale is primarily a research tool, it was designed so that it could be used in an ordinary clinical setting. Under no circumstances should sick people who have come for treatment be led to feel that their rights and privileges are being made subservient to their use as "clinical research material". Aside from technical considerations, this meant that the scale should be short enough to avoid interfering with the clinical interview and its contents should be such that the information required would be obtained during its course.

It was decided that the scale would be concerned with symptoms of the type described in the textbooks and which are, or should be, taught in the course of clinical training. The technical terms are therefore not only familiar but acceptable to the clinician. Even more important, they are what the patients complain about and for which they seek relief. This is an essential part of "face validity".

Items in a scale should be clearly defined, should be distinguishable from others, should be relevant to the purpose of the scale, i.e. to the condition which is being assessed, and should deal with the common symptoms. Items dealing with rare symptoms should be omitted. They improve the assessment of only a tiny minority of patients while lengthening the scale unnecessarily for the overwhelming majority. As most patients score zero on rare items, the distributions of scores are severely skewed (left sloping curve) and this makes the analysis difficult. For these reasons, the three symptoms: depersonalisation and derealisation, obsessional symptoms and paranoid symptoms were withdrawn from the set of items which are used to make a total score. Two other symptoms, hypersomnia and gain in weight, are so rare (they did not appear once in the first 100 patients assessed) that they were omitted entirely.

The number of grades of severity to be used was considered very carefully. Seven grades are about the maximum which can be differentiated, and for most symptoms this is too much. Five would be practical, but this is a number which has a serious disadvantage. It has a midpoint of three, which encourages the error of "central tendency". Inexperienced raters go for the middle point when they are in doubt and once there, they are reluctant to move away. It was therefore decided to have only four grades. Four grades of severity are a little lacking in discriminating capacity, but the ease with which they can be used is shown by their general acceptance.

For some symptoms it became quickly obvious that it was extremely difficult and even almost impossible to distinguish between different grades of severity. It was not so much that the distinction could not be made as that the patients had great difficulty in providing the necessary information. It was therefore decided to abandon grades of severity for them. This would give a zero-one scoring, but this has the disadvantage that it provides the maximum opportunity for bias: when in doubt, the rater tends to score a zero or one according to how he or she thinks it *should* be scored (halo effect). The scoring was therefore provided with an intermediate point, giving three grades.

Baumann has complained that whereas grades of 2 and upwards are related to the severity of a symptom, a score of 1 signifies a subjective state of the rater [1]. However, the use of a grade for "doubtful" is in accord with psychophysical measurement principles.

Description of the Scale

In addition to its specific use, the scale can be, and has been, used for other purposes but in all such cases it must be validated first. It contains 21 items, of which only 17 are used to give a total score of severity.

The items are concerned with symptoms of illness and not with traits of personality. Three items are excluded from the total score because they occur too infrequently, though they may be of great importance in special situations. Another symptom (diurnal variation of symptoms) is also excluded, on the grounds that it describes the characteristics of other symptoms and is not by itself an additional burden or source of suffering to the patient.

There are two types of items according to the method of grading. Those with three grades are scored on the basis of absent (0), doubtful or trivial (1), and present (2). For the items with five levels, the last level is split into three grades of mild (2), moderate (3), and severe (4). It is important for the rater to recognize that "severe" (four points) covers all grades of severity. There should be no hesitation in using this grade for a particular patient because it is thought that a more severe symptom could be found in other patients.

Characteristics of the Scale

A very detailed review has been made by Hedlund and Vieweg [10], so it will not be necessary to give more than a brief account of the work on the scale.

Validity

Validity of the scale has usually been assessed by comparing it with clinical "global" judgements. Bech et al. found that the interrater reliability of global judgements was 0.88 and therefore this sets an upper limit to validity measured in this way [2]. Zealley and Aitken similarly found a correlation of 0.90 for newly admitted patients, but this fell to 0.55 on discharge [17]. Bech et al. [2] found that the scale did not differentiate adequately between the more severe levels of illness, but as their global judgements were on an 11-point scale, and they confined their assessments to here-and-now, it is difficult to judge how relevant these findings are to ordinary usage. Snaith (personal communication) used a four-point scale of global judgement and found that the ratings gave much better differentiation at the more severe levels. Montgomery and Åsberg have claimed that their scale is more sensitive to improvement arising from treatment, but this has not yet been confirmed [13]. Kearns et al. found that its construct validity was as good as the Hamilton scale, but pointed out that it gave less information [11].

Concurrent validity is based on the correlation between the scale and others. Very few other observer-rating scales for depression are in current use, but they have in general shown a lower validity than this scale. Their correlations with it are fairly high. Self-assessment scales have a lower concurrent validity among themselves than with observer scales and even this is not high [7]. Zealley and Aitken found that the scale correlated 0.79 with the Visual Analogue Scale for patients on admission, but this fell to 0.06 on discharge [17].

Reliability

Interrater reliability for the total score ranges from 0.87 [3] to 0.95 [15]. Reliability for individual items ranges from 0.45 to 0.78 [16].

Two experienced raters working together will generally not differ by more than two points on the total score. For a mean score of about 20 points, this comes to a difference of 10%.

Factor Structure

As with all work on factor analysis, the results obtained by different investigators show considerable discrepancies. This is because the factors obtained are very sensitive to the mode of selection of patients and the types of patients included. Principal component analysis (and its simplified version of "simple summation") yields a general factor of severity and bipolar factors. If the range of severity of illness in the patients is small, then the general factor diminishes in size and the number of bipolar factors increases. Rotation to simple structure eliminates a general factor.

The number of other factors obtained has shown much variation. Hamilton obtained six factors, using Kaiser's criterion, though it was considered that the last two or three were too unstable to be considered seriously [6]. Hamilton and White found that the fourth factor had clinical meaning [9]. The second factor usually differentiates between the syndromes of "retarded" or "vital" depression and "anxious-agitated" or "neurotic" depression. Mowbray found that agitation did not appear at the anxious pole of this factor [14]. Baumann [1] came to the conclusion that the scale was unifactorial, though this must be regarded as an extreme view. Most investigators would accept two factors in the scale. I have not found that any of the factor scores have a distribution significantly different from normal (Gaussian).

Use of the Scale

During the past 25 years, many clinicians have written to me querying various matters concerning the method of use of the scale, both in regard to general and specific points. I have also had many opportunities to discuss the use of the scale with those involved in carrying out clinical trials. The following account takes into consideration the questions and problems raised.

Raters should have adequate clinical experience so that they can recognize the symptoms, even in the mildest forms. They should understand how scales are used and, if necessary, receive some training therein. It is absolutely fundamental to recognize that a rating scale is no more than a record of a clinical judgement. The fact that the judgement is recorded in numbers instead of adjectives does not increase its value. The numbers serve only to make the judgement more convenient for statistical analysis. If it is unsatisfactory, e. g. from ignorance or lack of information, then the scores are unsatisfactory, and no manipulation can improve them. Raters should use their clinical skill and experience in taking into account the complexity of the phenomena and the individuality of the patient.

The scale was designed so that the information required could be acquired during the course of a customary easygoing clinical interview. The patients should be allowed to have their say but should be guided back gently if they stray into irrelevancies. In general, depressive patients give a fairly accurate account of themselves. If the information provided is insufficient, they should be questioned. If necessary, direct questions may be asked (though such questions should be kept to a minimum) as depressives are not really suggestible. The patients' statements should be checked in the usual way, and the raters should use their judgement in evaluating the answers. For example, if a patient denies suicidal ideas, the statement does not have to be accepted at its face value; the manner in which this question is answered may give more information than the words.

When the patient is first seen, it is customary to interview a near relative or other appropriate persons as well. The information obtained should be used in filling in the scale. For patients in hospital, information should be obtained from the nurses. The scale is a record of the opinion of the physician and, as always, that opinion should be based on the best and most complete information available. The first assessment is best done against the background of the patient's history, and raters should evaluate the symptoms on the basis of the changes which have occurred since the patient fell ill. This is particularly important for such symptoms as sleep, appetite, constipation, hypochondriasis and libido.

In making the assessment the rater should not be confined to the current state (here-and-now). The judgement should be based on the condition of the patient during the past week or 10 days. In this way, short fluctuations are smoothed out. This is in accord with clinical tradition. This is particularly important for such symptoms as depressed and anxious mood, and also disturbance of sleep. Short-term assessment of libido and weight has no clinical meaning.

When a patient scores 2 for an item at first interview, and subsequently shows partial improvement, the item should then be scored 1 to indicate the change. It will not be scored zero until the symptom disappears.

Information which is used for the rating of one item should not be used in the rating of another one. The score on one item should not influence the scores on adjacent ones. Logical errors must be avoided: because a patient has lost weight, it cannot be assumed that his or her appetite has decreased; because the patient is suicidal, it cannot be assumed that he or she is very depressed. The ratings on two items should be based only on information pertaining to each. Raters should avoid "central" and "extreme" biases, i.e. the tendency to prefer either middle or extreme scores.

I have always recommended that when patients are rated on a scale, two interviewers should be present. The first interviews the patient and the second adds such questions as are thought fit to provide the information required. The raters complete their forms independently and afterwards compare their scores and discuss the differences. A difference of one point usually signifies only that the symptom lies close to the junction between two grades, but a difference of two points or more signifies that there is a real difference in interpretation between the two interviewers. Double interviews have two advantages. In the first place, if a rater is not available, a colleague who rates in the same way can act as substitute. In the second, the mean of the two sets of scores improves reliability and makes for finer differentiation. When the scale was first introduced, I recommended that the sum of the two scores should be used, rather than the mean, but this was merely to avoid fractional scores, a great convenience in the days when data were generally put onto punched cards.

Some of the clinical aspects of depressive symptoms, with regard to their rating, are dealt with by Hamilton [8], and are supplementary to the account given below.

In a clinical trial, raters may use the scale in any way they wish, provided they do so for all the patients. However, unless they conform to customary usage, they cannot compare their findings with those of anybody else.

Specific Symptoms

Depressed Mood

At the first assessment, it is necessary to direct the attention of the patient to the changes which have occurred since the onset of the illness. The assessment of depressed mood is based not only on the patients' statement about their mood but also on their feelings of helplessness and hopelessness. A tendency to weep is typical and occurs in women and men, though the latter may be reluctant to admit to it. In the milder grades, the weeping relieves the patient, but not with more severe depressed mood. When the symptom becomes severe, the patient may go "beyond weeping".

Guilt

Despite popular belief, this symptom is very common, though it may not be clearly expressed. It ranges from vague feelings that the patient is, somehow or other, responsible for his or her state. It is very characteristic that patients feel that they have let themselves, or their families, down in some way. The rater should not be deceived by the patient's justifications. For example, a patient may reproach himself for having been unkind or even cruel to his wife. He may indeed have been, but he cannot explain why he should be feeling guilty about it only since the onset of his illness. Delusions of guilt should not be confused with persecutory delusions. For example, a patient may declare that he is being pursued by the police who want to arrest him and punish him but adds that this is because of the wicked crimes he has committed.

Suicide

This ranges from vague feelings that life is not worth living to a serious attempt at suicide. Patients who have attempted to kill themselves may express great regret at having done so, but may still contemplate doing it again. Although patients may say that an attempt at suicide was made as a sudden spontaneous action without previous warning, this is very rarely true. Parasuicide in depressives is much more a gamble with death than a "cry for help" and must be evaluated just as in ordinary clinical circumstances.

At a first interview, a serious attempt at suicide during the past week or so should be rated as 4, even if the symptom has become less severe. At subsequent assessments this symptom is rated at its actual level of the past week.

Insomnia

Older people sleep less well than younger people and this symptom must be evaluated against what is normal for the patient. When questioned about sleep, patients are apt to consider only the previous night, and it may be necessary to ask details for every night for the past week or so. Account must be taken not only of the severity of the disturbance but also of its frequency. Disturbed sleep during the night (middle insomnia) can occur as the only form of sleep disturbance. Nurses' reports on a patient's sleep may be inaccurate if the patient is seen lying quietly in bed with eyes closed, yet wide awake. Hypersomnia is uncommon and usually signifies only that a patient who has slept badly during the night then dozes off during the day.

Work and Interests

It is difficult to distinguish between loss of interest and diminution of working capacity, which is why these two symptoms are combined. Loss of interest is most easily detected in men by asking about their hobbies. Loss of working capacity may not be obvious; a man's colleagues may help him because they realise that he is ill. A patient may say that his work has deteriorated, but this may be only an expression of his self-accusation.

If a patient is admitted to hospital because of the severity of illness, this item should be rated 4 points. If the symptom improves it should be given a lower score, even if the patient is still in hospital, e.g. to complete a course of treatment or because of extraneous reasons for delay in discharge. Difficulties arise when a patient makes a good recovery, but is unable to return to work because of its nature. Workers at the coalface in a mine or at a blast furnace cannot return to work until they are quite fit, whereas an office worker can return to work before recovery is complete. An attempt should be made to take these individual points into consideration in the rating.

Retardation

In the mildest forms, this symptom is difficult to recognize. One has to look for slight immobility of facies, monotony of voice, lack of gestures or slight hesitation before answering even simple questions.

Agitation

The more extreme forms described in the textbooks are now rarely seen except where adequate facilities for treatment are not available. In its mildest forms, patients sit restlessly in their chairs, fidget with a handkerchief, clothes or a cigarette. A more obviously agitated patient may suddenly stand up and sit down again.

Anxiety

The symptoms of anxiety, both psychic and somatic, are well known and need not be described. They have been fairly well documented in the description of a rating scale for anxiety states [4].

Somatic Symptoms

The somatic symptoms of the depressions should be distinguished from those related to anxiety. Loss or diminution of appetite is very common, and should be rated even if patients force themselves to eat a normal amount. Overeating is a symptom of anxiety, not of depression. Constipation as a depressive symptom is not common. Increased fatigability and constant weariness is common and may sometimes be a dominant symptom.

Loss of libido is typical and very common, though patients may be very reluctant to admit to it. Women who declare that normally they are frigid may find, when this symptom appears, that sexual intercourse, which had previously been accepted as one of the chores of married life, has now become repugnant and intolerable. When no information is available, as with older patients living alone, the symptom should be rated zero. When disturbances of menstruation appear with the illness they should be rated with this symptom.

Hypochondriacal thoughts, etc., occur only in the more severe depressions. The symptom should not be confused with the trait of personality.

Loss of Insight

This symptom has been a source of confusion to many raters. Insight does not mean an understanding of the illness in psychodynamic terms. In the mild form, the patient will admit that he or she is ill, but insists that there is something more to it, without being able to explain further. When patients make a complete recovery and then declare that they are not ill, they have not lost insight; on the contrary. They should be asked if they understand that they have *been* ill.

Loss of Weight

This would best be rated on actual measurements, but few patients know their normal weight. Patients should be asked if they have noticed that their face has become thinner or their clothes looser, or if anybody has remarked on this. A difficulty arises when the patient admits to having lost weight but claims that this is a result of a reducing diet. It will help to inquire about the effect of previous bouts of dieting. Loss of weight can occur independent of loss of appetite and vice versa. Some patients gain weight from overeating; this symptom should then be scored zero and a note made in the patient's records.

Other Symptoms

When patients are asked about depersonalisation and derealisation, they may have difficulty in answering and then agree that they have the symptom. In such cases, they should be asked to describe what they mean. Usually they will describe preoccupation with their illness which prevents them paying attention to other matters, feelings of guilt which cut them off from people, inability to concentrate, etc. The patient who has this symptom recognizes immediately what the question is about and is usually relieved to discover that it is not a sign of impending insanity.

Obsessional thoughts should not be confused with preoccupations. True obsessional thoughts are accompanied by anxiety and by attempts to resist them. A difficulty arises with thoughts of suicide, which may be rejected on moral or other grounds. Adequate clinical experience helps to make the distinction easy.

Paranoid thoughts should not be confused with guilt feelings. Paranoid mood should be included here, though I have never met it without paranoid thoughts (in depressives).

If diurnal variation is recorded at the first interview, it should not be altered at subsequent ones. This makes clinical sense. It is one of the reasons why this item is not included in a total score of severity.

References

1. Baumann, U. 1967. Methodische Untersuchungen zur Hamilton-Depression-Skala. Arch. Psychiatr. Nervenkr. 222: 359–375.
2. Bech, P., Gram, L. F., Dein, E., Jacobsen, O., Vitger, J., and Bolwig, T. G. 1975. Quantitative rating of depressive states. Correlation between clinical assessment, Beck's self-rating scale and Hamilton's objective rating scale. Acta Psychiatr. Scand. 51: 161–170.
3. Burrows, G. D., Foenander, G., Davies, B., and Scoggins, B. A. 1976. Rating scales as predictors of response to tricyclic antidepressants. Aust. N. Z. J. Psychiatr. 10: 53–56.
4. Hamilton, M. 1959. The assessment of anxiety states by rating. Br. J. Med. Psychol. 32: 50–55.
5. Hamilton, M. 1960. A rating scale for depression. J. Neurol. Neurosurg. Psychiatry 23: 56–62.
6. Hamilton, M. 1967. Development of a rating scale for primary depressive illness. Br. J. Soc. Clin. Psychol. 6: 278–296.

7. Hamilton, M. 1976. Comparative value of rating scales. Br. J. Clin. Pharmacol. 3 (suppl.): 58-60.
8. Hamilton, M. 1980. Rating depressive patients. J. Clin. Psychiatry 41: 21-24.
9. Hamilton, M., and White, J. M. 1959. Clinical syndromes in depressive states. Journal of Mental Science 105: 985-998.
10. Hedlund, J. L., and Vieweg, B. W. 1979. The Hamilton rating scale for depression: A comprehensive review. Journal of Operational Psychiatry 10: 149-162.
11. Kearns, N. P., Cruickshank, C. A., McGuigan, S. A., Riley, S. A., Shaw, S. P., and Snaith, R. P. 1982. A comparison of depression rating scales. Br. J. Psychiatry 141: 45-49.
12. Kim, K. I. 1977. Clinical study of primary depressive symptoms. Part 1: Adjustment of Hamilton's rating scale for depression. Neuropsychiatry (J. Korean Neuropsychiatr. Assoc.) 16: 36-60.
13. Montgomery, S., and Åsberg, M. 1979. A new depression scale designed to be sensitive to change. Br. J. Psychiatry 134: 382-389.
14. Mowbray, R. M. 1972. The Hamilton rating scale for depression: A factor analysis. Psychol. Med. 2: 272-280.
15. Robins, A. H. 1976. Depression in patients with Parkinsonism. Br. J. Psychiatry 128: 141-145.
16. Schwab, J. J., Bialow, M. R., and Holzer, C. E. 1967. A comparison of two rating scales for depression. J. Clin. Psychol. 23: 94-96.
17. Zealley, A. K., and Aitken, R. C. P. 1969. Measurement of mood. Proceedings of the Royal Society of Medicine 62: 993-996.

Chapter 15   The Development of Four Self-Assessment Depression Scales

R. P. SNAITH

Introduction

One of the major impediments to progress in psychiatry is the confusion which surrounds the instruments with which the severity of disorders is assessed [9]. The choice of a rating scale is usually an arbitrary decision; it is determined by local preference and custom, and frequently no thought is given to the characteristics of the scale or whether it is the most suitable one for the particular study [3]. For instance, in the particular field of depression, if a scale purports to be a measure of that disorder and, particularly if it is well known and widely used, then it is frequently assumed that it will be a suitable instrument for the study.

Rating scales may be designed for use as screening instruments, as instruments which delineate the characteristics of a particular patient or sample or as instruments to quantify the severity of a particular disorder. Scales to be completed by the patients themselves may fulfil all of these functions and are finding an increasing use in clinical practice and research; nonetheless they suffer from certain inevitable defects since they can only be expected to be reliable when used by cooperative patients, patients who are literate, who are not too ill to complete the scale, who are able to comprehend the purpose of the scale and who are unlikely to wish to present a faulty or misleading assessment of their state.

The development of a number of self-assessment scales undertaken by myself, Hamilton and other colleagues will now be described in the light of the foregoing principles.

The Wakefield Inventory [11]

At the time this scale was developed, the scale designed by Zung [16] was the most widely used self-assessment scale for depression available in the English language. The reasons for the need to design a new scale arose chiefly from what we considered to be a defect of Zung's scale. The Zung scale is composed of 20 items referring to symptoms which occur in depressive disorders, on each of which the patient has to assess him- or herself according to the following four responses: "a little of the time", "some of the time", "a good part of the time" or "most of the time". It therefore appeared that the orientation of the scale is toward *persistence* of the disorder rather than *severity* of the disorder; moreover, on some occasions the response categories appear to be irrelevant, for instance, in reply to the item: "I notice that I am losing weight".

The Wakefield Inventory is therefore based upon Zung's scale and was developed in an attempt to improve upon it. The reason for the reduction of the number of items from 20 to 12 is given in the original paper and was not based on arbitrary selection but upon an independent study which examined which of the Zung scale items were most responsive to change in severity. The response categories to each item were also changed to "yes, definitely", "Yes, sometimes", "No, not much" and "No, not at all"; this was judged to allow for the expression of both persistence of the symptom and its severity.

The validation of the Wakefield Inventory as a screening instrument was evaluated by comparing the scores of 100 depressed patients with 200 healthy people and there was found to be a satisfactory degree of separation between the two samples. The concurrent validity of the Wakefield Inventory was examined by comparing scores of a sample of depressed patients who were also independently rated on the Hamilton Depression Rating Scale [5]; a correlation of high statistical significance ($r+0.87$, $P<0.001$) was obtained, and it was therefore considered that the Wakefield Inventory was also an instrument for the assessment of severity of depressive illness.

All the preliminary work on the Wakefield Inventory was carried out on depressed patients referred to the psychiatric services, and there is still no information available concerning the validity of the instrument for studies in the community.

The Leeds Scales for Depression and Anxiety [12]

This development of the Wakefield Inventory was undertaken because of the increasing need to distinguish between the concepts of depression and anxiety, both in research and in clinical practice. Inspection of the items composing the Wakefield Inventory showed that several of them were as likely to be scored highly by anxious as by depressed patients and it was therefore likely that the scores on the Wakefield Inventory would not differentiate between the two disorders.

As a preliminary to the development of the Leeds Scales, a further aspect of item selection, neglected in earlier work on rating scales, was considered to be necessary: this was the examination of the influence on an individual item of age and sex; it was reasoned that if an item (symptom) is strongly related to age or sex then it should not be included in a scale which is proposed for general use. Accordingly, ten further items were added to the twelve items of the Wakefield Inventory and correlations of each item with age and sex were carried out in a population of patients between the ages of 16 and 85 years. The result was that three items were rejected because they correlated significantly with female sex; these referred to the symptoms of headache, weeping and fatigue. These items were excluded from the further analysis. No item had a significant correlation with age.

The next stage in the construction of the Leeds Scales was carried out with patients who had been diagnosed as suffering either from a primary depressive illness or an anxiety state. These patients completed the remaining items and were independently rated by research interviewers who used two scales which were derived from Hamilton's Depression and Anxiety Scales [4, 5] and which were judged to represent independent concepts of depression and anxiety. Full details of this procedure appear in the original paper. The result was that six items were selected as relating to depressive illness in contrast to anxiety state and these were concerned with the symptoms of depressed mood, lack of energy, loss of pleasure response, loss of interest in activities, delayed insomnia and suicidal thinking. The items which were found to be related to anxiety state rather than depressive illness were concerned with the symptoms of panic, fear of leaving the house unaccompanied, palpitations, dizziness, fearful mood and feeling tense. These two six-item scales were therefore considered to assess the severity of depressive illness and anxiety states in patients who had been diagnosed as suffering from one of those disorders and were designated as the Leeds Specific Depression Scale and the Leeds Specific Anxiety Scale respectively.

The next stage was to determine whether the same sets of items would serve to distinguish depression from anxiety in psychiatric patients who had not been specifically diagnosed as suffering from depressive illness or anxiety state but in whom depression and anxiety were prominent features of their illness; patients suffering from organic syndromes and psychoses were excluded and the research proceeded on patients suffering from a variety of neurotic disorders. The result was that the Leeds General Depression Scale was constructed from the same six items as the Specific Depression Scale, with the exception of the item referring to lack of energy, which was replaced by one referring to loss of appetite. Similarly, for the Leeds General Anxiety Scale, two items in the Specific Scale ("dizziness" and "feeling tense") were replaced by items concerned with the symptoms of irritability and of restlessness.

The last stage in the development of the Leeds Scales was to show that the Specific Scales could be used to some extent as a diagnostic device and the details of this procedure may be found in the original paper. (The Leeds scales are available from Psychological Test Publications, 107 Pilton Street, Barnstaple, Devon, England.)

The Irritability-Depression-Anxiety Scale [13]

This scale, referred to as the IDA Scale, was developed because of the need to incorporate a means of assessing a third important parameter of mood disorder, i.e. irritability. At the time the new scale was being planned there existed a few scales to assess aspects of aggression and hostility but these did not seem to assess precisely the aspect of mood disorder in which we were interested, i.e. a temporary psychological state characterised by impatience, intolerance and poorly controlled anger. The reason for the need to include a measure of irritability together with measures of depression and of anxiety arose from research planned in the field of postnatal depression and the frequent observation that irritability in the sense as defined above is an important component of mood disorder in these patients [8]. It was considered that the assessment of irritability might also be more useful if it took into account the direction of the expression of irritability, i.e., outward towards others or inward towards oneself.

Details of the construction of the four subscales (depression, anxiety, outward irritability and inward irritability) may be found in the original paper. There was found to be a satisfactory degree of concurrent validity for each of the subscales with the appropriate interviewer assessment for the aspects of mood disorder and it was therefore concluded that the subscales of the IDA Scale could each be used as a measure of the severity of the appropriate mood disorder. Cutoff points and score ranges distinguishing morbid and healthy degrees for each of the subscales are given in the original paper. Further work on the validity of the IDA Scale in screening for mood disorder in a sample of postnatal women was later presented [10]; for depression there were 10% false positives and no false negatives, for anxiety 12% false positives and no false negatives and for outward irritability no false positives and 17% false negatives.

Translations of the IDA Scale are available, on request to the author, in the following languages: Arabic, Bulgarian, Czech, Dutch, French, German, Hebrew, Italian, Portuguese, Spanish and Russian and translations into several languages of the Indian subcontinent are planned.

The Hospital Anxiety and Depression (HAD) Scale [15]

All the foregoing scales were developed in the setting of psychiatric services. The need became clear for a self-assessment mood scale for use in a general medical setting. It was considered that the provision of a reliable mood scale would assist the detection and management of depression and anxiety in nonpsychiatric medical services. Accordingly, research was carried out in general medical outpatient clinics at St.James's University Hospital, Leeds, and a scale to be known as the HAD Scale was developed; it consists of two subscales, each with eight items, one relating to depression and the other to anxiety. Care was taken to exclude from the scale all items which might relate either to the somatization of mood or to physical illness, such as headaches, dizziness and loss of appetite.

Full details of the development of the HAD Scale appear in the original paper. Both subscales were found to be valid as screening instruments for the appropriate mood: in 100 patients the depression subscale revealed 1% false positives and 1% false negatives and the anxiety subscale revealed 5% false positives and 1% false negatives. Both subscales had highly significant correlations with the independent measure of the appropriate mood (depression/scale depression $r = +0.70$, anxiety/scale anxiety $r = +0.74$, $P < 0.001$ for both) and it was therefore established that the subscales could be used to assess the severity of the appropriate mood disorder. Finally, evidence was provided that each subscale was relatively specific to the appropriate disorder of mood and further data were provided to show that the subscale scores of the HAD Scale were relatively little affected by physical illness.

As with the IDA Scale the original paper publishes the full scale together with details for scoring and range values for normality and morbidity of the moods. Translations of the HAD Scale are available, on request to the author, in the following languages: Arabic, Chinese, Czech, Danish, Dutch, French, German, Hebrew, Hungarian, Italian, Japanese, Polish, Russian, Spanish, and Swedish. (Translations into Bengali, Hindi, and Urdu are in preparation.)

Comparison Study [6]

The study was carried out in order to compare the performance of the first three scales described above, together with a number of other scales, in a sample of inpatients who had been diagnosed as suffering from primary depressive illness. The scales involved in the study were therefore the Wakefield Inventory, the Leeds Specific Depression Scale, the depression subscale of the IDA Scale, and three interviewer scales: the Hamilton Depression Scale [5], the Montgomery-Åsberg Depression Scale [7], and Bech's Melancholia Scale [1]; the well-known interviewer-assisted patient-rated scale, the Depression Inventory [2], was also included. Details of this study may be found in the original paper but to summarise the findings it was concluded that, among the self-assessment scales, the Leeds Specific Depression Scale and the IDA depression subscale should be retained for use but that the Wakefield Inventory should now be abandoned.

The findings suggest that a larger number of items does not necessarily increase efficiency since the Wakefield Inventory contained twelve items in contrast to six items for the Leeds Specific Depression Scale and five items for the depression subscale of the IDA Scale. A similar observation regarding numbers of items in interviewer scales was made in the work on the revision of the Hamilton Anxiety Scale [14].

It would appear that careful analysis of the items to be included in a scale is of far greater importance than their number. What the optimum number may be is not known; we did consider that five items may turn out to be too low for reliable use of a scale but the findings of this study suggest that this is not the case.

References

1. Bech, P., Gram, L. F., Dein, E., Jacobsen, O., Vitger, J., and Bolwig, T. G. 1975. Quantitative rating of depressive states. Acta Psychiatr. Scand. 51: 161-170.
2. Beck, A. T., Ward, C. H., Mendelson, M., Mock, J., and Erbaugh, J. 1961. An inventory for measuring depression. Arch. Gen. Psychiatry 4: 561-571.
3. Carrol, B. J., Fielding, J. M., and Blashki, T. G. 1973. Depression rating scales. Arch. Gen. Psychiatry 28: 361-366.
4. Hamilton, M. 1959. The assessment of anxiety states by rating. Br. J. Med. Psychol. 32: 50-55.
5. Hamilton, M. 1967. Development of a scale for primary depressive illness. Br. J. Soc. Clin. Psychol. 6: 278-296.

6. Kearns, N.P., Cruickshank, C.A., McGuigan, K.J., Riley, S.A., Shaw, S.P., and Snaith, R.P. 1982. A comparison of depression rating scales. Br. J. Psychiatry 141: 45–49.
7. Montgomery, S.A., and Åsberg, M. 1979. A new depression scale designed to be sensitive for change. Br. J. Psychiatry 134: 382–389.
8. Pitt, B. 1968. 'Atypical' depression following childbirth. Br. J. Psychiatry 114: 1325–1335.
9. Snaith, R.P. 1981. Rating scales. Br. J. Psychiatry 138: 512–514.
10. Snaith, R.P. 1982. Postnatal depression: its detection and management. Psychiatry in Practice 1: 10–18.
11. Snaith, R.P., Ahmed, S.N., Mehta, S., and Hamilton, M. 1971. Assessment of the severity of depressive illness: the Wakefield self-assessment depression inventory. Psychol. Med. 1: 143–149.
12. Snaith, R.P., Bridge, G.W.K., and Hamilton, M. 1976. The Leeds Scales for the self-assessment of anxiety and depression. Br. J. Psychiatry 128: 156–165.
13. Snaith, R.P., Constantopoulos, A.A., Jardine, M.Y., and McGuffin, P. 1978. A clinical scale for the self-assessment of irritability, depression and anxiety. Br. J. Psychiatry 132: 164–171.
14. Snaith, R.P., Baugh, S., Clayden, A.D., Hussain, A., and Sipple, M. 1982. The Clinical Anxiety Scale: a modification of the Hamilton Anxiety Scale. Br. J. Psychiatry 141: 518–523.
15. Zigmond, A.S., and Snaith, R.P. 1982. The Hospital Anxiety and Depression Scale. Acta Psychiatr. Scand. 1983: 67: 361–370.
16. Zung, W.W.K. 1965. A self-rating depression scale. Arch. Gen. Psychiatry 12: 63–70.

Chapter 16 Assessment of Depression Using the Brief Psychiatric Rating Scale

J. E. OVERALL and L. E. HOLLISTER

Introduction

The Brief Psychiatric Rating Scale (BPRS), initially developed for efficient evaluation of treatment response in clinical psychopharmacology research, has been widely used for the assessment of severity of depression and for the descriptive classification of depressive disorders. The initial version of the BPRS, which was published in 1962, consisted of 16 symptom-rating constructs representing distinct aspects of manifest psychopathology that had been identified in a series of factor analyses of larger item pools [21]. Interest in use of the BPRS for descriptive classification of psychiatric patients, as well as for rapid and efficient assessment of treatment response in selected target populations, prompted the addition in 1966 of two rating constructs to better delineate excited states and organic brain syndromes. That resulted in the current form of the instrument, which has been reproduced in numerous previous publications [8, 9, 18, 19, 20].

The BPRS, as widely used today, thus consists of 18 symptom constructs, each of which is rated on a seven-point scale of severity ranging from "not present" to "extremely severe." The brevity of the instrument permits inclusion of a brief definition of each symptom construct in a single-page format, as illustrated in Fig. 16.1.

The copyright, which was originally held by authors Overall and Gorham, is no longer invoked. Anyone desiring to use the BPRS is encouraged to reproduce it in any format desired. Language translations can be identified in the psychiatric literature of Belgium, Czechoslovakia, Chile, France, Germany, Italy, Japan, Mexico, Netherlands, Russia, Spain, and other countries. Out of the desire to retain the identity of the BPRS as a standard instrument for which a wealth of background data has accumulated, it is requested that the 18-symptom constructs be retained as a separate and integral set with the designation of Brief Psychiatric Rating Scale (BPRS) when referenced.

The Clinical Interview and Observational Mode

The BPRS is designed for recording the kinds of judgments about psychopathology that should be a natural consequence of any good clinical interview, such as an initial history and mental status examination. It has been widely used to describe manifest psychopathology observed in routine clinical practice, and the ratings in such

Fig. 16.1. Brief Psychiatric Rating Scale of Overall and Gorham

Directions: Place an X in the appropriate box to represent level of severity of each symptom.

Patient _____
Rater _____
No. _____
Date _____

Symptom	Not Present	Very Mild	Mild	Moderate	Mod. Severe	Severe	Extremely Severe
1. Somatic Concern - preoccupation with physical health, fear of physical illness, hypochondriasis.	☐	☐	☐	☐	☐	☐	☐
2. Anxiety - worry, fear, overconcern for present or future.	☐	☐	☐	☐	☐	☐	☐
3. Emotional Withdrawal - lack of spontaneous interaction, isolation, deficiency in relating to others.	☐	☐	☐	☐	☐	☐	☐
4. Conceptual Disorganization - thought processes confused, disconnected, disorganized, disrupted.	☐	☐	☐	☐	☐	☐	☐
5. Guilt Feelings - self-blame, shame, remorse for past behavior.	☐	☐	☐	☐	☐	☐	☐
6. Tension - physical and motor manifestations or nervousness, overactivation, tension.	☐	☐	☐	☐	☐	☐	☐
7. Mannerisms and Posturing - peculiar, bizarre, unnatural motor behavior (not including tics).	☐	☐	☐	☐	☐	☐	☐
8. Grandiosity - exaggerated self-opinion, arrogance, conviction of unusual power or abilities.	☐	☐	☐	☐	☐	☐	☐
9. Depressive Mood - sorrow, sadness, despondency, pessimism.	☐	☐	☐	☐	☐	☐	☐
10. Hostility - animosity, contempt, belligerence, disdain for others.	☐	☐	☐	☐	☐	☐	☐
11. Suspiciousness - mistrust, belief others harbor malicious or discriminatory intent.	☐	☐	☐	☐	☐	☐	☐
12. Hallucinatory Behavior - preceptions without normal external stimulus correspondence.	☐	☐	☐	☐	☐	☐	☐
13. Motor Retardation - slowed, weakened movements or speech, reduced body tone.	☐	☐	☐	☐	☐	☐	☐
14. Uncooperativeness - resistance, guardedness, rejection of authority.	☐	☐	☐	☐	☐	☐	☐
15. Unusual Thought Content - unusual, odd, strange, bizarre thought content.	☐	☐	☐	☐	☐	☐	☐
16. Blunted Affect - reduced emotional tone, reduction in normal intensity of feelings, flatness.	☐	☐	☐	☐	☐	☐	☐
17. Excitement - heightened emotional tone, agitation, increased reactivity.	☐	☐	☐	☐	☐	☐	☐
18. Disorientation - confusion or lack of proper association for person, place or time.	☐	☐	☐	☐	☐	☐	☐

Drugs continued: _____ New drugs: _____

circumstances have been found to be reliable enough to reveal important relationships to personal, environmental, and treatment variables [14, 15, 18, 24, 45]. Psychiatrists or clinical psychologists have most often served as interviewers and raters, although the BPRS has been used successfully by nurses and specially trained research assistants [37, 41].

Whereas the BPRS can be used to record observations of psychopathology made in the course of routine clinical practice, a brief, efficient, semistructured interview is recommended for more formal research. The original 1962 article by Overall and Gorham describes an 18- to 20-min interview that has been found adequate for gathering information required to complete the ratings [21]. The recommended apportionment of time is as follows: 3-5 min of introduction and explanation of the purpose of the interview (which explanation of purpose should satisfy current ethical standards for informed consent), 10 min of nondirective discussion of the patient's perceptions of his or her problems, and a final 5 min of follow-up questioning on specific issues not adequately covered in the more spontaneous portion of the interview.

In considering the nondirective portion of the interview, it is relevant to note that more than half of the BPRS rating constructs pertain to behavior or manner of verbalization and do not depend on the specific content that is discussed. Ratings of emotional withdrawal, tension, mannerisms and posturing, motor retardation, uncooperativeness, blunted affect, and excitement depend almost entirely on observation of the behavior of the patient during the interview. In addition, conceptual disorganization is a construct that pertains to the logic and syntax of verbal communication, not to the specific topics discussed. Thus, it can also be rated on the basis of verbalizations spontaneously produced during the nondirective portion of the interview. The nondirective portion of the interview provides the best opportunity for the interviewer to attend to such phenomena in relative freedom from attention to the strategy of interviewing. Nevertheless, the stress produced by direct questioning on sensitive issues may evoke pathological phenomena not otherwise apparent, making careful observation of the patient important throughout the interview.

Several of the BPRS symptom constructs, which do depend on the verbalized content, can be judged best from the topics emphasized by the patient during the nondirective portion of the interview. These include anxiety, guilt feelings, grandiosity, depressive mood, hostility, suspiciousness, and somatic concern. In general, the severity of symptoms such as these can be judged better from spontaneous verbal productions than from responses to specific queries. All of this is simply to emphasize that most of the information required to complete BPRS ratings is best obtained in a flexible clinical interview situation in which an experienced clinician pursues a general line of inquiry with questions such as:

> How have you been feeling about yourself lately?
> What is it that bothers you most?
> What about health problems during the past year? Any current concern?
> How have you been getting along with other people? Any particular problems?
> How have things been going at work (home or school)?
> Anything about the past that continues to bother you?
> What are your plans now? What about the future?

After each general question, the patient should be allowed to respond in his or her own time and extent. Prompts such as "Can you tell me more about that?" should be used when needed for clarification. Leads to subject matter pertinent to BPRS symptom constructs should be pursued at the time or reopened in subsequent direct questioning. The interview should then conclude with inquiry into areas not touched on spontaneously during the nondirective portion. Tact should be used in approaching sensitive material about which a patient may well be defensive. It is frequently useful to begin with general questions about the more distant past and then to proceed in steps to clarify recent presence and severity. Questions such as the following can serve as leads into current symptomatology in specific areas:

Have you ever had any unusual experiences such as seeing or hearing things that others do not?
Many people who are nervous or depressed have such experiences at times.
When was the last time that it happened to you?
Tell me more about what you thought while that was going on.

The interview should be concluded with (honest) assurances that the information the patient has provided will be kept confidential, and that should be followed by appropriate encouragement about the outlook for treatment.

In formal clinical investigations, such as double-blind drug trials, the use of two raters for each interview has been frequent practice with the aim of increasing reliability. One of the raters conducts most of the interview, allowing the other to ask about issues about which he or she is uncertain. The usual pairing of raters has involved psychiatrists and/or clinical psychologists, but any trained mental health professionals should provide satisfactory ratings. In some cases, the cost of having two independent raters participate in each interview is excessive. Comparative analyses have indicated that the same level of precision in treatment evaluations can be achieved by a single rater with a moderate increase in sample size [35]. Even where only one rater interviews each patient, it is good research design to have several different interviewers interviewing different patients in a study sample. Where the design requires repeated assessments, the same rater or raters should interview each patient on the different occasions.

As discussed in the introduction to this chapter, the rating constructs in the BPRS were chosen to represent relatively independent aspects of manifest psychopathology which, for the most part, had been identified in previous factor analyses of larger item pools. For this reason, it is meaningful to consider each symptom separately in order to provide detailed characterization of differences among patients within, as well as between, major diagnostic categories. Certain symptoms are obviously more relevant for assessment of depression than are others; however, the presence of specific associated symptoms or the absence of atypical symptoms can be important for fully characterizing depressive syndromes in clinical research.

Ratings are recorded by checking one of the seven categories of severity for each of the 18 BPRS symptom constructs. As shown in Fig. 16.1, the categories of severity are labeled: not present, very mild, mild, moderate, moderately severe, severe, and extremely severe. For numerical analysis, the seven ordered categories are coded 0, 1, 2, ..., 6. This 0-6 numerical scoring is considered preferable to the 1-7 scoring that has been recommended elsewhere [8]. The "not present" rating represents a meaningful origin or zeropoint, and that facilitates analyses of profile patterns which will be discussed in later sections of this chapter. If two raters independently rate symptom severity, their ratings, scored on the 0-6 scales, can be summed or averaged to provide measurements with increased reliability. In addition, the summing or averaging of two ratings produces finer gradation (13 steps rather than 7) along the severity continuum, and that also has advantages for statistical analyses that assume continuous, normally distributed, quantitative measurements.

The ratings of severity of symptoms should be recorded on the BPRS immediately upon completion of the interview. Where two raters participate in the interview, each should record his or her judgments of symptom severity independently of the other. When independent ratings derive from a joint interview, the reliability of the combined scores on individual BPRS items should range upward from 0.75, and the interrater reliability of factor scores should exceed 0.85. In most cases, the practice has been to sum (or average) the ratings by two independent raters; however, an alternative procedure requires raters to discuss their observations and to agree on a consensus rating. For symptom constructs on which the difference between raters is no more than two scale units, the average can be accepted. When a difference is greater than two scale units, discussion of the reasoning that went into the different judgments will usually result in a consensus. One rater may have observed something that the other missed. Whether the averaging or consensus method is used, a single score on each of the 18 BPRS symptom constructs is provided for subsequent analyses.

Symptom Clusters and Factor Scoring

Numerous factor analyses of intercorrelations among BPRS symptom ratings have revealed a generally consistent pattern of four or five clusters of related symptoms which form the major dimensions of difference in profile patterns. Several of the earlier factor analyses were accomplished on the 16 variables of the original 1962 version of the BPRS. In the absence of ratings of "excitement" and "disorientation," the factor structure is quite stable across different patient populations [22, 36, 38]. Factor analyses of the current 18-item version have generally produced five factors, with some variation in results depending on the diagnostic composition of the patient samples [8, 9]. The following five symptom clusters appear most consistently to relate to separate factors:

Thinking disturbance
    Conceptual disorganization
    Hallucinatory behavior
    Unusual thought content

Withdrawal retardation
    Emotional withdrawal
    Motor retardation
    Blunted affect

Anxious depression
    Anxiety
    Guilt feelings
    Depressive mood

Hostile suspiciousness
    Hostility
    Suspiciousness
    Uncooperativeness

Agitation excitement
   Tension
   Excitement

Factor scores can be calculated by summing the severity ratings for the BPRS symptoms in each cluster. This grouping of items differs somewhat from the factor scoring proposed by Guy, Cleary, and Bonato [8], but is not inconsistent with the pattern of factor loading resulting from their analysis. There is some advantage, we feel, to defining each factor in terms of a same number of variables. If one accepts only the three highest loading variables on each of the five factors resulting from the Guy, Cleary, and Bonato analysis and requires a minimum loading of 0.60 in order for a variable to be considered adequately related to a factor, the factor scoring would correspond precisely to that indicated above. This factor scoring of the BPRS symptom ratings is also consistent with results that have been reported from numerous other analyses [9].

Before leaving the topic of factor scoring, it should be mentioned that factor analyses of BPRS symptom ratings for elderly psychiatric patients suggest a different pattern of symptom correlations. Conceptual disorganization is related to cognitive dysfunction; depressive mood is more often associated with emotional withdrawal and motor retardation; and anxiety moves towards tension and excitement. Recommendations for factor scoring of the BPRS in psychogeriatric research are contained in a separate publication [33].

For assessment of treatment response of depressed patients, change in the total score summed across all 18 symptom ratings is recommended as the most sensitive single variable. This is because depression tends to present with several different combinations of associated symptoms, a fact that will be elaborated in the discussion of phenomenological subtypes of depressive disorder. The total score captures improvement in whatever particular symptoms characterize the depressed patient at the outset of treatment. Percentage change has been found to control better for individual differences in initial severity than does analysis of simple difference scores [16]. A 50% reduction in total score is characteristic of active antidepressant drugs in short-term treatment of 4–6 weeks duration [16]. A regression correction for initial levels of severity, as in the analysis of covariance, is also commonly used to correct differences in initial severity.

Phenomenological Classification of Depressions

Depressive mood is the one BPRS symptom that is ordinarily required as a manifestation of depressive disorder; however, depressive mood alone is not sufficient to define the syndrome. Anxiety almost always accompanies depressive mood as a basic symptom complex, with somatic concern and guilt feelings also often present. This basic complex may or may not be accompanied by motor retardation, hostility, or tension/excitement to define alternative phenomenological types.

The large number of different labels that have been used to describe the clinical picture strongly suggest that depression is a heterogeneous illness. Thus, one of the earliest directions that research with the BPRS took was to investigate whether a relatively few distinct profile patterns adequately represent most depressed patients. That is, do most depressed patients belong to one of a few distinct phenomenological types? Empirical cluster analysis methods were used to investigate this question [4, 25].

Cluster analysis methods were first applied to BPRS profiles of clinically depressed patients in an effort to identify types of depressed patients that responded best to imipramine and thioridazine treatment [34]. The BPRS profiles that were available for cluster classification at that time were recorded on the original 16-item version [21], and the empirical analysis resulted in identification of three distinct profile patterns that recurred in a similar form among depressed patients in the drug treatment groups.

They were described as *anxious depression, retarded depression,* and *hostile depression*. Later, after the addition of scales for rating "excitement" and "disorientation" (numbers 17 and 18 in Fig. 16.1), and with a much larger combined sample of French and American patients, the anxious, retarded, and hostile subtypes were confirmed and a distinct *agitated depression* pattern was also identified [17]. The BPRS profiles that have served as prototypes for the four empirically identified phenomenological types are displayed in graphic form in Fig. 16.2.

The combined French and American sample from which the four depression types shown in Fig. 16.2 were derived represented the general psychiatric populations of those countries. The empirical cluster analyses resulted in identification of eight distinct BPRS profile patterns – the four depression patterns and four other

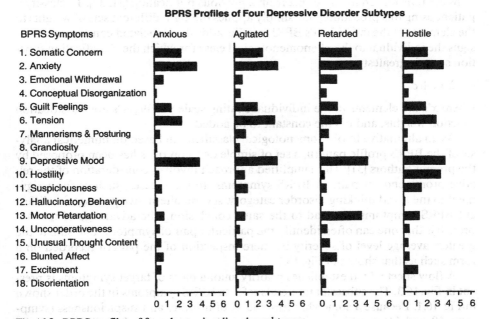

Fig. 16.2. BPRS profiles of four depressive disorder subtypes

patterns described as *florid thinking disorder, withdrawn-disorganized thinking disturbance, paranoid-hostile-suspiciousness,* and *agitation-excitement* syndrome [17]. Recently, the availability of a large psychopharmacology data bank provided an opportunity to verify and refine the prototype patterns for those eight phenomenological types [32]. The mean BPRS profile patterns for the eight phenomenological types, as defined in the large psychopharmacology data bank, are reproduced in numerical form in Table 16.1. These profiles can be the basis for classifying new patients, as described above, using any one of several numerical indices of profile similarity [4, 25].

Although alternative indices of profile similarity produce generally similar results, the recommended scoring of 0 for "not present" provides a meaningful origin for the numerical representation of individual symptom ratings that is particularly suited to calculate the "normalized vector product" index. The present authors prefer this index because it emphasizes shape rather than overall severity. Given prototype profiles and patient profiles in which symptom severity is scored 0 for "not present" to 6 for "extremely severe," the normalized vector product index of similarity between a patient profile x and a prototype profile y can be calculated as follows:

$$\Sigma xy \Big/ \sqrt{\Sigma x^2 \Sigma y^2}$$

where summation is across all 18 elements of the BPRS profile.

An alternative approach utilizes classification functions which maximally separate each group from the mean profile for all groups. Each classification function is defined by a set of weighting coefficients to be applied to the elements of an individual's BPRS profile. The weights defining phenomenological classification functions are reproduced in Table 16.2 from a previous publication [31, 32]. To classify a patient using this procedure, one simply applies the eight different sets of weights to the elements of the individual's BPRS profile, adds the associated constants, and assigns the individual to the phenomenological class for which the classification function score is greatest:

$$\Sigma wx + c$$

where x's are elements in the individual's rating scale profile, w's are classification function weights, and c is the constant to be added.

As an alternative to phenomenological classification based on numerical analysis of the BPRS profile pattern, a set of simple decision rules has been proposed by the present authors [31]. This simplified approach involves consideration of the relative prominence of pairs of BPRS symptoms. In some cases, such as for assignment to the florid thinking disorder category, several alternative pairings for different BPRS symptoms can lead to the same conclusion. The advantage of this approach is that one can often identify the particular pair of symptoms that sum to the greatest average level of severity by mere inspection of the pattern recorded on a form such as that shown in Fig. 16.1.

A flow sheet which establishes priority among pairs of target symptoms is present in Fig. 16.3. The subscript numerals refer to BPRS symptoms in the order shown in Fig. 16.1. Because a somewhat lesser level of hostility and suspiciousness (symptoms 10 and 11) combined with symptoms of thinking disorder still suggests the

Table 16.1. Mean BPRS profiles for eight phenomenological types

BPRS symptom rating constructs	Anxious depression	Retarded depression	Agitated depression	Hostile depression	Florid thinking disorder	Withdrawn-disorganized	Agitation-excitement	Hostile-suspiciousness
Somatic concern	2.42	2.80	2.41	2.10	1.09	0.63	1.84	2.19
Anxiety	3.89	3.59	3.83	3.60	1.74	0.99	2.56	3.11
Emotional withdrawal	0.82	1.49	0.61	0.78	3.14	3.88	1.66	3.02
Conceptual disorganization	0.26	0.60	0.45	0.29	3.62	2.79	2.43	2.17
Guilt feelings	1.57	1.55	1.93	2.01	0.37	0.11	0.73	0.95
Tension	2.39	1.94	3.59	3.02	2.24	1.51	3.74	2.77
Mannerisms and posturing	0.40	0.79	0.87	0.30	2.33	2.22	2.36	1.93
Grandiosity	0.09	0.10	0.31	0.27	1.19	0.11	1.48	0.90
Depressive mood	4.04	4.30	3.80	3.81	0.81	0.65	1.13	2.12
Hostility	0.37	0.37	0.76	3.37	0.98	0.39	2.39	2.61
Suspiciousness	0.58	0.49	1.07	1.61	2.06	0.39	2.24	3.79
Hallucinatory behavior	0.16	0.14	0.21	0.10	3.42	0.85	1.65	1.63
Motor retardation	0.74	3.70	0.77	1.27	1.24	1.92	0.44	1.94
Uncooperativeness	0.25	0.55	0.42	0.54	1.18	1.43	1.87	2.20
Unusual thought content	0.37	0.70	0.61	0.43	4.15	0.87	2.54	3.01
Blunted affect	0.61	1.43	0.36	0.51	2.82	3.74	1.19	2.72
Excitement	0.38	0.25	3.41	1.27	1.42	0.68	4.20	1.44
Disorganization	0.06	0.34	0.18	0.08	1.54	2.39	1.14	0.48

Table 16.2. Weighting coefficients defining classification functions for eight phenomenological types

BPRS symptom rating constructs	Anxious depression	Retarded depression	Agitated depression	Hostile depression	Florid thinking disorder	Withdrawn-disorganized	Agitation-excitement	Hostile-suspiciousness
Somatic concern	0.264	0.302	0.270	0.117	0.023	−0.102	0.228	0.296
Anxiety	0.940	0.592	0.465	0.628	0.191	0.331	0.673	0.740
Emotional withdrawal	0.294	0.490	−0.058	0.134	0.495	1.136	0.005	0.521
Conceptual disorganization	−0.156	−0.405	−0.381	−0.369	0.555	0.142	0.160	0.058
Guilt feelings	0.333	0.168	0.549	0.722	−0.71	−0.198	0.016	−0.075
Tension	0.629	0.513	0.835	0.766	0.453	0.251	0.656	0.458
Mannerisms and posturing	−0.146	−0.006	−0.354	−0.142	0.170	0.378	0.250	0.102
Grandiosity	0.290	0.444	0.220	−0.012	0.244	0.302	0.466	0.055
Depressive mood	2.012	1.874	1.886	1.558	−0.351	−0.107	−0.023	0.237
Hostility	−0.057	0.101	−0.208	2.156	−0.048	−0.221	0.573	0.732
Suspiciousness	−0.142	−0.260	−0.142	−0.158	0.139	−0.140	0.209	1.105
Hallucinatory behavior	−0.297	−0.360	−0.336	−0.367	0.451	−0.180	−0.198	−0.410
Motor retardation	−0.506	0.929	−0.201	0.089	−0.013	0.262	−0.407	0.145
Uncooperativeness	0.193	−0.111	−0.151	−0.399	−0.625	−0.424	−0.138	0.064
Unusual thought content	−0.251	−0.279	−0.016	−0.211	1.256	−0.350	0.677	0.664
Blunted affect	0.086	0.241	0.029	−0.065	0.523	1.044	0.098	0.459
Excitement	−0.377	−0.425	1.723	−0.242	−0.056	−0.346	1.361	−0.282
Disorganization	−0.045	0.091	−0.123	−0.026	−0.241	0.418	−0.310	−0.391
Constant	−8.755	−9.631	−11.153	−11.386	−8.590	−7.344	−9.375	−9.503

A. Hostile Suspiciousness

$$x_{10} + x_{11} + 1.0$$
$$x_{10} + x_{14} + 1.0$$
$$x_{11} + x_{14} + 1.0$$

B. Florid Thinking Disorder

$$x_4 + x_{12}$$
$$x_4 + x_{15}$$
$$x_{12} + x_{15}$$
$$x_{11} + x_{15}$$

C. Withdrawn Disorganized

$$x_3 + x_4$$
$$x_3 + x_{16}$$
$$x_4 + x_{16}$$

D. Retarded Depression

$$x_3 + x_9$$
$$x_9 + x_{13}$$

E. Agitated Depression

$$x_9 + x_{17}$$

F. Hostile Depression

$$x_9 + x_{10}$$

G. Anxious Depression

$$x_2 + x_9 - 1.0$$

H. Agitation-Excitement

$$x_6 + x_{17}$$

Sum ratings for pairs of symptoms as indicated. Add 1.0 to the sum of pairs in frame A, and subtract 1.0 from the sum of the pair in frame G. Consider the resulting sums in order from A to H. If any sum is equal to or greater than the sums for all pairs of symptoms listed below it in the ordering, assign the patient to the indicated category.

Fig. 16.3. Flow sheet for phenomenological classification of Brief Psychiatric Rating Scale (BPRS) profile

"hostile suspiciousness" classification, a constant +1 is added to the sum of paired symptoms in frame A. Similarly, because anxiety commonly accompanies depressive mood in all subtypes of depressive disorder, the constant −1 is subtracted from the sum of those two symptoms in frame G. To classify a patient, sums of pairs of symptoms as indicated are entered in the blanks on the right. Next, beginning at the top and going down, the first sum that is equal to or greater than the sums for all pairs listed below it in the priority sequence is identified and the patient assigned to the phenomenological type indicated on the left.

In concluding this discussion of phenomenological classification of depressive disorders, it is important to emphasize that phenomenological classification is not equivalent to diagnosis and is not intended to supplant diagnostic considerations. Previous studies have shown that, even among patients who meet the diagnostic criteria, almost complete heterogeneity with respect to phenomenological classifications exists [19, 30]. Thus, phenomenological classification can provide a valid and meaningful way to stratify patient samples in an effort to reduce error variance and to identify important treatment interactions.

Diagnostic Profiles

The BPRS has also been used to obtain profiles of major diagnostic groups [13, 23] and to compare diagnostic concepts of psychiatrists in different countries [5, 6, 26, 39]. Several early studies asked psychiatrists to provide BPRS rating-scale descriptions of "typical" patients in different major diagnostic categories. Most of that earlier work was done, however, with the original 16-item BPRS and will not be emphasized here.

As large data banks accumulated from use of the BPRS in clinical research, a statistical approach to diagnosis was possible [3, 18, 20, 27]. Mean BPRS profiles for groups of patients with clinical diagnoses of depression, mania, schizophrenia, and organic brain syndrome are contrasted in Fig. 16.4. Although it would be possible to employ these mean profiles as prototypes to which individual patient profiles can be compared for classification purposes, the primary interest in presenting them here is to illustrate the adequacy of BPRS profile patterns for characterizing differences among major syndromes of psychopathology. The profile patterns which are

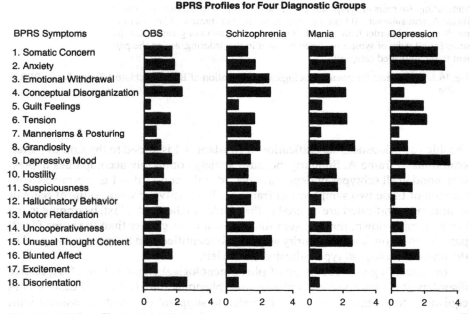

Fig. 16.4. BPRS profiles for four diagnostic groups

shown in Fig. 16.4 give means of ratings for the indicated diagnostic groups in a sample of 563 patients previously utilized in a study of diagnostic criteria [20].

Whereas current trends in research diagnosis emphasize more restrictive criteria [2, 7, 42], the actual clinical management of patients tends to correspond to major drug groups: antipsychotics for thinking disorders, antidepressants for depressive disorders, lithium for mania, and (at present) no specific drug for brain syndromes [24]. If the aim is to constitute groups corresponding to those major divisions, classification of BPRS profiles based on numerical similarity to the four major diagnostic prototypes may be useful. Numerical methods for assessing similarity of an individual's profile to each of several prototype patterns were discussed earlier in this chapter and have been discussed elsewhere in greater detail [25].

The Texas Actuarial Criteria provide an objective basis for establishing a diagnosis of depressive disorder in a way consistent with treatment practices [19, 20]. Based on accumulated data, statistical weighting of both history and background information and BPRS symptom ratings lead to diagnostic decisions that agree with clinical diagnoses [18, 19, 20] and which have greater interrater reliabilities than do diagnoses based on less information [37]. Because more items of information are considered, the total accuracy of each observation is not as critical.

The BPRS ratings, as well as history and background information, are treated as categorical data for calculating three diagnostic indices of the Texas Actuarial Criteria. For the purpose of statistical weighting, the seven levels of severity on which each BPRS symptom is rated are reduced to four categories: (1) *not present,* (2) *mild* including BPRS ratings of very mild and mild, (3) *moderate* corresponding to BPRS ratings of moderate, and (4) *severe* including BPRS ratings of moderately severe, severe, and extremely severe. Three sets of scoring weights for the 9 background variables and the 18 BPRS symptom-rating variables are represented in Table 16.3. Three index scores are calculated by summing weights corresponding to the category of each variable to which an individual belongs. Thus, each diagnostic index (schizophrenia, depression, other) is the sum of 27 statistically derived weights corresponding to his/her status on nine background variables plus 18 BPRS symptom ratings. A patient is then assigned to the schizophrenia, depression, or other diagnostic category indicated by the largest of the three scores.

A sample of 150 consecutive new admissions to the general adult psychiatry unit of the teaching hospital (Hermann Hospital) of the University of Texas Medical School at Houston was interviewed by a specially trained psychiatric research assistant. Among other data, history and background information were recorded on a standard checklist [20] and BPRS symptom ratings were based on an interview similar to that described above. The three diagnostic indices of the Texas Actuarial Criteria were calculated by summing weights associated with selected background and BPRS data, as indicated in Table 16.3. Comparison of the actuarial diagnosis with the final clinical diagnosis revealed 95% agreement. Of the 76 patients in the sample of 150 who were diagnosed as having a depressive disorder, 72 were assigned to the depression category by the actuarial criteria. Accepting the independently derived clinical diagnosis as a (fallible) criterion, the actuarial classification produced four false positives and four false negatives. The size of the depression population de-

Table 16.3. Scoring weights for nine background variables and 18 BPRS symptom ratings

	Schizophrenia	Depression	Other
Variable			
Age (years)			
20	10	0	20
20-29	6	0	4
30-39	6	10	0
40-49	0	3	2
50+	0	0	15
Sex			
Male	2	0	4
Female	2	4	0
Marital status			
Never married	10	0	3
Married or widowed	0	6	3
Divorced or Divorced- and -remarried	0	2	4
Work level			
Unskilled	3	0	3
Skilled or housewife	0	3	1
Alcohol abuse			
Not problem	7	7	0
Problem	0	10	30
Drug abuse			
Not problem	4	4	0
Problem	0	3	15
Sleep difficulty			
Not problem	4	0	5
Problem	0	5	0
Previous psychiatric hospitalization			
None	0	4	4
One	3	3	0
Multiple	5	0	0
Family history			
No	0	0	0
Yes	7	7	0
Sign/Symptom			
Somatic concern			
Not present	10	0	10
Mild	0	2	4
Moderate	0	10	6
Severe	0	5	0
Anxiety			
Not present	8	0	3
Mild	5	0	10
Moderate	0	5	2
Severe	5	10	0
Emotional withdrawal			
Not present	0	4	8
Mild	0	0	0
Moderate	4	0	0
Severe	6	4	0

Table 16.3 (continued)

	Schizophrenia	Depression	Other
Conceptual disorganization			
Not present	0	12	15
Mild	0	2	5
Moderate	10	0	0
Severe	15	0	0
Guilt feelings			
Not present	3	0	0
Mild	0	1	2
Moderate	0	8	6
Severe	8	10	0
Tension			
Not present	3	0	3
Mild	1	0	4
Moderate	1	2	0
Severe	5	8	0
Mannerisms, posturing			
Not present	0	2	4
Mild	4	1	0
Moderate	8	0	0
Severe	10	0	0
Grandiosity			
Not present	0	1	2
Mild	8	0	8
Moderate	6	0	8
Severe	4	0	8
Depressive mood			
Not present	7	0	5
Mild	3	0	8
Moderate	0	4	0
Severe	0	10	0
Hostility			
Not present	0	1	1
Mild	1	1	0
Moderate	1	0	0
Severe	7	0	0
Suspiciousness			
Not present	0	4	6
Mild	0	3	0
Moderate	5	2	0
Severe	10	0	0
Hallucinatory behavior			
Not present	0	5	5
Mild	8	1	0
Moderate	12	0	12
Severe	16	0	6
Motor retardation			
Not present	0	1	0
Mild	3	1	3
Moderate	0	6	0
Severe	0	0	0
Uncooperativeness			
Not present	0	3	3
Mild	0	0	0
Moderate	8	0	0
Severe	10	0	0

Table 16.3 (continued)

	Schizophrenia	Depression	Other
Unusual thought content			
Not present	0	10	13
Mild	0	1	2
Moderate	10	4	0
Severe	18	2	0
Blunted affect			
Not present	0	6	9
Mild	2	0	0
Moderate	4	1	0
Severe	15	8	0
Excitement			
Not present	0	0	0
Mild	3	0	3
Moderate	3	3	4
Severe	6	3	6
Disorientation			
Not present	0	1	1
Mild	2	0	8
Moderate	3	0	8
Severe	10	0	15

fined by the actuarial criteria was thus identical to that defined by hospital diagnosis. Full results of this study, including comparisons with other more restrictive research criteria for diagnosis of depressive disorder, are contained in a previous report [3].

In another previously reported study of 563 patients in which BPRS ratings were completed by psychiatric residents as a part of routine clinical duties, the Texas Actuarial Diagnosis agreed with final clinical diagnosis in 81% of the cases [20]. Of the 115 patients who were assigned to the depression category by the actuarial criteria, 84% received a final clinical diagnosis of depressive disorder. The lower agreement in this study is attributed to the fact that the BPRS symptom ratings were not a primary part of patient evaluation but were done after-the-fact by psychiatric residents who interviewed the patients as part of routine intake procedure. Even with a reasonable lack of research motivation on the part of those who completed the BPRS, the agreement of 84% between actuarial and clinical diagnoses is higher than the agreement previously reported in comparison of clinical diagnoses made independently and without the use of specified criteria [43]. In the case of Texas Actuarial Criteria, reliability is not achieved by artificially narrowing the boundaries for the major diagnostic entities.

An investigation of reliability of diagnoses of depressive disorder based on alternative research diagnostic criteria has also favored the lengthier Texas Actuarial Criteria [37]. Two specially trained psychiatric research assistants jointly interviewed and then independently rated 100 consecutive new admissions to the adult psychiatry inpatient service of the teaching hospital of the University of Texas Medical School at Houston. This was a different series of patients from the 150 patients included in the comparison of actuarial and clinical diagnosis discussed earlier [3].

The two observers, in this instance, independently recorded symptom ratings on the BPRS, history and background information on the Brief Psychiatric History Form (BPHF), and information pertinent to evaluation of several different criteria for schizophrenia and depression on appropriate composite checklists [28, 30]. Agreement on a diagnosis of depressive disorder was higher for the Texas Actuarial Criteria than for the more restrictive Research Diagnostic Criteria (RDC). Specifically, the diagnosis of depression was agreed upon in 48 cases, a diagnosis other than depression was agreed upon in 42 cases, and the independent observers disagreed in 10 cases. This level of agreement resulted in a *kappa* coefficient of 0.80, which was higher than the corresponding value for the New York RDC or the Feighner (Saint Louis) criteria. This also represents a higher concordance than has generally been reported in the literature for clinical diagnosis [43].

Depression in the Elderly

As indicated in the discussion of factor scoring for the BPRS, symptom profile patterns tend to be somewhat different in an eldery psychiatric population. Because separation of depression from organic dysfunction is a difficult and critical problem, a brief look at the most representative profile patterns in an elderly patient population in which both depressive reactions and organic brain syndromes are common will be provided.

The factor structure of the BPRS in a group of elderly people suffering from different psychiatric disorders reveals that depressive mood more often occurs in association with motor retardation, emotional withdrawal, and blunted affect, whereas it is usually accompanied by anxiety in younger patients [33]. This is not to say that simple anxious depression profile patterns do not occur. They are just relatively less common in older patients. Also, conceptual disorganization is qualitatively different in the younger and older patient populations, although it registers on the same BPRS scale. Whereas conceptual disorganization represents looseness of association and communication difficulties evidenced by younger schizophrenic patients, ratings of conceptual disorganization and disorientation form a separate BPRS dimension that correlates with externally assessed cognitive dysfunction and memory loss in elderly patients. The independence of withdrawn depression, agitation excitement, and cognitive dysfunction factors in the symptom profiles of elderly patients suggests that the BPRS should be a useful tool for assessment and classification of depression in that population.

A recent investigation of the most frequently occurring profile patterns in a sample of 88 patients who were newly admitted to an inpatient psychogeriatric treatment unit revealed the presence of five distinct phenomenological types [1]. They are characterized as *agitated dementia, retarded dementia, anxious depression, withdrawn depression,* and *paranoid psychosis.*

Mean BPRS profiles for the five empirically defined phenomenological types within the psychogeriatric population have been included in the referenced publication. They can be a basis for classification of new patients, using one of the numerical indices of profile similarity. Because larger data bases are needed to provide more reliable definitions of prototype patterns, those tentative prototypes will not be reproduced here. The purpose of this brief section is to alert the reader to differences that he/she should expect to encounter in the use of the BPRS for assessing psychopathology in the elderly patient population.

Of the five empirically identified psychogeriatric patterns, as one might expect, the most difficult to distinguish are the withdrawn depression and the retarded dementia. The distinction rests primarily on higher levels of conceptual disorganization and disorientation in the retarded dementia profile, with a higher level of anxiety in the withdrawn depression profile. The two dementia patterns (agitated and retarded) and the two depression patterns (anxious and withdrawn) are rather clearly different, and the paranoid psychosis pattern is clearly different from the others. Although larger samples are required to define precisely the prototype patterns, the results obtained so far confirm that elderly patients do appear in relatively distinct phenomenological types and that the BPRS holds promise for classification research within the psychogeriatric population.

Conclusion

The use of the BPRS for evaluation and classification of depressions has evolved gradually over time. Initially, it was used primarily to provide a numerical assessment of the overall severity of depressive illness. The further isolation of primary factors and the definition of factor scores consisting of related items on the BPRS led to more specific assessment of depressive illness, especially in relation to other psychiatric disorders. The BPRS was next employed in the search for primary, distinct phenomenological types with resulting recognition that most depressed patients tend to present with one of four typical profile patterns. Methods for classification of depressed patients were made available and have been found to have heuristic value in the clinical evaluation of antidepressant drugs. Actuarial and statistical approaches have resulted in diagnostic categorization of depressed patients based on a combination of BPRS symptom ratings and selected background data. The validity of BPRS diagnostic categorization has been evaluated by comparison to clinical diagnoses and somewhat narrower Research Diagnostic Criteria. Recent work has focused on differential diagnoses of dementia and depression in the elderly. Thus, the BPRS has found applications in assessment, classification, and diagnosis of depression and depressive disorders in a variety of different patient populations.

References

1. Beller, S. A., and Overall, J. E. 1983. The Brief Psychiatric Rating Scale (BPRS) in geropsychiatric research: Representative profile patterns. Geropsychiatry, In press.
2. Carpenter, W. T., Strauss, J. S., and Bartko, J. J. 1973. Flexible system for the diagnosis of schizophrenia: Report from the WHO International Pilot Study of Schizophrenia. Science 182: 1275-1278.
3. Cobb, J. C., and Overall, J. E. 1981. Computer simulation and comparison of specific diagnostic concepts for schizophrenia and depression. In: H. G. Hefferman (ed.), Proceedings of the Fifth Annual Symposium on Computer Applications in Medical Care, pp. 412-416. IEEE, Washington, D.C.
4. Cronbach, L. J., and Gleser, G. C. 1953. Assessing similarities between profiles. Psychol. Bull. 50: 456-473.
5. Delmonte, P., Gabrielli, F., Giberti, F., Overall, J. E., and Rossi, R. 1970. Concetti classificationi diagnostici tra gli psychiatri italiani. Archivio Di Psicologia Neurologia E Psichiatria 6: 531-555.
6. Engelsmann, F., Pichot, P., Rossi, R., Hippius, H., and Overall, J. E. 1970. International comparison of diagnostic patterns. Transcultural Psychiatric Research 7: 130-137.
7. Feighner, J. P., Robins, E., Guze, S. B., Woodruff, R. A., Winoku, G., and Munoz, R. 1972. Diagnostic criteria for use in psychiatric research. Arch. Gen. Psychiatry 26: 57-63.
8. Guy, W. 1976. ECDEU Assessment Manual for Psychopharmacology (DHEW no. 76-338). National Institute of Mental Health, Rockville, MD.
9. Hedlund, J. L., and Vieweg, B. W. 1980. The Brief Psychiatric Rating Scale (BPRS): A comprehensive review. Journal of Operational Psychiatry 11: 48-65.
10. Hollister, L. E., Bennett, J. L., Kimbell, I., Jr., Savage, C., and Overall, J. E. 1963. Diazepam in newly admitted schizophrenics. Diseases of the Nervous System 24: 1-4.
11. Hollister, L. E., Overall, J. E., Kimbell, I., Jr., Bennett, J. L., Meyer, F., and Caffey, E. 1963. Oxypertine in newly admitted schizophrenics. Journal of New Drugs. 3: 26-31.
12. Hollister, L. E., Overall, J. E., Bennett, J. L., Kimbell, I., Jr., and Shelton, J. 1965. Triperidol in schizophrenia: Further evidence for specific patterns of action of antipsychotic drugs. Journal of New Drugs. 5: 34-42.
13. Overall, J. E. 1963. A configural analysis of psychiatric diagnostic stereotypes. Behav. Sci. 8: 211-219.
14. Overall, J. E. 1968. Historical and sociocultural factors related to the phenomenology of schizophrenia. In: D. V. Siva Sankar (ed.), Schizophrenia, Current Concepts and Research. pp. 36-43. PJD Publications LTD, Hicksville, NY.
15. Overall, J. E. 1971. Association between marital history and the nature of manifest psychopathology. J. Abnorm. Psychol. 78: 213-221.
16. Overall, J. E. 1974a. Rating scales in the measurement of change. In: Neuropsychopharmacology, pp. 208-212. Excerpta Medica International Congress Series no. 359. Excerpta Medica, Amsterdam.
17. Overall, J. E. 1974b. The brief psychiatric rating scale in psychopharmacology research. In: P. Pichot and R. Oliver-Martin (eds.), Psychological Measurements in Psychopharmacology: Modern Problems in Pharmacopsychiatry, pp. 67-78. Karger, Basel.
18. Overall, J. E. 1977. Actuarial methods in the diagnosis of schizophrenia. In: E. Fann, I. Karacan, A. D. Pokorny, and R. L. Williams (eds.), Phenomenology and Treatment of Schizophrenia. Spectrum, Jamaica.
19. Overall, J. E. 1978. Critères de diagnostic et de classification des dépressions. In: P. Pichot and C. Pull (eds.), La Symptomatologie Dépressive: Enregistrement et évaluation, pp. 15-30. Editions Spire, Paris.
20. Overall, J. E. 1981. Criteria for the selection of subjects for research in biological psychiatry. In: H. M. Van Praag, M. H. Lader, O. J. Rafaelsen, and E. J. Sachar (eds.), Handbook of Biological Psychiatry, Part VI, Practical Applications of Psychotropic Drugs and Other Biological Treatments, pp. 359-404. Dekker, Basel.
21. Overall, J. E., and Gorham, D. R. 1962. The brief psychiatric rating scale. Psychol. Rep. 10: 799-812.

22. Overall, J. E., and Porterfield, J. 1963. The powered vector method of factor analysis. Psychometrika. 28: 415-422.
23. Overall, J. E., and Hollister, L. E. 1967. Studies of quantitative approaches to psychiatric classification. In: J. Cole and W. Barton (eds.), The Role and Methodology of Classification in Psychiatry and Psychopharmacology, pp. 277-299. U. S. Department of Health, Education, and Welfare, Washington, D. C.
24. Overall, J. E., and Henry, B. W. 1972. Decisions about drug therapy I: Selection of treatment for psychiatric outpatients. Arch. Gen. Psychiatry. 26: 140-145.
25. Overall, J. E., and Klett, C. J. 1972. Applied Multivariate Analysis. McGraw-Hill, New York.
26. Overall, J. E., and Hippius, H. 1974. Psychiatric diagnostic concepts among German-speaking psychiatrists. Compr. Psychiatry 15: 103-117.
27. Overall, J. E., and Higgins, C. W. 1977. An application of actuarial methods in clinical diagnosis. J. Clin. Psychol. 33: 973-980.
28. Overall, J. E., and Hollister, L. E. 1979. Comparative evaluation of research diagnostic criteria for schizophrenia. Arch. Gen. Psychiatry 36: 1198-1207.
29. Overall, J. E., and Hollister, L. E. 1980. Phenomenological classification of depressive disorders. J. Clin. Psychol. 36: 372-377.
30. Overall, J. E., and Zisook, S. 1980. Diagnosis and the phenomenology of depressive disorders. J. Consult. Clin. Psychol. 48: 626-634.
31. Overall, J. E., and Hollister, L. E. 1982. Decision rules for phenomenological classification of psychiatric patients. J. Consult. Clin. Psychol. 50: 535-545.
32. Overall, J. E., and Rhoades, H. M. 1982. Refinement of phenomenological classification in clinical psychopharmacology research. Psychopharmacology 77: 24-30.
33. Overall, J. E., and Beller, S. A. The brief psychiatric rating scale in geropsychiatric research. I: Factor structure. Geropsychiatry. In press.
34. Overall, J. E., Hollister, L. E., Johnson, M., and Pennington, V. 1966. Nosology of depression and differential response to drugs. Journal of the American Medical Association 195: 946-948.
35. Overall, J. E., Hollister, L. E., and Dalal, S. N. 1967. Psychiatric drug research: Sample size requirements for one vs. two raters. Arch. General Psychiat. 16: 151-161.
36. Overall, J. E., Hollister, L. E., and Pichot, P. 1967. Four dimensional model of major psychiatric disorders. Arch. Gen. Psychiatry 16: 146-151.
37. Overall, J. E., Cobb, J. C., and Click, M. A., Jr. 1982. The reliability of psychiatric diagnoses based on alternative research criteria. Journal of Psychiatrical Treatment Evaluation. 4: 209-220.
38. Pichot, P., Overall J. E., Samuel-Lajeunesse, B., and Dreyfus, J. F. 1969. Structure factorielle de l'échelle abrégée d'appréciation psychiatrique (B. P. R. S.). Revue de Psychologie Appliquée. 19: 217-232.
39. Pichot, P., Bailly, R., and Overall, J. E. 1966. Les stéréotypes diagnostiques des psychoses chez les psychiatres français: Comparaison avec les stéréotypes américains. In: Proceedings of IV World Congress of Psychiatry, pp. 16-26. Excerpta Medica International Congress Series no. 129. Excerpta Medica, Amsterdam.
40. Prusmack, J. J., Hollister, L. E., Overall, J. E., and Shelton, J. 1966. Mesoridazine (TPS-23). A new antipsychotic. Journal of New Drugs. 6: 182-188.
41. Rubin, R. T., and Overall, J. E. 1970. Manifest psychopathology and urine biochemical measures. Multivariate analyses in manic depressive illness. Arch. Gen. Psychiatry 22: 45-57.
42. Spitzer, R. L., and Fleiss, J. L. 1974. A re-analysis of the reliability of psychiatric diagnosis. Br. J. Psychiatry 125: 341-347.
43. Spitzer, R. L., Endicott, J., and Robins, E. 1975. Research diagnostic criteria (RDC). Psychopharm. Bull. 11: 22-24.
44. Tryon, R. C., and Bailey, D. E. 1970. Cluster Analysis. McGraw-Hill, New York.
45. Woodward, J. A., and Overall, J. E. 1975. Patterns of symptom change in anxious depressed outpatients treated with different drugs. J. Nerv. Ment. Dis. 36: 125-129.
46. Zisook, S., Overall, J. E., and Click, M. A., Jr. 1981. Treatment validity of different diagnostic concepts of depression. Psychiatry Research. 5: 77-85.

Chapter 17   The Brief Depression Rating Scale

R. KELLNER

The uses and characteristics of rating scales for depression have been discussed by several authors [3, 4, 8, 17, 21]. The main aims in designing the Brief Depression Rating Scale (BDRS) were to construct a scale which sensitively measures changes in depression, detects small differences between the effects of two treatments, and takes a short time to administer.

The studies in this chapter and the scales have been described in greater detail elsewhere [11, 12]. The scales are available from the author. All correlation coefficients in this paper indicate the Spearman *rho* [18]. Results at or below the 5% level of probability (two-tailed) were regarded as significant.

Description of the Scales

The BDRS is one of three scales of a set of the Rating Scales of Depression, Anxiety and Somatic Symptoms (RDAS). The BDRS consists of eight items:

1. Depressive mood, feeling of despair
2. Psychophysiologic somatic symptoms
3. Lack of interest, initiative, and activity
4. Sleep disturbance
5. Anxiety
6. Appearance
7. Depressive beliefs
8. Suicidal thoughts and behavior

(The scale and scoring instructions are given in Appendix A)

The items for the Anxiety Rating Scale are:

1. Anxious mood
2. Psychophysiologic somatic symptoms
3. Thought content
4. Sleep disturbance
5. Depressive mood, feeling of despair
6. Concentration and memory
7. Feeling of physical tension and observed restlessness
8. Irritability

The items for the Somatic Symptoms Rating Scale are:

1. Gastrointestinal, e.g., stomach upset, colic, diarrhea
2. Appetite
3. Cardiac symptoms, e.g., heart racing, pounding, awareness of heartbeat
4. Feeling of instability, e.g., faint, dizziness, vertigo
5. Headaches, including feelings of pressure or tightness
6. Muscular pains and aches, e.g., limbs, chest, and back
7. Fatigue without physical exertion
8. Sexual function and interest

Each item is rated on a nine-point scale. The cues range from "totally absent" to "incapacitating". Five of the rating cues for each item are clearly defined; the remaining cues are intermediate and should be used only if the main cues do not adequately express the rater's opinion.

Development of the Scale

The Brief Depression Rating Scale (BDRS) evolved from a series of studies. The initial stages consisted of reviews of symptoms in the populations studied; for the BDRS these were several groups of inpatients and outpatients suffering from primary depression diagnosed by Research Diagnostic Criteria [6] and the symptoms and the behaviors were selected as items for the scales. The scales were validated by methods which are suitable for the validation of scales purporting to measure changes, and appropriate reliability studies were carried out [9, 10]. The scales were tested in drug trials and their performances compared with those of other scales. The procedure adopted for improving the sensitivity of the scales was validation against an external chemical criterion [5, 9], that is, validating the scales in double-blind drug trials with psychotropic drugs. The aim was to construct scales which could detect the effect of the smallest dose of a psychotropic drug when compared with placebo, or the smallest difference between two doses of the same active psychotropic drug, or differences in a drug trial with the smallest possible number of patients.

The items were reviewed after the validation of studies and deleted or modified if they were unsuitable for the scale; for example, if an item did not discriminate adequately between an active psychotropic drug and placebo. Similarly, the cues for raters were modified when it was found that the interrater reliability was inadequate. Finally, only those items which were either a part of factors in published factor analyses of symptoms and signs or occurred consistently in the same sample studies were retained. Item VIII of the BDRS (suicidal thoughts or behavior) was added subsequently because of the frequency of occurrence in depressed inpatients and because of its clinical and research importance.

The validation studies on which the self-rating scales were constructed have been described in greater detail elsewhere [9, 13, 14]. In a large proportion of these studies self-rating scales and observer-rating scales were validated together.

Reliability, Validity, and Sensitivity

Reliability

The interrater reliability between two psychiatrists assessing depressed inpatients ($N = 32$) at various stages of treatment was 0.94. When the ratings were carried out by one psychiatrist and one research assistant ($N = 28$) the correlation was 0.91. In another study of depressed inpatients ($N = 22$), the correlation between two psychiatrists was 0.89. In depressed outpatients who were at various stages of treatment ($N = 26$), the correlation with the Hamilton Depression Rating Scale [7] was 0.83.

Tests of reliability of rating scales which purport to measure changes have been discussed elsewhere [9]. The split half reliability and the split half reliability changes are not suitable for scales which have only a few items. The test-retest reliability in psychiatric outpatients ($N = 24$) at various stages of treatment (time interval between test and retest ranging between 1 and 2 weeks) was 0.85.

The BDRS was used in a multicentred drug trial in the United States and in Europe. The drugs compared were imipramine and pridefine, an experimental pyrolidine derivative. The mean scores of American raters (37 patients) were 42 before treatment and 29 after treatment: the corresponding scores by German raters (28 patients) were 40 and 30 [1]. Thus, the changes in ratings were almost identical on two continents by raters using different languages. Although it is not certain whether the actual degree of change was the same, the close similarity of the changes in ratings suggests reliability of the scale.

Validity

In all studies the ratings changed in the expected direction. Depressed outpatients ($N = 22$) suffering from a major depression [2] were compared with nonpsychotic outpatients who suffered from anxiety disorders, somatoform disorders, or personality disorders ($N = 36$) who were not substantially depressed. The comparison was limited to the scores of the pure depressive items of the BDRS (depressed mood, loss of interest and initiative, psychomotor retardation, depressive beliefs, and suicidal ideation). The ratings for these items clearly differentiated between the two groups of patients except for three highly anxious patients who scored in the depressive range. A group of recently admitted severely depressed inpatients ($N = 20$) were rated and the scores of these five items were compared with those of outpatients. Except for one, all inpatients scored higher than outpatients ($P < 0.001$).

In a multicenter drug trial in which one of the drugs used was imipramine, the ratings were correlated with blood levels of imipramine in a central laboratory. The correlation of the total BDRS score with imipramine levels was 0.37 ($P < 0.05$) [20].

Sensitivity

In several placebo-controlled studies the BDRS discriminated sensitively between treatments. In a study with depressed inpatients, two doses of imipramine (150 mg vs 300 mg daily) were compared. A large number of rating and self-rating scales were used: The BDRS, The Hamilton Rating Scale for Depression [7], the Zung Self-Rating Depression Scale [22], the Symptom Rating Test [14], and the Brief Distress Scales and Global Scales. Several individual items of the various scales showed significantly more improvement with 300 mg imipramine than with 150 mg. Of the *total* scores only the BDRS discriminated significantly between the treatments. (In this study the scale was referred to by its previous name: The Physician Rating Scale for Depressed Patients [19].)

In a crossover study of high doses of chlordiazepoxide (CDP) and placebo with nonpsychotic anxious and depressed outpatients ($N=22$) who suffered largely from depressive neurosis (dysthymic disorder) and anxiety disorders [16] the decrease of self-rated depression was about equal to the decrease in self-rated anxiety. A subsample of 14 patients were also administered the Hamilton Rating Scale for Depression (HAM-D) and the BDRS. The total score of the BDRS discriminated significantly between the effects of CDP and placebo even when the anxiety item and somatic items were excluded from the scale, whereas the HAM-D failed to discriminate at a significant level [12]. The scales were used in two intensive design [15] placebo-controlled studies; the BDRS tended to be more sensitive than other rating scales. Some of these and other findings on the comparison of ratings were not included in the original papers (which dealt largely with self-rating scales) but they have been described elsewhere [12].

The findings are not conclusive because the number of double-blind drug trials in which the BDRS was compared with other scales is small and the number of patients in the studies was small. However, the findings suggest that the BDRS is as sensitive or more sensitive in discriminating between the effects of treatments than other scales with which it had been compared.

Discussion

The cues in the BDRS are clearly defined and the items are suitable for examining changes in individual symptoms such as impaired activity or depressive beliefs. The clear definition of cues promotes a high interrater reliability. Since the scale is short, it can be included in studies when also more elaborate assessments are made without unduly encroaching on the patients' and investigators' time. It is suitable for frequent repeated assessments of progress, for example, daily ratings of hospitalized patients when it is desirable to measure changes from day to day. Because of the scale's sensitivity it appears to be particularly useful when changes to be measured are small, or when the difference between two treatments is small; a less sensitive scale might fail to detect existing differences between treatments. The scale appears to be suitable for measuring changes in a few patients when these changes are correlated with other measures such as changes in medication or findings of biochemical studies.

The BDRS resembles the Montgomery-Åsberg Depression Scale (MAS); however, the items and the cues of these two scales are somewhat different. The BDRS has six items of depressive symptoms or signs, one item of anxiety, and one of symptomatic symptoms; the MAS has nine depressive items and one item pertaining to appetite. The two scales were designed for the same purpose, that is for the measurement of changes in the severity of depression; they were developed independently by different methods, and yet the results obtained with the two scales are likely to be similar. The MAS was published first; however, the BDRS had been used in earlier published research (the old name was Physician Rating Scale of Depression) [11, 12, 19]. The BDRS, because of the smaller number of items, is somewhat less time consuming than the MAS; this does not apply to the full scale (RDAS), in which anxiety and somatic symptoms are rated in detail.

Appendix A Brief Depression Rating Scale

Circle the appropriate number

I Depressive mood. Feeling of despair	Incapacitating 9	Severe distress 8 7	Moderately distressed 6 5	Slight 4 3	Cheerful* 2 1
II Psychophysiologic somatic symptoms**	Incapacitating 9	Severe symptoms or impairment 8 7	Moderate 6 5	Slight 4 3	Completely absent or normal functions 2 1
III Lack of interest, initiative, and activity	Totally inactive 9	Severe apathy, very few activities 8 7	Moderately impaired interest and initiative 6 5	Slight loss of interest and initiative 4 3	Interested and energetic 2 1
IV Sleep disturbance***	Apparently sleeping 1 h or less 9	Sleeping about 2 h a night 8 7	Sleeping 4–5 h 6 5	Slight sleep disturbance 4 3	Sleeping well* 2 1
V Anxiety, worry, tension	Incapacitating 9	Severe distress 8 7	Moderate tension or anxiety 6 5	Slight 4 3	Calm and relaxed 2 1
VI Appearance	Continuous expression of utmost despair 9	Sad appearance, does not smile at all 8 7	Sad appearance, but can be made to smile 6 5	Sad appearance at times 4 3	Appears cheerful* 2 1

The Brief Depression Rating Scale

VII Depressive beliefs	Most thoughts are delusional 9	Has some depressive psychotic delusions 8 7		Frequent beliefs of no hope or unworthiness 6 5		Occasional brief depressive beliefs 4 3		Confident* and optimistic 2 1
VIII Suicidal thoughts or behavior	Evidence of serious suicide risk and a recent suicide attempt 9	Frequent suicidal preoccupations and wishes to die 8 7		Intermittent thoughts of suicide. No plans 6 5		Occasional thoughts of suicide. Does not want to die 4 3		No suicidal thoughts 2 1

* If excessive, please comment
** Including appetite, sexual interest, gastric symptoms, etc. Rate the symptom which is most severe
*** If any of the following is reported: difficulty in falling asleep, waking up early, restless sleep, or nightmares, rate the sleep disturbance as "slight", "moderate", or "severe" even if the total number of hours slept is adequate

Appendix B Guide for Rating

If in doubt whether to rate *severity* of the symptoms or behavior or *frequency* of occurrence, rate *severity* of the symptom or behavior.

The usual period rated is the *past week;* the rating period can be made longer or shorter, depending on the design of the study.

If the symptoms varied in intensity (some days good, some days bad) and it is difficult to find the appropriate cue, the most severe symptom during the last 2 days should be rated.

For the symptoms which do not have specific rating instructions the rating cues should be interpreted as follows:

9 – Incapacitating – The patient is unable to carry out everyday tasks (not only related to his or her occupation) because of the severity of his or her symptoms.

7 – Severe – The patient is severely distressed and/or his or her performance is substantially impaired but not to the point of incapacity.

5 – Moderate – This rating is made when neither "severe" nor "slight" is applicable.

3 – Slight – The patient either mentions spontaneously or replies to questioning that the symptom is not troublesome with statements such as "slight" or "only a little."

1 – Absent – Total absence of the symptom during the period covered by rating.

Intermediate ratings – (Scores 2, 4, 6, and 8) should be used only if the main cues (1, 3, 5, 7, and 9) do not adequately express the rater's opinion.

References

1. A. H. Robins Company. 1979. Symposium on AHR-1118, Santa Monica. A. H. Robins Data, on file.
2. American Psychiatric Association. 1980. Diagnostic and Statistical Manual of Mental Disorder. 3rd Ed. American Psychiatric Association, Washington.
3. Åsberg, M., Kragh-Sorensen, P., Mindham, R. H. S., and Tuck, J. R. 1973. International reliability and communicability of a rating scale for depression. Psychol. Med. 3: 458–465.
4. Carroll, B. J., Fielding, J. M., and Blashki, T. G. 1973. Depression rating scales. Arch. Gen. Psychiatry 28: 361–366.
5. Clyde, D. J., 1960. Self-ratings. In: L. Uhr and J. G. Miller (eds), Drugs and Behavior, Wiley, New York.
6. Feighner, J. P., Robins, E., Guze, S. B., Woodruff, R. A., Winokur, F., and Munoz, R. 1972. Diagnostic criteria for use in psychiatric research. Arch. Gen. Psychiatry 26: 57–63.
7. Hamilton, M., 1960. A rating scale for depression. J. Neurol. Neurosurg. Psychiatry 23: 56–62.
8. Hamilton, M. 1976. Comparative value of rating scales. Br. J. Clin. Pharmacol. 3: 58–60.
9. Kellner, R. 1971. Part 1. Improvement criteria in drug trials with neurotic patients. Psychol. Med. 1 (5): 416–425.
10. Kellner, R. 1972. Part 2. Improvement criteria in drug trials with neurotic patients. Psychol. Med. 2 (1): 73–80.
11. Kellner, R. 1976. Physician's Rating Scale for Depression, Anxiety and Somatic Symptoms. University of New Mexico, Albuquerque (mimeographed).
12. Kellner, R. 1982a. Abridged Manual of the Rating Scale of Depression, Anxiety and Somatic Symptoms. University of New Mexico, Albuquerque (mimeographed).

13. Kellner, R. 1986. A symptom questionnaire. J. Clin. Psychiatry (in press)
14. Kellner, R., and Sheffield, B. F. 1973. A self-rating scale of distress. Psychol. Med. 3 (1): 88-100.
15. Kellner, R., Uhlenhuth, E. H., and Glass, R. M. 1977. Clinical evaluation of antianxiety agents: Subjects-own-control design. In: M. A. Lipton, A. DeMascio, and K. F. Killam (eds.), Psychopharmacology: A Generation of Progress. Raven Press, New York.
16. Kellner, R., Rada, R., Andersen, T., and Pathak, D. 1979. The effects of chlordiazepoxide on self-rated depression, anxiety, and wellbeing. Psychopharmacology 64: 185-191.
17. Montgomery, S. A., and Åsberg, M. 1979. A new depression scale designed to be sensitive to change. Br. J. Psychiatry 134: 382-389.
18. Siegel, S. 1956. Nonparametric Statistics for the Behavioral Sciences. Mc Graw Hill, New York.
19. Simpson, G. M., Lee, H. J., Cuculic, Z., and Kellner, R. 1976. Two dosages of imipramine in hospitalized endogenous and neurotic depressives. Arch. Gen. Psychiatry 33: 1093-1102.
20. Simpson, G. M., White, K. L., Boyd, J. L., et al. 1982. Relationship between plasma antidepressant levels and clinical outcome for inpatients receiving imipramine. Am. J. Psychiatry 139 (3): 358-360.
21. Snaith, R. P., Bridge, G. W. K., and Hamilton, M. 1976. The Leeds scale for the assessment of anxiety and depression. Br. J. Psychiatry 128: 156-165.
22. Zung, W. W. K. 1965. A self-rating depression scale. Arch. Gen. Psychiatry 12: 63-70.

Chapter 18   The Carroll Rating Scale for Depression

M. FEINBERG and B. J. CARROLL

Introduction

Research studies of depression require a measure of the severity of illness, and various rating scales or inventories have been designed in attempts to meet this need. Ratings by clinicians were introduced first, and these were complemented later by self-rating scales. The performance of these two types of rating has been compared extensively in recent years. Self ratings generally have highly significant overall correlations with clinician ratings, but some significant disagreements have been described. For example, Carroll et al. [5] found that the Hamilton Rating Scale (HAM-D) [11] completed by clinicians was superior to the Zung Self-Rating Depression Scale (SDS) [19] in discriminating global severity of depression across three treatment settings (inpatient, day hospital, general practice). Bailey and Coppen [2] found satisfactory and significant correlations between the HAM-D and the self-rated Beck Depression Inventory (BDI) [4] in only two-thirds of patients: the results in the remaining third were often very divergent. Neither type of rating scale should be used for making a diagnosis of depression [11, 5, 13], although the self-rating scales are often used as screening instruments.

The general problems of concordance between clinician ratings and self ratings were discussed by Prusoff et al. [15] and by Carroll et al. [5]. While some of these problems (such as denial, exaggeration, and loss of insight) are unavoidable, at least the content of the two types of rating can be controlled. The HAM-D is weighted towards the behavioral and somatic features of depression, whereas the BDI is weighted more towards the psychological and cognitive features. The Zung SDS contains a broad sample of features but is limited in its access to information about several items because of the way it was constructed [5]. Since the Hamilton scale is the most widely used clinician-rating instrument for depression, a self-rating version of the HAM-D could be useful, especially if it were designed to match closely the item content of the HAM-D. Work on the development of such a scale [Carroll Rating Scale (CRS)] has begun in 1969. After several modifications, the final form of the CRS was published recently [7]. Translations of the CRS in French, Italian and Chinese [8] have since been developed.

We addressed several of the issues described above in a study of depressed outpatients, discussed below. Specifically, we wanted to determine whether a self-rating instrument could accurately assess the intensity of depression, as well as its presence or absence. We also wished to determine the effect of diagnosis on the self-rating scales by comparing observer ratings and self ratings in patients with endogenous and nonendogenous depression.

We compared not only the HAM-D and CRS but also compared these two structured rating scales with two more global ones [9]. The "global" ratings used include Clinicians' Global Ratings of Depression (CGRD) and the Visual Analogue Scale (VAS) originally described by Aitken [1]. This ingeniously simple instrument is a 10-cm line accompanied by a question asked of the respondent, who answers by marking a point on the line. The answer is scored by measuring the distance of the mark from the left end of the line.

Methods

Design of the Carroll Rating Scale

The CRS was designed as a direct self-rated adaptation of the original 17-item HAM-D. Items in the HAM-D that are scored 0-4 are represented in the new scale by four statements denoting progressively increasing severity of illness. Similarly, items scored 0-2 in the HAM-D are represented by two statements in the new scale. Thus, the maximum possible score is 52, as in the HAM-D. The form that patients complete contains the 52 statements in random order (Appendix A). Because of the large number of statements, patients are asked simply to answer "yes/no" to each statement. The direction of a response indicative of depression is "yes" for 40 statements, "no" for 12 statements. We avoided constructing double-negative responses. Each statement is scored as one point toward the total score. While the logic of the set of statements for each item should require that patients answering positively to statement 4 also answer positively to statements 1, 2, and 3, we have not complicated the scoring procedure by assigning different weights to the statements. Using a scoring key, one can easily determine the total CRS score and the scores for the 17 HAM-D items.

Reliability and Validity

We tested the face validity of the CRS by having 119 adults, aged 18-64 years, complete the scale [7]. To preserve confidentiality, we did not know the sex of the respondents or whether a respondent was receiving psychiatric treatment. The 119 respondents were a reasonably representative sample of the population in this area and covered a range of socioeconomic status. In a separate study [9], we obtained global ratings of severity of depression by psychiatrists concurrently with CRS ratings of patients being treated for depression. These concurrent ratings were obtained on 1191 occasions for over 200 patients. The global rating of severity of depression was made on a four-point (0-3) scale.

The concurrent validity of the CRS was estimated by comparing CRS scores with HAM-D scores in patients with the clinical diagnosis of endogenous depression. The clinical diagnoses were made as described by Carroll et al. [6] and were supported in 98% of cases by the Research Diagnostic Criteria [17]. The two scores were obtained on the same day in each patient, HAM-D ratings being made by psychiatrists trained in the use of this scale.

We also compared the CRS with the BDI [7]. For this comparison, HAM-D, CRS, and BDI ratings were obtained from 279 inpatients representing a range of psychiatric diagnoses, similar to the range employed by Beck [3] for his validation of the BDI. We calculated correlations and partial correlations among the three severity scales.

The internal consistency of the CRS was examined in patients with endogenous depression by correlating individual item scores with the total score, in parallel with an identical analysis of matched HAM-D ratings. We tested the split-half reliability of the CRS by correlating the sums of odd- and even-numbered statements with each other, and with the total score. Similarly, we examined the effect of direction of response by correlating the sums of "yes" and "no" response items with each other and with the total score. For these analyses we used all available ratings, including sequential ratings in many patients. Separate analyses (below) revealed only minor changes in correlations within subjects compared with correlations across subjects.

The data for the second study [9] were gathered in an outpatient clinic concentrating on research and treatment of patients with affective disorders. All patients in this study had significant affective symptoms and carried a diagnosis of unipolar endogenous depression (UP), bipolar affective disorder (BP), schizophrenia, schizoaffective psychosis, or nonendogenous depression (usually with a primary diagnosis of neurosis or personality disorder). The diagnoses were made as described in detail elsewhere [6].

Patients completed the two self ratings (CRS and VAS) at each visit, before seeing a clinician, who completed the CGRD. The clinician also completed the HAM-D if the patient was significantly depressed, or was recovering from an episode of depression. The clinicians rarely knew the CRS or VAS scores before completing their ratings of the patients. The CGRD was a four-point scale (0–3), with $0=$ not depressed and $3=$ severely depressed.

The question asked for the VAS was "How are you feeling today?" The 10-cm line was labeled "worst ever" on the left end, and "best ever" on the right. This scale is scored in a direction opposite to the other ratings used, with zero being "worst ever" and 99 being "best ever." As a result, correlation coefficients involving the VAS which are conceptually "positive" are numerically negative.

Results

General Population Scores

The mean CRS score of 119 subjects from the general population was 4.6 (SE = 0.4). The distribution of these scores was skewed heavily towards low values, with the median score being 3 (Fig. 18.1). In 91% of cases the score was <10. From inspec-

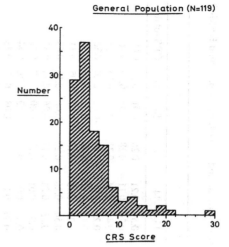

Fig. 18.1. CRS scores obtained from 119 persons in the general population

tion of Fig. 18.1 we would propose a score of 10 as a reasonable cutoff point if the CRS is to be used as a screening for depression. The higher scores reflect significant depressive symptoms in at least 9% of this general population sample. This rate may be compared with a rate of 17% found by Weissman and Myers [18], using another self-report instrument, in a United States urban community survey. For comparison, analysis of the 1191 concurrent global ratings and CRS ratings of patients revealed that 80% of global ratings >0, and 99% of global ratings >1, were associated with CRS scores >10.

Split-Half Reliability

The split-half reliability was calculated with a total of 3725 CRS ratings. The sum of the odd-numbered statements correlated well with the sum of the even-numbered statements ($r = +0.87$, $P<0.001$). The sum of each half-set of statements correlated highly with the total score ($r = +0.97$, $+0.96$, respectively). The sum of "yes" statements correlated highly with the sum of "no" statements ($r = +0.74$, $P<0.001$) in the same set of 3725 CRS ratings. The sum of the 12 "no" statements correlated $+0.87$ with the total score, while the sum of the 40 "yes" statements correlated $+0.98$ with the total score.

Correlation with HAM-D

The matrix of correlations between items and total scores for 278 matched HAM-D-CRS ratings in 97 patients with endogenous depression is presented in Table 18.1. The correlations of individual HAM-D items with the CRS total are listed in the

Table 18.1. Correlations for pairs of CRS and HAM-D items, correlations for particular CRS items and HAM-D total, and correlations for particular HAM-D items and CRS total

	Carroll item																	
	1	2	3	4	5	6	7	8	9	10	11	12	13	14	15	16	17	CRS total
Hamilton item																		
1	0.67	0.43	0.48	0.25	0.34	0.28	0.51	0.46	0.42	0.55	0.21	0.30	0.51	0.21	0.26	0.01	0.17	0.68
2	0.48	0.48	0.31	0.15	0.10	0.05	0.40	0.39	0.26	0.35	0.11	0.12	0.26	0.11	0.28	0.05	0.06	0.46
3	0.69	0.46	0.72	0.15	0.21	0.11	0.48	0.46	0.39	0.49	0.21	0.32	0.41	0.24	0.21	−0.02	0.16	0.65
4	0.08	0.09	0.02	0.73	0.43	0.36	0.16	0.15	0.24	0.31	0.23	0.26	0.23	0.06	0.10	−0.02	0.20	0.36
5	0.12	0.09	0.02	0.47	0.67	0.49	0.22	0.17	0.27	0.24	0.26	0.27	0.17	0.10	0.09	0.02	0.16	0.38
6	0.06	0.05	−0.03	0.37	0.57	0.68	0.14	0.07	0.20	0.25	0.20	0.12	0.24	0.05	0.13	0.11	0.05	0.31
7	0.57	0.40	0.37	0.27	0.30	0.30	0.64	0.54	0.44	0.53	0.25	0.37	0.54	0.26	0.22	0.06	0.16	0.68
8	0.21	0.17	0.18	0.05	0.08	0.06	0.32	0.27	0.21	0.26	0.11	0.13	0.23	0.24	0.13	0.06	0.16	0.31
9	0.12	0.11	0.05	0.38	0.26	0.23	0.16	0.16	0.23	0.29	0.18	0.22	0.09	0.01	0.15	0.00	0.17	0.29
10	0.30	0.19	0.09	0.31	0.25	0.26	0.24	0.23	0.38	0.52	0.28	0.28	0.35	0.07	0.27	0.09	0.10	0.44
11	0.35	0.15	0.13	0.28	0.28	0.30	0.31	0.24	0.37	0.47	0.41	0.33	0.39	0.15	0.23	0.08	0.15	0.48
12	0.32	0.15	0.22	0.18	0.30	0.29	0.40	0.37	0.42	0.43	0.36	0.63	0.34	0.26	0.17	0.16	0.42	0.54
13	0.40	0.30	0.26	0.21	0.22	0.25	0.40	0.38	0.33	0.46	0.21	0.20	0.60	0.22	0.25	0.10	0.12	0.53
14	0.30	0.30	0.18	0.10	0.07	0.02	0.25	0.33	0.12	0.25	0.01	0.13	0.29	0.53	0.23	−0.00	0.14	0.35
15	0.04	0.04	−0.04	0.16	0.23	0.25	0.07	0.03	0.11	0.18	0.27	0.14	0.15	0.20	0.28	0.03	0.16	0.22
16	0.02	−0.07	0.01	0.07	0.12	0.11	−0.01	0.05	0.06	0.08	0.08	0.06	−0.04	0.04	−0.13	−0.06	0.03	0.04
17	0.05	0.06	0.04	0.14	0.18	0.19	0.20	0.19	0.21	0.20	0.12	0.44	0.11	0.07	0.09	0.20	0.60	0.28
HAM-D total	0.57	0.40	0.36	0.48	0.51	0.47	0.56	0.52	0.53	0.67	0.38	0.47	0.57	0.32	0.34	0.09	0.30	0.80

right-hand column, while the corresponding correlations of CRS items with the HAM-D total are along the bottom row. The correlation of HAM-D total with CRS total was highly significant ($r = +0.80$, $P<0.001$). Those CRS items strongly correlated with the HAM-D total (e.g., items #1, 7, 10) also were strongly correlated with several HAM-D items. Conversely, those CRS items only weakly correlated with the HAM-D total (e.g., items #14, 15, 16, 17) were only weakly correlated with HAM-D items. The same comment applies to HAM-D items and the CRS total. The matching items for the two scales (the principal diagonal terms) were generally more highly correlated than other pairs of items. These correlations between matching items ranged from -0.06 (item #16) to $+0.73$ (item #4), indicating that the design of the CRS items was not uniformly successful in matching the content of HAM-D items. The median correlation of the matching items was $+0.60$ ($P < 0.001$).

We calculated the correlation matrices of HAM-D items and of CRS items to evaluate the internal consistency of the two scales. We found that those CRS items which were strongly correlated with the CRS total (e.g., items #1, 7, 8, 10) were generally also strongly correlated with other CRS items, the converse was true for those CRS items that were weakly correlated with the CRS total. There was a similar profile of internal correlations for the HAM-D items. Individual CRS items exhibited correlations with the CRS total of between $+0.05$ and $+0.78$ (median $r = +0.55$). Similarly, individual HAM-D items exhibited correlations with the HAM-D total of between $+0.19$ and $+0.78$ (median $r = +0.54$). The rank order of CRS item-CRS total correlations was similar to the rank order of HAM-D item-HAM-D total correlations ($r_s = +0.72$, $P<0.001$). In addition, the rank order of HAM-D item-HAM-D total correlations was similar to the rank order of CRS item-HAM-D total correlations ($r_s +0.67$, $P<0.01$). We conclude from these results that (1) the total scores of the CRS and HAM-D correlated well; (2) matching items of the two scales correlated to a variable degree; (3) the internal consistency of the CRS was similar to that of the HAM-D; (4) the least informative items for the HAM-D total score also tended to be the least informative items for the CRS total score; and (5) the clinician-rated items that were least predictive of the total HAM-D score tended to be the same items, upon translation into the CRS format, that were still least predictive of the HAM-D score. Thus, certain items (#14, 15, 16, 17) may be so weakly correlated with global severity (either because they contribute so little to the total variance or because they are difficult to rate reliably) that they have low predictive utility in either their HAM-D or CRS versions. A further factor analysis of the patterns of responses to items in the two scales is presented elsewhere [16].

Comparison with BDI and HAM-D

Same-day ratings of severity of depression by the HAM-D, CRS, and BDI were obtained on 279 occasions with inpatients representing a range of psychiatric diagnoses. Each scale correlated highly with each of the other two. The two self-rating instruments (CRS and BDI) had the strongest correlation ($r = +0.86$). The correlation of the CRS with the HAM-D (0.71) was somewhat better than that of the BDI with the HAM-D (0.60). The partial correlation was significant for HAM-D-CRS (0.49) and for CRS-BDI (0.77), but not for HAM-D-BDI (-0.03). These results indicate that the BDI did not contain information about the HAM-D beyond that present in the CRS, while the CRS did contain information about the HAM-D beyond what could be predicted from the BDI scores. These findings confirm the value of the complementary use of both a clinician rating and a self rating for assessing the severity of depression (see Hedlund and Vieweg [13]).

Outpatient Study

The data from all patient visits (Table 18.2) showed that the rating scale scores were highly correlated. The severity of depression as measured by the HAM-D accounted for over half of the variance in the CRS score. The high correlation (0.774) between the HAM-D score and the CGRD provides confirmation of earlier validations of the HAM-D (see Hedlung and Vieweg [13] for a review). Our results also validated the VAS (10-cm line) as a rating scale for global severity of depression, confirming the earlier work of Folstein and Luria [10] and of Luria [14].

Because the major affective disorders are recurrent illnesses, we have been following some of our patients for many years. We were concerned that these patients with many visits, and many ratings, might bias our data. Therefore, we used each patient's data only once, in a separate set of analyses. We selected the earliest occurrence of each rating scale pair from each patient's data and repeated the analyses described above. The correlation coefficients did not decrease when only one data point per patient was used; four of the six correlations increased. We decided, therefore, to do all further analyses on the full data set.

The ability of the HAM-D and CRS to distinguish among patients with varying degrees of severity of depression is shown diagrammatically in Fig. 18.2. The means and standard deviations of the rating scale scores are plotted against severity of depression as measured by the CGRD. The lines of best fit are also plotted and the slopes and intercepts of the regression lines are given. The slopes of the lines were different ($P<0.05$), while the intercepts were not. The difference in the slopes suggests that the difference between HAM-D and CRS scores will increase with increasing severity of illness. For both rating scales, each of the four points differed significantly from the others ($P<10^{-4}$, analysis of variance and Scheffe's test).

Table 18.2 Correlations among four ratings of depressed mood. Data from all visits were used

	CRS	CGRD	VAS
HAM-D	0.752[a] (865)	0.774 (284)	-0.645 (750)
CRS		0.634 (2331)	-0.711 (2394)
CGRD			-0.555 (2335)

[a] Correlation coefficients (Pearson's r) and number of data points
All correlation coefficients are significant, $P<10^{-4}$

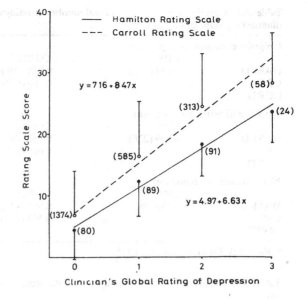

Fig. 18.2. Hamilton Rating Scale and Carroll Rating Scale scores in relation to Clinicians' Global Rating of Severity scores. Mean values and standard deviations are shown with the number of observations *in parentheses*. The calculated regression lines, intercepts, and slopes are shown. The two slopes were significantly different ($P<0.05$)

Differences Among Diagnostic Groups

In order to compare the performance of these rating scales across diagnostic categories, we selected those groups which were best defined and largest in our clinic: patients with unipolar endogenous depression (UP), patients with bipolar endogenous depression (BP), and those with nonendogenous depression. We found several differences among diagnostic groups in the correlations among the rating scales (Table 18.3). The correlations among the rating scales were, on the whole, higher in the UP and BP groups than in the nonendogenous group. (The pattern of correlation coefficients in Table 18.3 was repeated when only the earliest ratings obtained from each patient were analyzed). The differences between diagnostic groups were most apparent in the correlations of self ratings with observer ratings. The HAM-D-CRS correlation and the CGRD-VAS correlation were highest in the UP group and lowest in the nonendogenous group.

The differences among the correlation coefficients reflect, we believe, a difference in self-perception between endogenous and nonendogenous depressed patients. We examined this difference in another way. Regression analysis of CRS score, with HAM-D score as the independent variable, will give as the y-intercept the CRS score at a HAM-D rating of zero. As shown in Table 18.4, the intercept for the nonendogenous group was significantly higher than that for the unipolar and bipolar groups, which did not differ statistically from each other. There were no significant differences among the slopes calculated for the three diagnostic groups. These results suggest that patients with nonendogenous depression report more symptoms than UP- and BP-depressed patients when they are considered not depressed by clinicians. The equal slopes calculated for increasing CRS scores against

Table 18.3. Correlations (Pearson's r) and number of ratings for four ratings of depression in three diagnostic groups of outpatients

Unipolar endogenous depression			
	CRS	CGRD	VAS
HAM-D	0.834 (278)	0.818 (96)	−0.731 (239)
CRS		0.686 (681)	−0.816 (688)
CGRD			−0.648 (669)
Bipolar endogenous depression			
	CRS	CGRD	VAS
HAM-D	0.749 (236)	0.850 (91)	−0.644 (220)
CRS		0.669 (555)	−0.703 (578)
CGRD			−0.619 (563)
Nonendogenous depression			
	CRS	CGRD	VAS
HAM-D	0.655 (97)	0.905 (15)[a]	−0.657 (77)
CRS		0.567 (279)	−0.603 (290)
CGRD			−0.513 (279)

[a] $P = 0.003$; for all others, $P < 10^{-4}$

Table 18.4. Results of regression analysis of CRS score, with HAM-D score as independent variable

Diagnostic Group	N	Slope ± SE	Intercept ± SE
Unipolar	278	1.015 ± 0.040	3.752 ± 0.627
Bipolar	237	1.060 ± 0.061	4.510 ± 0.760
Nonendogenous	97	0.981 ± 0.116	7.707 ± 1.632[a]

[a] Differs from unipolar ($P < 0.025$); differs from bipolar ($P < 0.05$); (Student's t-tests, one-tailed)

increasing HAM-D scores indicate that patients with nonendogenous depression will be likely to report relatively more symptoms than expected across a wide range of HAM-D scores.

Discussion

The overall performance of the CRS was consistent with the purposes for which it was designed. As a free-standing self-rating scale for severity of depression it yielded low scores in the general population. Virtually all patients with a global rating of more than mild depression recorded CRS scores greater than the cutoff score of 10 derived from the general population study. The split-half reliability of the CRS was acceptable, being equal to that reported for the BDI [3]. The subsets of "yes" and "no" response statements showed a less strong but still acceptable correlation in a very large set of ratings.

The correlation of CRS total with HAM-D total scores in patients with endogenous depression was high. This result compares favorably with correlations reported between the HAM-D and the BDI or Zung SDS [13]. Some of the CRS items failed to match the information content of the corresponding HAM-D items, despite the overall good agreement for total scores. Nevertheless, the internal consistency of the CRS was very similar to that of the HAM-D. Both scales showed a wide and comparable range of correlations of individual items with total scores, both within scales and across scales. Further, the same items tended to be the least correlated with the total score in both the CRS and HAM-D. The internal consistency of the HAM-D in our sample was as good as that reported by Hamilton [12]. He found item correlations with total score ranging from +0.11 to +0.69 (median +0.39) in women and similar figures in men. By comparison, we found item correlations with total score ranging from +0.19 to +0.78 (median +0.54) for the HAM-D. For the CRS, the corresponding figures were +0.05 to +0.78 (median +0.55). These results indicate acceptable cross-validation between the CRS and HAM-D, which is most obvious when the total scores are considered.

The results obtained on comparing the CRS with both the HAM-D and BDI were of interest. The primary correlations of each scale with the two others were highly significant. When the partial correlations were examined, however, the HAM-D-BDI correlation dropped to zero, while the others remained significant. Apparently, the BDI did not contribute information predictive of the HAM-D score, beyond what was already contained in the CRS. On the other hand, the CRS did correlate significantly with the HAM-D, after their intercorrelations with the BDI were partialled out. Furthermore, the self ratings were significantly correlated (0.77) after their intercorrelations with the HAM-D were partialled out. Thus, both the CRS and BDI seem to have access to a subjective dimension of depression that is not predicted by the HAM-D. These results suggest that the CRS may be a useful alternative to the BDI as a self-rating scale, with the additional advantage of closer correspondence to the HAM-D.

Appendix A

Name:

Reg no.:

Date:

How are you feeling today? Please answer by marking a point on the line below.

Worst ever ——————————————————————————— Best ever

Answer the following questions in terms of how you have felt in the *last few days*, circle your answers and please do not leave any questions unanswered.

I feel just as energetic as always	yes	no
I am losing weight	yes	no
I have dropped many of my interests and activities	yes	no

Since my illness I have completely lost interest in sex	yes	no
I am especially concerned about how my body is functioning	yes	no
It must be obvious that I am disturbed and agitated	yes	no
I am still able to carry on doing the work I am supposed to do	yes	no
I can concentrate easily when reading the papers	yes	no
Getting to sleep takes me more than half an hour	yes	no
I am restless and fidgety	yes	no
I wake up much earlier than I need to in the morning	yes	no
Dying is the best solution for me	yes	no
I have a lot of trouble with dizzy and faint feelings	yes	no
I am being punished for something bad in my past	yes	no
My sexual interest is the same as before I got sick	yes	no
I am miserable or often feel like crying	yes	no
I often wish I were dead	yes	no
I am having trouble with indigestion	yes	no
I wake up often in the middle of the night	yes	no
I feel worthless and ashamed about myself	yes	no
I am so slowed down that I need help with bathing and dressing	yes	no
I take longer than usual to fall asleep at night	yes	no
Much of the time I am very afraid but don't know the reason	yes	no
Things which I regret about my life are bothering me	yes	no
I get pleasure and satisfaction from what I do	yes	no
All I need is a good rest to be perfectly well again	yes	no
My sleep is restless and disturbed	yes	no
My mind is as fast and alert as always	yes	no
I feel that life is still worth living	yes	no
My voice is dull and lifeless	yes	no
I feel irritable or jittery	yes	no
I feel in good spirits	yes	no
My heart sometimes beats faster than usual	yes	no
I think my case is hopeless	yes	no
I wake up before my usual time in the morning	yes	no
I still enjoy my meals as much as usual	yes	no
I have to keep pacing around most of the time	yes	no
I am terrified and near panic	yes	no
My body is bad and rotten inside	yes	no

I got sick because of the bad weather we have been having	yes	no
My hands shake so much that people can easily notice	yes	no
I still like to go out and meet people	yes	no
I think I appear calm on the outside	yes	no
I think I am as good a person as anybody else	yes	no
My trouble is the result of some serious internal disease	yes	no
I have been thinking about trying to kill myself	yes	no
I get hardly anything done lately	yes	no
There is only misery in the future for me	yes	no
I worry a lot about my bodily symptoms	yes	no
I have to force myself to eat even a little	yes	no
I am exhausted much of the time	yes	no
I can tell that I have lost a lot of weight	yes	no

References

1. Aitken, R. C. B. 1969. Measurement of feelings using visual analogue scales. Proceedings of the Royal Society of Medicine 62: 989-993.
2. Bailey, J., and Coppen, A. 1976. A comparison between the Hamilton rating scale and the Beck inventory in the measurement of depression. Br. J. Psychiatry 128: 486-489.
3. Beck, A. T. 1967. Depression. Clinical, Experimental and Theoretical Aspects. Harper and Row, London.
4. Beck, A. T., Ward, C. H., Mendelson, M., Mock, J., and Erbaugh, J. 1961. An inventory for measuring depression. Arch. Gen. Psychiatry 4: 561-571.
5. Carroll, B. J., Fielding, J. M., and Blashki, T. G. 1973. Depression rating scales: A critical review. Arch. Gen. Psychiatry 28: 361-366.
6. Carroll, B. J., Feinberg, M., Greden, J. F., Haskett, R. F., James, N. McI., Steiner, M., and Tarika, J. 1980. Diagnosis of endogenous depression: Comparison of clinical research and neuroendocrine criteria. J. Affective Disord. 2: 177-194.
7. Carroll, B. J., Feinberg, M., Smouse, P. E., Rawson, S. G., and Greden, J. F. 1981. The Carroll Rating Scale for Depression. I. Development, Reliability and Validation. Br. J. Psychiatry 138: 194-200.
8. Dunner, D. L., Zheng, Y., Quijie, S., and Dunner, P. Z. 1983. Clinical Studies of Affective Disorder in the People's Republic of China. Presented at the Annual Meeting of the Society of Biological Psychiatry, New York.
9. Feinberg, M., Carroll, B. J., Smouse, P., and Rawson, S. G. 1981. The Carroll rating scale for depression III. Comparison with other rating instruments. Br. J. Psychiatry 138: 205-209.
10. Folstein, M. F., and Luria, R. E. 1973. Reliability, validity, and clinical application of the visual analogue mood scale. Psychol. Med. 3: 479-486.
11. Hamilton, M. 1960. A rating scale for depression. J. Neurol. Neurosurg. Psychiatry 23: 56-62.
12. Hamilton, M. 1967. Development of a rating scale for primary depressive illness. Br. J. Soc. Clin. Psychol. 6: 278-296.

13. Hedlund, J. L., and Vieweg, B. W. 1979. The Hamilton rating scale for depression: A comprehensive review. J. Operational Psychiatry 10: 149-165.
14. Luria, R. E. 1975. The validity and reliability of the visual analogue mood scale. J. Psychiatr. Res. 12: 51-57.
15. Prusoff, B. A., Klerman, G. L., and Paykel, E. S. 1972. Concordance between clinical assessments and patients' self-report in depression. Arch. Gen. Psychiatry 26: 546-552.
16. Smouse, P. E., Feinberg, M., Carroll, B. J., Park, M. H., and Rawson, S. G. 1981. The Carroll rating scale for depression II. Factor analyses of the feature profiles. Br. J. Psychiatry 138: 201-204.
17. Spitzer, R. L., Endicott, J., and Robins, E. 1975. Research Diagnostic Criteria (RDC) for a Selected Group of Functional Disorders. 2nd Ed. New York State Psychiatric Institute, New York.
18. Weissman, M. M., and Myers, J. K. 1978. Rates and risks of depressive symptoms in a United States urban community. Acta Psychiatr. Scand. 57: 219-231.
19. Zung, W. W. K. 1965. A self-rating depression scale. Arch. Gen. Psychiatry 12: 63-70.

Chapter 19 The Newcastle Scale

M. W. P. CARNEY

The classification of depressive disorders has aroused interest and controversy ever since Kraepelin [40] defined melancholia and manic-depressive illness, and distinguished a distinct subgroup of psychogenic depressives. He was followed in this by Lange [43] and Gillespie [24] and more recently by Roth [65], Kalinowsky [32], Kiloh and Garside [37], Kay et al. [33], Teja et al. [73] and Venkoba Rao [75]. Mapother [46], however, held that manic-depressive illness was but a quantitative variation from normal. Lewis [44, 45] and later authors [14, 15, 19, 74] followed him in maintaining that all variation in affective illness was solely quantitative. More recently, Sandifer et al. [69] applied a diagnostic index to North Carolina depressives and his results supported the two-type hypothesis. Garside et al. [23], re-examining this material, reached the same conclusion. Eysenck [17] and Mendels and Cochrane [50], summarizing the statistical work up till then, concluded that there was more than one type of depression, though whether it could be explained on a categorical, dimensional or some other basis was unclear. Later studies [4, 39], however, have supported a compromise solution – an endogenous depressive category and a neurotic depressive dimension. Further statistical evidence against the unitary view of depression stems from multivariate analytical work [49], numerical taxonomy [18, 60] and cluster analysis [1, 59, 60].

There is also an impressive accumulation of data correlating biochemical, physiological and therapeutic findings with the endogenous-neurotic dichotomy [36, 67]. In recent years, the controversy has reappeared in the guise of an all-embracing bipolar-unipolar classification of affective disorders, unipolar covering both anxiety states and depression.

When I started working with Sir Martin Roth in Newcastle-upon-Tyne, we were both impressed with the work of Crooks et al. [13] on diagnostic indices for the separation of thyrotoxicosis and euthyroid patients. Simultaneously, Professor Kiloh and his colleagues were applying multivariate analysis to the problem of predicting imipramine response [38]. Following a suggestion from Roth, I compiled a list of features culled from the literature credited with having significance in the differential diagnosis of these two subtypes of depression, and weighted them in proportion to their apparent importance in making this distinction. I then used these weighted features to analyse retrospectively the records of inpatients at Newcastle General Hospital, admitted and treated with ECT over a 3-year period. I found a good separation between endogenous depressives, who seemed mostly to have responded to ECT, and neurotic depressives, most of whom had responded poorly.

Thus encouraged, I carried out a prospective investigation of depressives admitted to all the psychiatric facilities in Newcastle-upon-Tyne. From statistical analyses of these data Garside devised two sets of weighted features, the one for differential diagnosis and the other for predicting ECT response [5].

Subsequently, Gurney and her co-workers [2] produced a set of weighted features to differentiate between depression and anxiety state. All three sets of weights have been called the "Newcastle Index" but in this paper I have reserved the title for the diagnostic inventory of Carney, Roth and Garside [5], unless otherwise stated.

Description of the Newcastle Index

Carney et al. [5] rated 129 depressed inpatients admitted for ECT for the presence or absence of 35 clinical features. The 129 were followed up for 3 months after discharge; and 108 were followed for 6 months. A principal component analysis of the features shown by all 129 patients revealed a bipolar factor corresponding to the endogenous and neurotic distinction and a general factor for depression. The bipolar factor supported the two-type hypothesis of depression. A multiple regression analysis yielded 3 series of 18 weighted coefficients for making the differential diagnosis between the two varieties of depression and the prediction of response to ECT at 3 months and 6 months respectively. As the weights based on the 18 features were complex, the following two sets of weighted items were selected in simplified form for use in making the differential diagnosis and the prediction of response to ECT:

Diagnosis weights

Adequate personality	+1
No adequate psychogenesis	+2
Distinct quality	+1
Weight loss – exceeding 7 lbs	+1
Previous episode	+1
Depressive psychomotor activity	+2
Anxiety	−1
Nihilistic delusions	+2
Blame others	−1
Guilt	+1

A score of 6 or more indicates endogenous depression and 5 or less, neurotic depression

ECT prediction weights

Weight loss – exceeding 7 lbs	+3
Pyknic physique	+3
Early waking	+2
Anxiety	−2
Somatic delusions	+2
Paranoid delusions	+1
Worse p.m.	−3
Self-pity	−1
Hypochondriacal	−3
Hysterical	−3

A score of 1 or more suggests a good result with ECT whereas a score of 0 or less suggests a poor result

Definitions

Most items are self-explanatory but some require further explanation:

Adequate Personality. This describes subjects free from any history of neurotic breakdown and chronic disabling neurotic symptoms or serious social maladjustment.

No Adequate Psychogenesis. No psychological stress or difficulty continuing to operate after the onset of symptoms and adequate to explain perpetuation of the symptoms.

Distinct Quality. Some patients may describe their depression as similar to normal sadness or gloom, differing in degree only; others describe their mood as having a quality distinct from the depression with which they normally respond to adversity. It is to this latter type of depression that this feature refers.

Pyknic Physique. The assessment of physique was made according to criteria described by Kretschmer [41].

Depressive Psychomotor Activity. This term is used inclusively to describe objective evidence of retardation, stupor or agitation.

Nihilistic Delusions. Delusions of doom and imminent destruction, somatic dissolution or poverty of the patient and/or the patient's family.

Somatic Delusions. Delusions of bodily change or disease, usually of a bizarre nature.

Hypochondriasis. Excessive or morbid preoccupation with bodily sensations which have little or no organic basis.

It was suggested [4] that the definition of quality of depression be expanded by adding "patients may even deny depression despite ample evidence to the contrary, and instead refer to an indescribable mood state". This redefined item has been shown to be helpful in clinical practice [2, 4].

Because of occasional difficulty experienced in distinguishing between nihilistic delusions and feelings, and in view of the finding of Paykel et al. [59] that "feelings of hopelessness" were positively correlated with endogenous depression, Carney and Sheffield [4] suggested that "feelings of hopelessness" be substituted for "nihilistic delusions" but further work on this remains to be done.

Validity

The evidence that the Newcastle Scales are valid comes from several sources:

1. Statistical
2. Biochemical
3. Differential results of treatment
4. Other physiological evidence
5. Cerebral tomography

Statistical

A rating scale is validated if the original results are replicated by different investigators at different times with patients of various ages, cultures and regions. By these criteria Newcastle Indices are valid though there are insufficient studies from different regions. One of the earlier validating studies was that of Kendell and Post [35]. They can hardly be said to have shared the alleged nosological preconception of the Newcastle school. Nevertheless, by means of the Kendell scale and the Newcastle Index they confirmed the presence of an endogenous-neurotic "dimension" in Kendell's material, varying qualitatively, and meaningful in terms of treatment and prognosis. They failed, however, to show a similar bimodality in their data as did Post [61], after using the Newcastle Index with data from 92 elderly depressives. Both investigators argued that these results invalidated the two-type thesis of depression, and, by implication, the Newcastle studies giving rise to the Index. Roth and Garside [22, 66] contended that bimodality, no matter how the means of finding it are derived, always favours two distinct populations whereas a unimodal distribution either supports a homogeneous population or a bimodal distribution obscured by other factors. Moreover, distribution of the scores of Kendell's group B were later found to depart significantly from normality. Garside [20] and Hope [28] confirmed that the balance of evidence was in favour of bimodality. Mowbray [56] replicated Kendell's discriminate function analysis and concluded that his findings supported a bimodal distribution of his patient's scores.

Garside [21], finding similarities between Kendell's and Post's patients, pooled their data. The frequency distribution of the combined scores departed significantly from normal, with a dip in the middle. He interpreted this finding as supporting the original study [5]; Kendell and Post [35] then applied the Newcastle Index to a larger group of 271 patients, demonstrating a trimodal distribution. They believed this conflicted with the Newcastle findings but Roth and Garside [66] pointed to an inflection at score 5 – the same as in the distribution curves of the original work [5] and Kendell [34].

Carney and Sheffield [4] applied the diagnosis index to a group of Lancashire depressives, inpatients and outpatients, all given ECT. They replicated the original Newcastle curve [5], one "hump" comprising mainly endogenous patients responsive to ECT and the other, neurotics, poorly responsive to ECT. Post [61], by means of features of the Newcastle Index was able to divide his patients into "severely psychotic", "intermediate psychotic" and "neurotic", differing in respect to the stability and neuroticism of the premorbid personality.

An inventory of items taken largely from the Newcastle Scales of Carney et al. [5] and Gurney et al. [26] was devised by Bech for comparison with the WHO's Schedule for the Standardized Assessment of Depressive Disorders (SADD) [2]. When applied to inpatients classified as endogenous by these scales a significant relationship between plasma levels of imipramine and clomipramine and antidepressant effect was achieved. On the other hand, in non-endogenous patients there was no such correlation. Montgomery et al. [54], working with mianserin, have reported a similar finding (see below). On the other hand, the initial severity of patients diagnosed as endogenous, non-endogenous and doubtful diagnosis did not differ in terms of the Hamilton Depression Scale. This replicated the findings of Carney and Sheffield [4]. Matthew et al. [48], reporting on the incidence of vegetative symptoms in 61 drug-free patients with affective features compared with the same number of untreated normal controls, found, on performing multiple regression analyses, that the features most predictive of depression were among those identified by Carney et al. [5], including sleep disturbance and weight loss. A more recent example of validation by other rating scales is the work of Feinberg and Carroll [18]. They separated the two depressive types, using discriminate function analysis and criterion diagnoses derived from two certainly diagnosed groups of depressives. They validated the scale thus obtained by applying it to a second group of depressives and achieved a similar separation.

Eighty per cent of these were correctly classified by this index, which has an agreement with initial clinical diagnosis of 90%. They also validated their index by means of the dexamethasone suppression test (see below). The authors commented on the similarity of this inventory with the Newcastle scale. In the Feinberg-Carroll work, however, delusional items were combined and anxiety was not prominent.

Carney and Sheffield [6] carried out, a month after ECT, a blind assessment of 165 patients who had participated in various research projects and were rated on the Newcastle Scale. There were 101 "good" (socially recovered) outcome patients and 64 "poor" (not fully socially recovered) patients. There was a striking difference ($P<0.001$) between the mean Newcastle Scale scores of the recovered and unrecovered patients, the higher figure representing the good-outcome patients. The Newcastle ECT scale was also validated by reference to mean fall in Hamilton score after ECT [4]. There was a significant rank order correlation between mean fall in Hamilton score and ECT prediction score.

Biochemical

Naylor et al. [57] measured erythrocyte sodium and potassium concentration in 11 neurotic and 14 psychotic depressives, diagnostic type being determined by the Newcastle and Kendell scales. There was complete agreement between the scales in allocating patients to one or other category. Though there was no change in sodium with recovery and no changes at any time in potassium, the mean erythrocyte sodium in the neurotic patients was lower than that of the psychotic depressives and remained so after recovery. Naylor and his colleagues [58] also applied the Newcastle Index to the assessment of 12 patients suffering from ICD 296.2 (endogenous depression), all with Newcastle and Kendell scores in the endogenous range. Their urinary cyclic AMP was estimated. The mean value increased with recovery, the urinary volumes being constant. In both studies good concordance of results in patients rated by the Newcastle and Kendell scales [34] was reported.

Montgomery et al. [54] measured plasma levels with mianserin in endogenous and neurotic depressives as defined by the Newcastle Scale. A significant relationship between plasma levels and response was only found in patients with endogenous depression but not in those with neurotic depression. Similarly, in 98 patients divided into endogenous and neurotic depressives by means of the Newcastle Scale, a significant relationship between plasma level and response to imipramine and clomipramine was found in endogenous depression but not in the neurotic group [2]. Both these sets of results suggest that inconsistencies in results concerning the correlation between response to antidepressants and their plasma levels will remain until the results are analysed by *type* of depression.

Holden [27] has reported the results of the dexamethasone suppression test (DST) in 41 depressives allocated to endogenous or neurotic categories by the Newcastle Scale. The results correlated highly with the Newcastle Diagnosis of endogenous depression, with a specificity of 89%, sensitivity of 82% and diagnostic confidence of 94%. Further validation of the Newcastle Scale comes from the use of DST with a larger number of patients with various diagnoses [12]. Eighty-nine per cent of those allocated to endogenous depression had an abnormal DST response compared with only 49% of those with Newcastle Scale scores indicating non-endogenous depression.

Physiological

Mirkin and Coppen [52] measured the electrodermal activity in 18 depressive patients to whom the Newcastle Scale had been applied and compared their responses to those of 15 controls. The endogenous depressives had significantly lower skin conductance and lower 5-HT platelet uptake than the non-endogenous depressives.

In two studies of depressed patients, the presentation of external information at a high rate was used to reduce the frequency of negative (depressing) thoughts [72]. There was a reduction in depressive thoughts which correlated significantly with Newcastle Score, being greater for neurotic than for endogenous depressives.

Cerebral Tomography

Jacoby and Levy [29], in the course of clinical and computed tomography investigations on a series of 41 elderly patients with affective disorders compared with 50 healthy controls, identified a subgroup of patients older than the rest and with a higher mean Newcastle Score and later onset of depression who had enlarged ventricles. It was thought that organic cerebral factors may have contributed to the development of their depressive illnesses. The same team [30] followed up these 41 patients for a year. This subgroup was found to be persistently depressed as measured by the Hamilton Depression Scale and had a higher mortality than the other patients.

Treatment

Carney and Sheffield [4], in a study of depressive patients, showed that those scoring 6 or more on the diagnostic scale (endogenous) did significantly better in terms of social and clinical recovery both immediately and 3 months after treatment than the remaining depressives treated with ECT. The same authors [6] subsequently carried out a blind assessment 1 month after ECT of 165 depressed patients who had been rated on the Newcastle Scale previous to treatment in the course of several research projects. There were 101 patients who had recovered socially and 64 patients who had not made a full social recovery. There was a striking difference between them in terms of mean results of ECT, those with the Newcastle Score > 6 (endogenous) doing better. The predictive value of the Newcastle Scale in depressed patients treated with ECT has also been confirmed by Vlissades and Jenner [76].

Carney and his colleagues [3, 7] used the Newcastle Scale to classify patients as endogenous or non-endogenous in an open trial of S-adenosyl methionine (SAM). Significantly more of the endogenous than the non-endogenous depressives responded as judged by Hamilton depression scores.

Slade and Checkley [70] tested the hypothesis that the antidepressant action of ECT is due to the enhanced responsiveness brought about by stimulation of monoamine receptors. In endogenous depressives (as defined by Newcastle Score) they measured pituitary hormone responses to test doses of clonidine and methylamphetamine. No enhancement was seen. Glass et al. [25] also investigated the effect of desipramine upon central adrenergic function in depressed patients, again defining diagnostic groups by means of Newcastle Scores. However, they do not comment on the relationship (if any) between type of depression and their findings. The investigations of Checkley and his colleagues [9, 10, 70] involved the administration of methylamphetamine and clonidine to endogenous depressives (defined as 6 or more on the Newcastle Scale). They attributed their findings to a deficiency of central alpha adrenoceptors. The implication of their results is as yet unclear but differences with respect to depressive diagnosis as made by reference to the Newcastle Scale have emerged.

Checkley et al. [10] found that the growth hormone response to clonidine was significantly less in ten drug-free patients with endogenous depression (by the Newcastle Scale) than in ten normal subjects matched for age and sex.

Reliability

It seems that there has been little investigation of the reliability of the Newcastle Scales, most reports being concerned with their validity or practical application. However, Carney and Sheffield [4], in a study of 11 depressed inpatients, reported complete concordance in decisions as to endogenous or non-endogenous illness. Each patient was rated by two to four briefly trained assessors. Martin and Nissenbaum (unpublished) – in part of an open trial of S-adenosyl methionine [3, 7] – also found complete agreement in their diagnostic decisions (endogenous or otherwise) when applying the scale to ten depressed inpatients. Obviously more work is needed in this field.

Newcastle Scale in Use

Rao and Coppen [62] rated 54 depressed inpatients on the scale before giving them amitriptyline. When the clinical response was assessed 6 weeks later patients scoring 4-8 did significantly better than those with higher or lower scores, a difference not accounted for by differences in pretreatment severity of depression as measured by the Hamilton Depression Scale.

Another investigation using the Newcastle Scale was the controlled comparison of simulated and real-pulse ECT in depression by Lambourn and Gill [42]. The results were inconclusive but the low-energy-pulse ECT used in this trial has more recently been shown to be relatively ineffective [63] in an investigation comparing the effects of low-energy ECT, high-energy pulses and pulse-current ECT. Both Newcastle diagnoses and ECT scales were employed. Most patients were endogenous depressives and did well whereas those given low-energy-pulse ECT did not. However, in a double-blind placebo controlled trial of phenelzine and amitriptyline in patients with a Newcastle Score exceeding 8, there was no clear evidence of clinical subgroups responding preferentially to one drug or the other [64]. Johnstone et al. [31] used the scale in the Northwick Park ECT trial of real and simulated ECT to define more exactly patients admitted to the trial. The Newcastle Scale has also been used in a placebo-controlled trial of lithium carbonate in the long-term continuation therapy of 38 depressed patients following ECT [11]. Both groups had very similar Newcastle Scores (in the endogenous range) and lithium was found to be significantly more effective than the placebo in preventing relapse.

Montgomery [53] examined the validity of several scales used in research in depression. He believed the MRC [51] criteria to be inadequate and unreliable. The Present State Examination (PSE) [77] failed to distinguish between primary depression and that due to alcohol, drugs, etc. On the other hand the Research Diagnostic Criteria [71] used a definition which leaned too heavily on endogenous depression. Neither did the DSM III [16] constitute an advance in this field. Montgomery [53] graded the Newcastle diagnosis scale [5] and that of Gurney et al. [26] as being adequate.

Conclusions

In the absence of a generally agreed morbid anatomy or pathophysiology, reliable valid rating scales easily handled by briefly trained observers are necessary in that large area of psychiatry concerned with functional conditions, especially depressive illness. There has to be a simple standardized way of transmitting clinical data, especially over linguistic and cultural boundaries if, in the present state of incomplete knowledge, further advances are to be made. Moreover, it is necessary to have standardized measures for defining the effects of treatment and the carrying out of clinical trials. This need is underlined by the fact that in no field of psychiatry has there been more disagreement than in depression, either clinically or in respect of biochemical findings.

There is continuing controversy over whether there is any relationship between plasma levels and the therapeutic effects of antidepressant drugs. Montgomery [53] has pointed out that this confusion is probably due to the absence from most research schemes of criteria for making this differential diagnosis. To say somebody is depressed is not enough. In addition degree of severity and type of depression should be specified. These parameters are not congruous but may well be orthogonally related. Thus, several investigators have found groups of endogenous and neurotic depressives to have the same mean Hamilton score. Regardless of disputes concerning aetiology and classification of depression, for the purposes of determining types of depression in the context of research as well as in clinical practice, the Newcastle Diagnosis Score of Carney et al. [5] has been shown to be a valid and reliable instrument.

The number of items is small and the method of scoring, relying as it does on the yes-no principle, is easily understood. Most of the items are virtually self-explanatory. As the original instrument was derived from a group of very severely depressed inpatients selected for ECT, it is not surprising that delusional items are included. Some of these items may not seem very relevant clinically when more mildly depressed patients are rated. In particular, the term "quality of depression" has been more fully defined and found to be useful. "Nihilistic delusions" may need to be modified to make it more appropriate for these conditions. It is suggested that "feelings of hopelessness" may be an acceptable alternative without loss of validity but fuller evidence is awaited.

It is sometimes suggested that efforts at a typological classification are sterile academic exercises and that instead attempts should be made to classify in terms of response to a particular treatment like tricyclic antidepressants or ECT. However, individual treatments tend to be transitory while systems of classification should be enduring. Recent advances in the biochemistry of depression should be matched by an increasing refinement of our diagnostic methods if the potential value of these findings is to be realized. It is in this process that the Newcastle Scale has a specific contribution to make.

The reliability of the scale has been recently confirmed by Bech and co-workers [2a].

References

1. Andreasen, W. C., Grove, W. M., and Maurer, R. 1980. Cluster analysis and classification of depression. Br. J. Psychiatry 137: 256-265.
2. Bech, P., Gram, L. F., Reisby, N., and Rafaelsen, O. J. 1980. The WHO depression scale; relationship to the Newcastle Scales. Acta Psychiatr. Scand. 62: 140-153.
2a. Bech, P., Gjerris, A., Anderson, J., Bojholn, S., Kamp, P., Kastrup, M., Clemmessen, L., and Rafaelsen, O. J. 1983. The Melancholia Scale and the Newcastle Scales. Item Combinations and Inter-Observer Reliability. Br. J. Psychiatry 143: 58-63.
3. Carney, M. W. P. 1983. S-Adenosyl methionine (SAM) in the treatment of depression. Symposium on antidepressant therapy, University of Cadiz, May 1983.
4. Carney, M. W. P., and Sheffield, B. F. 1972. Depression and the Newcastle Scale. Their relationship to Hamilton's Scale. Br. J. Psychiatry 121: 35-40.
5. Carney, M. W. P., Roth, M., and Garside, R. F. 1965. The diagnosis of depressive syndromes and the prediction of ECT response. Br. J. Psychiatry 111: 659-674.
6. Carney, M. W. P., and Sheffield, B. F. 1973. The depressive illnesses of late life. Br. J. Psychiatry 123: 723-725.
7. Carney, M. W. P., Martin, R., Bottiglieri, T., Toone, B. K., Nissenbaum, H., Reynolds, E. H., and Sheffield, B. F. 1983. The switch mechanism in affective illness and SAM. Lancet 1: 820-821.
8. Checkley, S. A. 1978. A new distinction between the euphoric and antidepressant effects of methylamphetamine. Br. J. Psychiatry 133: 416-423.
9. Checkley, S. A., and Crammer, J. L. 1977. Hormone responses to methylamphetamine in depression. Br. J. Psychiatry 131: 582-586.
10. Checkley, S. A., Slade, A. P., and Shur, E. 1981. Growth hormone and other responses to clonidine in patients with endogenous depression. Br. J. Psychiatry 138: 531-551.
11. Coppen, A., Abou-Saleh, P., Milln, P., Bailey, J., Metcalf, M., Burns, B. A., and Armond, A. 1981. Lithium continuation therapy following electro-convulsive therapy. Br. J. Psychiatry 139: 284-287.
12. Coppen, A., Abou-Saleh, P., Milln, P., Metcalf, M., Harwood, J., and Bailey, J. 1983. Dexamethasone suppression test in depression and other psychiatric illness. Br. J. Psychiatry 142: 498-504.
13. Crooks, J., Murray, I. P., and Wayne, E. J. 1959. Statistical methods applied to the clinical diagnosis of thyrotoxicosis. Q. J. Med. 28: 211.
14. Curran, D. 1937. The differentiation of neuroses and manic-depressive psychoses. Journal of Mental Science 83: 156.
15. Curran, D., and Mallinson, W. P. 1941. Depressive states in war. Br. med. J. 1: 305.
16. Diagnostic and Statistical Manual of Mental Disorder. 1979. 3rd Ed. American Psychiatric Association, Washington D. C.
17. Eysenck, H. J. 1970. The classification of depressive illness. Br. J. Psychiatry 117: 241-250.
18. Feinberg, M., and Carroll, B. J. 1982. Separation of the subtypes of depression using discriminant function analysis. Br. J. Psychiatry 140: 384-390.
19. Garmany, G. 1958. Depressive states: their aetiology and treatment. Br. Med. J. 2: 341.
20. Garside, R. F. 1967. Neurotic and endogenous depression. Br. J. Psychiatry 113: 924-925.
21. Garside, R. F. 1973. Depressive illness in late life. Br. J. Psychiatry 122: 118-119.
22. Garside, R. F., and Roth, M. 1978. Multivariate statistical methods and problems of classification in psychiatry. Br. J. Psychiatry 133: 53-67.
23. Garside, R. F., Kay, D. W. K., Wilson, I., Denton, I. B., and Roth, M. 1971. Depressive syndromes and classification of patients. Psychol. Med. 1: 333-338.
24. Gillespie, R. D. 1936. The clinical differentiation of types of depression. Guys Hospital Reports 79: 306.
25. Glass, I. R., Checkley, S. A., Shur, E., and Darling, S. 1982. The effect of desipramine upon central adrenergic function in depressed patients. Br. J. Psychiatry 141: 372-376.
26. Gurney, C., Roth, M., Garside, R. F., Kerr, T., and Schapira, K. 1972. Studies in the classification of depressive disorders. Br. J. Psychiatry 121: 162-166.
27. Holden, N. L. 1982. Depression and the Newcastle Scale; their relationship to the Dexamethasone Suppression Test. Br. J. Psychiatry 142: 505-507.

28. Hope, K. 1969. Review of "the classification of depressive illnesses" by R. E. Kendell. Br. J. Psychiatry 115: 731-734.
29. Jacoby, R. J., and Levy, R. 1980. Computed tomography in the elderly. Three affective disorders. Br. J. Psychiatry 136: 270-275.
30. Jacoby, R. J., Levy, R., and Bird, J. M. 1981. Computed tomography and outcome of affective disorder. A follow-up study of elderly patients. Br. J. Psychiatry 139: 288-292.
31. Johnstone, E. C., Deakin, J. F. W., Lawler, P., Frith, C. D., Stevens, M., McPherson, K., and Crow, T. J. 1980. The Northwick Park electroconvulsive therapy trial. Lancet 2: 1317-1320.
32. Kalinowsky, L. B. 1959. Organic (non-drug) therapy of depression. Can. Psychiatr. Assoc. J. (special suppl.) 4: 138.
33. Kay, D. W., Garside, R. F., Roy, J. R., and Beamish, P. B. 1969. Endogenous and neurotic syndromes of depression. Br. J. Psychiatry 115: 389-399.
34. Kendell, R. E. 1968. The problem of classification. In: A. Coppen and A. Walk (eds.), Recent Developments in Affective Disorder. Br. J. Psychiatry (special publication No. 1), London.
35. Kendell, R. E., and Post, F. 1973. Depressive illnesses in late life. Br. J. Psychiatry 122: 615-617.
36. Kiloh, L. G., and Garside, R. F. 1963. The independence of neurotic depression and endogenous depression. Br. J. Psychiatry 109: 451.
37. Kiloh, L. G., and Garside, R. F. 1979. Depression: a multivariate analysis of Sir Aubrey Lewis's data on melancholia. Aust. N. Z. J. Psychiatry 11: 149-156.
38. Kiloh, L. G., Ball, J. R. B., and Garside, R. F. 1962. Prognostic factors in the treatment of depressive states with imipramine. Br. med. J. 1: 12-25.
39. Kiloh, L. G., Andrews, G., Neilson, M., and Bianchi, G. N. 1972. The relationship of the syndromes called endogenous and neurotic depression. Br. J. Psychiatry 121: 183-196.
40. Kraepelin, E. 1923. Manic-depressive Insanity and Paranoia. Livingstone, Edinburgh.
41. Kretschmer, E. 1927. Physique and Character. Springer, Berlin Heidelberg New York.
42. Lambourn, J., and Gill, D. 1978. A controlled comparison of simulated and real ECT. Br. J. Psychiatry 133: 514-519.
43. Lange, J. 1926. Zeitschrift für die gesamte Neurologie und Psychiatrie, 101: 77 [Quoted by Gillespie, R. D. 1926. The clinical differentiation of types of depression. Guys Hospital Rep. 79: 306].
44. Lewis, A. J. 1934. Melancholia: a clinical survey of depressive states. Journal of Mental Science 80: 277.
45. Lewis, A. J. 1936. Melancholia: prognostic study and case material. Journal of Mental Science 82: 488.
46. Mapother, E. 1936. Discussion on manic depressive psychosis. Br. med. J. 2: 872.
47. Martin, R., and Nissembaum, H. 1983. Unpublished results.
48. Matthew, R. J., Swihart, A. A., and Weinman, M. L. 1982. Vegetative symptoms in anxiety and depression. Br. J. Psychiatry 141: 162-165.
49. Matussek, P., Soldner, M., and Nagel, D. 1981. Identification of the endogenous depressive syndrome based on the symptoms and characteristics of the course. Br. J. Psychiatry 138: 361-372.
50. Mendels, J., and Cochrane, C. 1968. The nosology of depression. The endogenous-reactive concept. Am. J. Psychiatry 124: 1-11.
51. Mental Research Criteria. 1965. Clinical trial of the treatment of depressive illness. Br. med. J. 1: 881-886.
52. Mirkin, A. M., and Coppen, A. 1980. Electrodermal activity in depression: clinical and biochemical correlates. Br. J. Psychiatry 137: 93-97.
53. Montgomery, S. A. 1981. Measurement of serum blood levels in the assessment of antidepressants. In: M. Lader and A. Richens (eds.), Central Nervous System, pp. 61-68. MacMillan, London.
54. Montgomery, S. A., Montgomery, D. B., McAuley, R., and Rani, S. J. 1978. Mianserin plasma levels and differential clinical response in endogenous and reactive depression. Acta Psychiatr. Belg. 78: 798-812.
55. Moran, B. O. P. 1966. The establishment of a psychiatric syndrome. Br. J. Psychiatry 112: 1165-1171.
56. Mowbray, R. M. 1969. Classification of depressive illness. Br. J. Psychiatry 115: 1344-1345.
57. Naylor, J. G., McNammee, H. B., and Moody, G. P. 1971. Changes in erythrocyte sodium and potassium on recovery from a depressive illness. Br. J. Psychiatry 118: 219-223.

58. Naylor, J. G., Stanfield, D. A., Whyte, S. F., and Hutchinson, F. 1974. Urinary excretion of adenosine 3: 5-cyclic monophosphate in depressive illness. Br. J. Psychiatry 125: 268–274.
59. Paykel, T. S., Prusoff, B. A., and Tanner, J. 1976. Temporal stability of symptom patterns in depression. Br. J. Psychiatry 128: 369–374.
60. Pilowsky, I., Levine, S., and Boulton, D. M. 1969. The classification of depression by numerical taxonomy. Br. J. Psychiatry 15: 927–945.
61. Post, F. 1972. The management and nature of depressive illness in late life: a follow through study. Br. J. Psychiatry 121: 393–404.
62. Rao, R., and Coppen, A. 1979. Classification of depression and response to amitriptyline therapy. Psychol. Med. 9: 321–325.
63. Robin, A., and DeTissera, S. 1982. Double blind controlled comparison of the therapeutic effects of low and high energy electro-convulsive therapies. Br. J. Psychiatry 141: 357–366.
64. Robinson, A., Nies, A., and Ravaris, L. 1973. The mono-amine oxidase inhibitor phenelzine in the treatment of depressive anxiety states: a controlled clinical trial. Arch. Gen. Psychiatry 129: 407–413.
65. Roth, M., 1959. The phenomenology of depressive states. Can. Psychiatr. Assoc. J. (special suppl.) 4: 532.
66. Roth, M., and Garside, R. F. 1973. Depressive illness in late life. Br. J. Psychiatry 123: 373–375.
67. Roth, M., and Barnes, T. R. E. 1981. The classification of affective disorders: the synthesis of old and new concepts. Compr. Psychiatry 22: 54–77.
68. Rowan, P. R., Paykel, E. S., and Parker, R. R. 1982. Phenelzine and amitriptyline: effects on the symptoms of neurotic depression. Br. J. Psychiatry 140: 475–483.
69. Sandifer, M., Wilson, I. C., and Green, L. 1966. The two-type thesis of depressive disorders. Am. J. Psychiatry 123: 93–97.
70. Slade, A. P., and Checkley, S. A. 1980. A neuroendocrine study of the mechanism of the action of ECT. Br. J. Psychiatry 137: 217–221.
71. Spitzer, R. L., and Endicott, J. 1978. Schedule for Affective Disorders and Schizophrenia: Biometric Research. New York State Psychiatric Institute, New York.
72. Teasdale, J. D., and Regin, V. 1978. The effects of reducing frequency of negative thoughts in the mood of depressed patients – tests of a cognitive model of depression. Br. J. Clin. Psychol. 17: 65–74.
73. Teja, J. S., Narang, R. I., and Aggarwal, A. K. 1971. Depression across cultures. Br. J. Psychiatry 119: 253–263.
74. Tredgold, R. F. 1941. Depressive states in the soldier. Br. med. J. 2: 109.
75. Venkoba Rao, A. 1966. Depression – a psychiatric analysis of 30 cases. Indian J. Psychiatry 8: 143–154.
76. Vlissades, B. N., and Jenner, F. A. 1982. The response of endogenously and reactively depressed patients to electroconvulsive therapy. Br. J. Psychiatry 141: 239–242.
77. Wing, J. K., Cooper, J. E., and Sartorius, N. 1974. The Measurement and Classification of Psychiatric Symptoms: An Instruction Manual for the PSE and Catego Programme. Cambridge University Press, Cambridge.

Chapter 20 The Symptom-Rating Test

R. KELLNER

The Symptom-Rating Test (SRT) was originally designed to measure changes in the symptoms of neurotic adults and in experiments in therapeutics, such as drug trials. After several stages of research, new versions were designed to make the scale more economical and sensitive to discriminate between the effects of psychotropic drugs and placebo, or between two drugs in double-blind drug trials. It has been found to be a measure of distress and it has been used effectively with depressed patients [5, 10, 19, 20, 24], in psychosomatic disorders [9-11, 21], in schizophrenics [15, 16], and in epidemiological studies [6, 7].

A large number of studies have been carried out with the SRT which have attested its reliability, validity, and sensitivity. Only some of the studies are summarized here; most of them have been listed elsewhere [15, 16]. All correlation coefficients listed refer to the Spearman *rho* [23], except where otherwise indicated. Results at, or below, the conventional 5% level of probability were regarded as statistically significant.

Development of the Scales

Each stage of the development of the scales was based on research findings. The initial checklist was compiled from the complaints of 100 consecutive neurotic patients; the aim was to compile a short, but comprehensive, checklist of symptoms, using expressions easily understood by most patients. Subsequent studies have shown that the symptoms were readily accepted and understood by patients in England and in various parts of the United States. Italian and Spanish translations have been validated [11, 22]. (Copies of the translations are available from the author.) After several item analyses based on sensitivity of the items in drug trials and on published factor analytic studies of symptoms, the list of symptoms was condensed and some symptoms were eliminated.

Initially, test cards were used for self-rating and each symptom was rated on three dimensions: intensity, duration, and frequency of occurrence, with a compound score taking into account all three dimensions. It was found that some scores were more sensitive than others [16] and the use of one scale for each symptom was as effective as the more time-consuming self-rating of three dimensions. Subsequent studies showed that no advantage was gained by increasing the number of items beyond a certain point and a short version was constructed. The short form of the SRT which contains the depression scale has 30 items; the expanded version which has seven scales (SRT-7) is described below; it has another 26 items [14].

A comparison of pencil and paper test and test cards showed that the pencil and paper version was almost as sensitive [3, 17] and for the sake of economy the checklist was omitted and the self-rating scales retained. Studies showed that most patients preferred a box scale to a continuous line [1]. The cues for self-rating were simplified and became similar to those used in several other self-rating scales of symptoms [16].

Reliability

The problems of testing reliability of a distress scale which measures a changeable state are different from those of a personality inventory which measures stable traits. These issues have been discussed elsewhere [13]. The function of the SRT is analogous to that of a clinical thermometer rather than to that of a tape measure.

Several tests of reliability were carried out. Test-retest reliabilities after short intervals ranged from 0.94 to 0.92. The conventional split half reliability test was not carried out because the items are not psychometrically equivalent. Using the test card version, the changes in scores of one-half of the scale were correlated with those of the other half; this split half reliability of *changes* of SRT scores in neurotic outpatients ($N = 40$) after 1 month was 0.89.

Validity and Sensitivity

A large number of conventional validity studies were carried out [15, 16]. The items of the checklist were administered to psychiatric patients and normals, both in England and in the United States, and in one of these studies only 2 of the 39 items failed to discriminate at a significant level. (These items have since been eliminated.) To date 17 comparisons between psychiatric patients and normals in various populations have shown that all four scales of the SRT discriminated significantly between patients and normals in all studies. The SRT tends to distinguish psychiatric patients from normal controls with greater accuracy than scales with which it has been compared with [6, 16]. In several studies, the SRT significantly discriminated between patients with somatic disorders such as psoriasis, duodenal ulcer and hypertension and control groups; in some of these disorders, previous studies using different scales failed to do so [9, 11, 18, 21]. For example, patients with confirmed peptic ulcers had higher total SRT scores than other patients with gastric symptoms [21]. Patients with psoriasis and chronic urticaria had higher depression scores than patients with fungal infections of the skin [9], and hyperprolactinemic women had higher depression scores than women attending a family practice clinic and normal controls [18].

The total SRT score was significantly correlated with the neuroticism scale scores of the Eysenck Personality Inventory [8], 0.70 in normals and 0.71 in psychiatric patients; and with the Taylor Manifest Anxiety Scale scores [25], 0.75 in normals and 0.72 in psychiatric patients [16]. Correlations with psychiatrists' ratings varied with the kind of populations studied, the kind of rating scales the psychiatrists used, and the individual scales of the SRT. For example, the depression scale of the SRT showed a correlation of 0.72 (Pearson's product moment method) with the Hamilton Depression Rating Scale [12] in depressed patients and 0.65 in normals. This is a higher correlation than usually found between ratings and self-ratings in depressed patients [10]. The correlation between psychiatrists' ratings and SRT scores in various studies ranged from 0.55 to 0.95, with a median correlation of 0.71.

The SRT has been found to be highly sensitive in discriminating between an active psychotropic drug and placebo in double-blind studies, and between the effects of two drugs. Generally, the sensitivity of the SRT in double-blind drug trials is similar to that of ratings by psychiatrists using standard rating scales such as the Hamilton Depression Rating Scale or the Hamilton Anxiety Rating Scale; it tended to be more sensitive than other self-rating scales included in the same drug trial [15, 19]. The SRT scales were found to be pure state measures [2, 3].

Studies in Depression

The depression level has been evaluated by administering the SRT in various populations in a large number of studies; a few of these have been listed above and others are described elsewhere [15, 16]. Some of these studies are described here in somewhat greater detail.

Fava and his associates administered the SRT to 40 consecutive depressed outpatients who had primary depressions or a major depressive disorder severe enough to require antidepressant treatment. This scale was also administered to a matched control group who were not patients. Both groups were also rated by the Hamilton Depression Rating Scale (HDRS) by a research psychiatrist in a diagnostic and research interview which covered the total duration of the depressive episode. The identification of patients by the SRT and HDRS was almost the same. With a cutoff point score of 7, the SRT misclassified 9 depressives and 4 controls and the HDRS with a cutoff point of 17 misclassified 10 depressives and 2 controls. Moreover, patients who were misclassified by the HDRS had significantly lower SRT depression scores than those who were classified correctly [10]. This finding suggests that the SRT depression score detects depressed patients in need of treatment as accurately as a research psychiatrist using the HDRS. However, the SRT should not be used as the only method for this purpose, and the findings should be confirmed by a clinician.

In a double-blind study Simpson and his associates compared the effects of 150 mg imipramine with those of 300 mg using several rating and self-rating scales. (This study is described in greater detail in Chap. 10). Of the various *total* scores, including the global scales, only the Brief Depression Rating Scale (see Chap. 10) discriminated significantly between the two treatment effects. The SRT depression scale was about as sensitive as the HDRS [24].

Carney and Sheffield compared the responses of ECT in 15 patients with endogenous depression and 14 patients with neurotic depression. The decrease in SRT scores was significantly greater in patients who had been diagnosed as having endogenous depression than in those diagnosed as having neurotic depression. The decrease in endogenous depression was two-thirds of the score before treatment, whereas the decrease in neurotic depression was not significant [5].

Loudon and his associates compared amitriptyline and zimelidine in a drug trial in general practice. The SRT and the HDRS were included among the outcome measures. The changes in scores of the HDRS and the SRT were similar [20].

In a study with nonpsychotic depressed and anxious outpatients, the effects of large doses of chlordiazepoxide were individually titrated. The depression score, as well as the anxiety score, decreased significantly more in the chlordiazepoxide group than in the placebo group [19].

Buckman and Kellner [4] compared changes in depression in hyperprolactinemic patients treated with bromocriptine. Before treatment and while on placebo, eight patients were substantially depressed. In a double-blind crossover study with bromocriptine, there was a significant decrease of the SRT depression scores. The decrease in depression was parallel with the decrease in prolactin levels and the scores after treatment with bromocriptine were in the normal range.

Thus, the findings in studies with depressed patients show that the depression scale of the SRT identifies depressed patients, discriminates between the level of depression and between various sociodemographic groups, and discriminates between the level of depression in patients with various psychosomatic disorders (some of these studies were briefly referred to in the paragraphs on validation studies). The depression score changes in response to treatment; it discriminates between the effects of treatments such as the effects of a psychotropic drug and placebo and in one study discriminated between responses to ECT in two diagnostic categories of depression.

Seven-Scale Version (SRT-7)

The SRT-7 is a modification and expansion of the short form. The depression scale, anxiety scale, and somatic symptom scale have remained unchanged. The inadequacy scale has been deleted because it was found that it did not consist of a factor and contained cognitive symptoms and feeling of inadequacy. The SRT-7 contains four additional scales: cognitive symptom scale, anger-hostility scale, paranoia - self-reference scale, and psychotic symptoms scale. The items of these scales are listed in Appendix A. These new scales, like the original scales of the SRT, are state measures.

The new scales of the SRT-7 have been developed and validated by the same methods as those which comprise the short form [14]. The studies show that the new scales are valid and sensitive to changes in treatment. In nonpsychotic depressives the scores on all scales were higher than in normals, except for the psychotic symptoms scale. (The failure of the psychotic symptom scale to differentiate between these groups was an expected result because this scale was designed to measure symptoms which largely do not occur in nonpsychotic patients.) The SRT-7 takes somewhat longer to administer, but leads to a more thorough screening and exploration of the psychopathology which tends to be associated with depression.

Uses in Clinical Work

In clinical work the SRT-7 can serve as a checklist of symptoms. A review of the symptoms that the patient has checked can save the clinician's time in that he need not repeat all the questions during the interview. Filled in before the interview, the scale can serve as a preliminary measure of the severity of distress by examining whether the patient has checked any symptoms as having troubled him "a great deal" or "extremely – could not have been worse". Some patients who are distressed will fail to reveal the extent of their suffering during an interview, but are willing to do so when filling in self-rating scales. The kind of symptoms which the patient has checked as troublesome or extremely distressing can guide the clinician's emphasis when exploring the psychopathology during the interview. Finally, repeated self-ratings over time can serve as a measure of progress. When treatments have been changed, for example, different medications have been used, the changes in self-ratings can help in assessing which of the drugs has led to the greatest relief of symptoms.

Conclusions

The Symptom-Rating Test (SRT – short form) consists of four self-rating scales: depression, anxiety, somatic symptoms, and inadequacy. The scale was designed for the measurement of changes in the symptoms in therapeutics such as in drug trials. In a large number of studies it was found to discriminate consistently between psychiatric patients and normals. In drug trials it was found to be sensitive in distinguishing between the responses to psychotropic drugs and placebo and between the responses to two drugs. Later findings suggest that the scales are measures of distress and their use is not limited to neurotic patients. The SRT has been used effectively in the measurement of changes in depression and changes in distress in schizophrenia and in the measurement of distress in various psychosomatic disorders. It identifies depressed patients about as accurately as a psychiatrist using a standard rating scale of depression and it has been used effectively in epidemiological research. The seven-scale version (SRT-7) also includes scales of anger-hostility, cognitive symptoms, paranoia-self-reference, and psychotic symptoms; it has been used effectively as a screening device and in the study of the psychopathology of depressed patients. In clinical work, if administered before the interview, it can help as a preliminary assessment of the severity of the patient's complaints, it can serve as a checklist of symptoms, it helps to assess which of the symptoms the patient finds most distressing, and, if the patient had several treatments, it can help to assess which of the treatments was the most effective.

Appendix A

Seven-scale version of the SRT (SRT-7)

The layout and instructions and examples for the patient are the same as those of the short form [16]. The cues for self-rating are at the top of the forms and the scores are as follows: not at all = 0; a little, slightly = 1; a great deal, quite a bit = 2; extremely, could not have been worse = 3. The score is the sum of the self-rating and each scale is scored separately. The items of the seven scales are listed below. On the form, the items are printed in numerical order.

Scales of the SRT-7

1. Anxiety
    3 Nervous
    5 Scared or frightened
    9 Restless or jumpy
    16 Trembling or shaking
    19 Feeling tense or "wound up"
    23 Thoughts which you cannot push out of your mind
    26 Attacks of panic
    29 It takes a long time to fall asleep, or restless sleep or nightmares

2. Depression
    2 Feeling tired or a lack of energy
    6 Poor appetite
    8 Feeling that there was no hope
    12 Feeling guilty
    18 Feeling unworthy or a failure
    24 Lost interest in most things
    25 Unhappy or depressed
    30 Awakening too early and not being able to fall asleep again

3. Somatic scale
    1 Feeling dizzy or faint
    4 Feelings of pressure or tightness in head or body
    7 Heart beating quickly or strongly without reason (throbbing or pounding)
    11 Chest pains or breathing difficulties or feeling of not having enough air
    14 Muscle pains, aches, or rheumatism
    21 Parts of body feel numb or tingling
    27 Parts of your body feel weak

4. Anger-hostility
   13 Feeling annoyed
   15 Angry
   22 Irritable
   34 Losing temper easily
   40 Furious
   44 Feeling hostile
   46 Feeling of hate

5. Cognitive symptoms
   10 Poor memory
   17 Difficulty in thinking clearly
   20 Mind wanders
   28 Cannot concentrate
   38 Forgetting important matters
   41 Easily distracted
   45 Attention poor

6. Paranoia – self-reference scale
   31 Feeling that people don't like you
   33 Feeling that people look down on you
   35 Feeling that people are hostile to you
   39 Feeling that people are trying to hurt you
   42 Feeling that people are saying bad things about you
   49 Feeling that people are persecuting you
   50 Feeling that people are laughing at you

7. Psychotic symptoms
   32 Strange experiences which others do not have
   36 Hearing voices which others cannot hear
   37 Seeing things others cannot see
   43 Feeling that your body is being influenced by someone
   47 Feeling that people can read your mind or hear your thoughts
   48 Feeling that you are getting messages from TV or radio
   51 Feeling that your thoughts are not your own

References

1. Battle, C. C., Imber, S. D., Hoehn-Saric, R., Stone, A. R., Nash, E. R., and Frank, J. D. 1966. Target complaints as criteria of improvement. Am. J. Psychother. 20: 184–192.
2. Bedford, A., McIver, D., and Pearson, P. R. 1978. A further test of Foulds' personality and personal illness differential in a psychiatric group. Psychol. Med. 8: 467–470.
3. Bedford, A., Edington, A., and Kellner, R. 1979. Changes in self-rating of symptoms: A comparison of questionnaire graphic scales with test cards. Br. J. Psychiatry 134: 108–110.
4. Buckman, M. T., and Kellner, R. 1985. Reduction of distress in hyperprolactinemia with bromocriptine. Am. J. Psychiatry 142: 242–244.
5. Carney, W. P., and Sheffield, B. F. 1974. The effects of pulse ECT in neurotic and endogenous depression. Br. J. Psychiatry 125: 91–94.

6. Cochrane, R. 1980. A comparative evaluation of the Symptom Rating Test and the Langner 22-item Index for use in epidemiological surveys. Psychol. Med. 10: 115-124.
7. Cochrane, R., and Stopes-Roe, M. 1981. Women, marriage and mental health. Br. J. Psychiatry 139: 373-381.
8. Eysenck, H. J., and Eysenck, S. B. G. 1964. Manual of the Eysenck Personality Inventory. University of London Press, London.
9. Fava, G. A., Perini, G. I., Santonastaso, P., and Fornasa, C. V. 1980. Live events and psychological distress in dermatologic disorders: Psoriasis, chronic urticaria and fungal infections. Br. J. Med. Psychol. 53: 277-282.
10. Fava, G. A., Kellner, R., Munari, F., and Pavan, L. 1982. The Hamilton depression rating scale in normals and depressives: A cross-cultural validation. Acta. Psychiatr. Scand. 66: 26-32.
11. Fava, G. A., Kellner, R., Perini, G. I., Fava, M., Michelacci, L., Munari, F., Evangelisti, L. P., Grandi, S., Bernardi, M., and Mastrogiacomo, I. 1983. Italian Validation of the Symptom Rating Test (SRT) and Symptom Questionnaire (SQ). Can. J. Psychiatry 28: 117-123.
12. Hamilton, M. 1960. A rating scale for depression. J. Neurol. Neurosurg. Psychiatry 23: 56-62.
13. Kellner, R. 1971. Improvement criteria in drug trials with neurotic patients. Part 1. Psychol. Med. 1: 416-425.
14. Kellner, R. 1982. Abridged Manual of the Symptom Rating Test - Seven Scale Version (SRT). University of New Mexico, Albuquerque. Mimeographed.
15. Kellner, R. 1982. Symptom Rating Test (SRT): A Survey of Studies. University of New Mexico, Albuquerque.
16. Kellner, R., and Sheffield, B. F. 1973. A self-rating scale of distress. Psychol. Med. 3 (1): 88-100.
17. Kellner, R., Sheffield, B. F., and Simpson, G. M. 1978. The value of self-rating scales in drug trials with nonpsychotic patients. Prog. Neuropsychopharmacol. 2: 197-205.
18. Kellner, R., Buckman, M. T., Fava, G. A., and Pathak, D. 1983. Hyperprolactinemia, distress and hostility. Am. J. Psychiatry. In press.
19. Kellner, R., Rada, R. T., Andersen, T., and Pathak, D. 1979. The effects of chlordiazepoxide on self-rated depression, anxiety, and well-being. Psychopharmacology 64: 185-191.
20. Loudon, J. B., Tiplady, B., Ashcroft, G. W., and Waddell, J. L. 1981. Zimelidine and amitriptyline in the treatment of depressive illness in general practice. Acta Psychiatr. Scand. 63 (suppl. 290): 454-463.
21. Magni, G., de Leo, D., and Salmi, A. 1982. The role of anxiety in duodenal ulceration. S. Afr. Med. J. 20: 262.
22. Perini, G. I., Fava, G. A., Kellner, R., Munari, F., Fava, M., Rossi, N., Grandi, S., Pasquali Evangelisti, L., Bernardi, M., and Zecchino, F. 1982. Validazione Italiana Del Symptom Rating Test (S. R. T.) Di Kellner E Sheffield. In: Canestrari, R. (ed.), Nuovi Metodi In Psicometria, pp. 41-50. Organizzazioni Speciali. Firenze.
23. Siegel, S. 1956. Nonparametric Statistics for the Behavioral Sciences. McGraw Hill, New York.
24. Simpson, G. M., Lee, H. J., Cuculic, Z., and Kellner, R. 1976. Two dosages of imipramine in hospitalized endogenous and neurotic depressives. Arch. Gen. Psychiatry 33: 1093-1102.
25. Taylor, J. A. 1953. A personality scale of manifest anxiety. J. Abnorm. Soc. Psychol. 48: 285-290.

Chapter 21   Zung Self-Rating Depression Scale and Depression Status Inventory

W. W. K. ZUNG

Introduction

Every classification of depressive disorders uses the "Linnaean" binomial approach to its nomenclature that is familiar in taxonomies of both plant and animal kingdoms. Thus, the endogenous-reactive depressions, neurotic-psychotic depressions, or unipolar-bipolar depressions become depression endogenous, depression reactive, depression neurotic, depression psychotic, depression unipolar, or depression bipolar. The term depression is used as an equivalent to the "genus" and is modified by a term that is equivalent to the "species" of the binomial nomenclature. Conceptualized in this manner, the genus denotes depression as a disorder with common characteristics of types or subtypes of depression. To be operationally effective, symptomatology that can be demonstrated in patients diagnosed as having depression (genus), regardless of the type or subtype (species), must have a high degree of universal agreement.

The purpose of my research was first to develop an operational definition of a depressive disorder, second to use the definition in the development of rating scales (both self-rated and interviewer-rated), and third to use the constructed scales to generate a quantifiable data base and test various hypotheses about the diagnosis of the disorder and its treatment.

Methods and Results

Planning an Operational Definition

The hundreds of symptoms and signs used in the vast psychiatric literature to characterize depressive disorders were analyzed and categorized into four basic disturbances: (1) psychic or affective, (2) physiological or somatic, (3) psychomotor, and (4) psychological. Within each category, specific characteristics were selected that could be tested heuristically on potential brain structure-function relationships.

The result of my effort is presented in Table 21.1 [22].

Table 21.1. Diagnostic criteria for a depressive disorder

1. Psychic-affective disturbance
    Depressed mood
    Crying spells
2. Physiological disturbance
    Diurnal variation
    Sleep disturbance
    Decreased appetite
    Decreased libido
    Decreased weight
    Constipation
    Tachycardia
    Increased fatigue
3. Psychomotor disturbance
    Psychomotor retardation
    Psychomotor agitation
4. Psychological disturbance
    Confusion
    Hopelessness
    Irritability
    Indecisiveness
    Personal devaluation
    Emptiness
    Suicidal rumination
    Dissatisfaction

Construction of Rating Scales

The Zung Self-Rating Depression Scale (SDS)

Goals and Construction

The goals in the construction of the SDS were that it should include all the symptoms of the illness; that it should be short and simple; that it should quantify rather than qualify; that it should be self-rated; and that it should indicate the patient's own response at the time the scale is used.

In preparation for constructing the scale, illustrative verbatim records were made from patient interviews. Included were examples that were most representative of a particular symptom. In using the actual scale (see Table 21.2), the patient is asked to rate each of the 20 items as to how they applied to him or her within the past week in the following four quantitative terms: "none or a little of the time," "some of the time," "good part of the time," and "most or all of the time." The SDS is constructed so that the more depressed patients will have higher scores. An index for the SDS was derived by dividing the sum of the values obtained on the 20 items (raw scores) by the maximum possible score of 80.

Table 21.2. The Zung Self-Rating Depression Scale

	None or a little of the time	Some of the time	Good part of the time	Most or all of the time
1. I feel downhearted, blue, and sad				
2. Morning is when I feel the best				
3. I have crying spells or feel like it				
4. I have trouble sleeping through the night				
5. I eat as much as I used to				
6. I enjoy looking at, talking to, and being with attractive women/men				
7. I notice that I am losing weight				
8. I have trouble with constipation				
9. My heart beats faster than usual				
10. I get tired for no reason				
11. My mind is as clear as it used to be				
12. I find it easy to do the things I used to				
13. I am restless and can't sleep				
14. I feel hopeful about the future				
15. I am more irritable than usual				
16. I find it easy to make decisions				
17. I feel that I am useful and needed				
18. My life is pretty full				
19. I feel that others would be better off if I were dead				
20. I still enjoy the things I used to do				

Copyright © W. Zung, 1965, 1974. All rights reserved.

Validity of the SDS

Validity of a scale is the extent to which the instrument actually measures what it seeks to measure. Validity itself can be divided into content validity, concurrent validity, and construct validity.

Content validity can be further divided into face and logical validity. A rating scale can be said to have face validity when the items in the scale are obviously related to the phenomenon measured, when the items are relevant to the stated purpose of the scale, and when they are based upon whatever knowledge is available at the time of the construction. The SDS fulfills this by virtue of its epistemological approach. Its contents are almost identical to those found in the Hamilton Rating Scale for depression [10] as shown in Table 21.3. In addition, it is comparable to later constructed definitions of depressive disorders such as those in the *American Psychiatric Association's Diagnostic and Statistical Manual,* 3rd edition [1], as shown in Table 21.4, and the U.S. Food and Drug Administration's definition for a depressive disorder as found in their guidelines for conducting clinical studies of antidepressants [7] as shown in Table 21.5.

A scale is said to have logical validity when the total area of interest has been defined and broken into categories, with sufficient numbers of items in each category to assess the individual parts of the whole. The SDS was constructed to categorize

Table 21.3. Comparison of the Zung and Hamilton operational definitions for depressive disorders

Zung scale		Hamilton scale	
Number	Item	Item	Number
I.	Pervasive psychic disturbance		
	1. Depressed mood	Depressed mood	1
	2. Crying spells	Depressed mood	1
II.	Physiological disturbance		
	3. Diurnal variation	Diurnal variation	18
	4. Sleep disturbance	Insomnia early, middle, late	4, 5, 6
	5. Decreased appetite	Somatic symptoms, gastrointestinal	12
	6. Decreased weight	Loss of weight	16
	7. Decreased libido	Genital symptoms	14
	8. Constipation	Somatic symptoms, gastrointestinal	12
	9. Tachycardia	Anxiety somatic	11
	10. Increased fatigue	Work and activities	7
		Somatic symptoms general	13
III.	Psychomotor disturbance		
	11. Psychomotor agitation	Agitation	9
	12. Psychomotor retardation	Retardation	8
IV.	Psychological disturbance		
	13. Confusion	Retardation	8
	14. Emptiness		
	15. Hopelessness		
	16. Indecisiveness	Work and activities	7
	17. Irritability		
	18. Dissatisfaction	Work and activities	7
	19. Personal devaluation		
	20. Suicidal rumination	Suicide	3
No corresponding items in Zung		Feelings of guilt	2
		Anxiety psychic	10
		Hypochondriasis	15
		Insight	17
		Depersonalization and derealization	19
		Paranoid symptoms	20
		Obsessional and compulsive symptoms	21

the psychopathology of depressive disorders into the four categories of affective, physiological, psychomotoric, and psychological disturbances.

The concurrent validity of a scale is concerned with the relationship between one scale and others that purport to have the same function. This is measured by the correlation between the scores on the scale with the scores of other scales, when used on the same or similar sample, all determined under the same conditions and in the same circumstances. This was demonstrated in several studies that correlated the SDS with other depression ratings made concurrently using the Hamilton scale [2, 17], the Beck scale [24], the "D" scale of the Minnesota Multiphasic Personality Inventory (MMPI) [23, 30], and the Depression Adjective Checklists [13].

Construct validity has been demonstrated in studies which showed that there was a change in item scores with changes in the depression: depressed patients have sleep disturbances which revert back to normal when their depression improves

Table 21.4. Comparison of the Zung and DSM III operational definitions for a depressive disorder

DSM III diagnostic criteria for major depressive disorder	Self-rating depression scale (Zung)	
	Item content	Number
A. Dysphoric mood:		
1. Depressed, sad, blue	Depressed mood	1
	Crying spells	3
2. Hopelessness	Hopelessness	14
3. Irritability	Irritability	15
B. At least four of the following:		
1. Poor appetite or significant weight loss	Decreased appetite	5
	Weight loss	7
2. Insomnia	Sleep disturbance	4
3. Psychomotor agitation or psychomotor retardation	Psychomotor agitation	13
	Psychomotor retardation	12
4. Loss of interest in usual activities	Emptiness	18
	Dissatisfaction	20
or decrease in sexual drive	Decreased libido	6
5. Loss of energy, fatigue	Fatigue	10
6. Feelings of worthlessness	Personal devaluation	17
7. Diminished ability to think, or indecisiveness	Confusion	11
	Indecisiveness	16
8. Suicidal thoughts, wish to be dead	Suicidal rumination	19

[25]; depressed patients have decreased eye contact which is related to intimacy and distance, which is increased after recovery from depression [11]; depressed patients have functional impairments which are reversible [12]; and depressed patients have an impaired ability to experience humor so that highly depressed patients would rate something humorous as less funny than would patients who were not depressed [21].

Reliability of the SDS

The reliability of a scale, that it measures dependably the same each time, and that it is free from random irrelevant sources of error can be determined by interrater reliability, which is not applicable to the self-rating version of the scale. Several methods are available in the case of self-rating forms of rating scales to determine their reliability. A split-half correlation for the even-odd SDS items was used initially, which yielded a statistically significant r value of 0.73 [28]. Statistical analysis in a later study using the alpha-coefficient calculation for reliability analysis yielded a coefficient alpha of 0.92, indicating high internal consistency for the depressive disorder as measured by the SDS.

Table 21.5. Comparison of the Zung and Food and Drug Administration (FDA) guidelines for psychotropic drugs definitions for depressive disorders

Zung Scale	FDA guidelines	
I. Pervasive psychic disturbance		
1. Depressed mood	Depressed mood	(a)
3. Crying spells		
II. Physiological disturbance		
2. Diurnal variation		
4. Sleep disturbance	Sleep difficulty	(d)
5. Decreased appetite	Poor appetite	(c)
6. Decreased libido	Decrease in libido	(h)
7. Decreased weight		
8. Constipation		
9. Tachycardia		
10. Increased fatigue	Loss of energy	(e)
III. Psychomotor disturbance		
12. Psychomotor retardation	Retardation	(g)
13. Psychomotor agitation	Agitation	(f)
IV. Psychological disturbance		
11. Confusion	Diminished thinking and concentration	(k)
14. Hopelessness	Helplessness/hopelessness	(m)
15. Irritability		
16. Indecisiveness	Work and activities	(i)
17. Personal devaluation	Self-reproach or guilt	(j)
18. Emptiness	Work and activities	(i)
19. Suicidal rumination	Thoughts of death/suicide	(l)
20. Dissatisfaction	Work and activities	(j)
	Anhedonia	(b)
No corresponding items in Zung	Anxiety or tension	(n)
	Bodily complaints	(o)

Establishing Baseline SDS Values

The fabric of normal emotions includes feelings of happiness and sadness together with other emotions. In a perusal of the signs and symptoms listed in any operational definition of depression, it becomes evident that most, if not all of them, are experienced by us, singly and in differing combinations, to varying degrees, and at various times. Therefore, it is important to establish normal baseline or reference values on any psychometric scale and show significant quantitative differences between scores of depressed patients and normal control individuals.

The SDS was administered to groups of normal subjects who were tested at school or at work, while carrying out the ordinary demands of their lives. Results of such studies conducted in the United States showed that controls between the ages of 20 and 64 years old had a mean SDS index of 39, while controls younger and older had higher mean SDS indices [26]. In addition to the normative data from the United States, data from normal control subjects from other countries of the world have been published. These include studies in Australia [3]; Czechoslovakia,

England, Germany, Spain, and Sweden [24]; India [14]; Japan [9]; Korea [19]; and the Netherlands [31]. Mean SDS indices from Czechoslovakia, Korea, and Sweden were higher than those from the other countries studied, which were comparable to the United States data, with mean SDS indices below 50.

SDS Results in Patients with Depressive Disorders

Results of the SDS given to groups of patients with diagnoses of depressive disorders in the United States as well as in other countries are shown in Table 21.6.

This cross-national comparison of psychiatric patients with diagnoses of depression permits evaluation of the effects of many variables. If depression has a biological basis of organic etiology (whether it be genetic, biochemical, neurophysiological, or any combination of factors), the resultant alteration of the central nervous system should produce behavioral (symptoms and signs), biochemical (levels of neurotransmitters, or endocrine production), neurophysiological (sleep electroencephalogram, photic arousal responses) and other changes that are independent of social and cultural influences, i.e., culture free.

To perform the studies, the SDS was translated into the native language of the patients. Presently, the SDS is available in 30 languages (Chinese, Czech, Dutch, English, Estonian, Finnish, French, German, Greek, Hmong, Hungarian, Italian, Japanese, Korean, Lao, Luganda, Marathi, Norwegian, Persian, Polish, Romanian, Russian, Serbo-Croatian, Slovakian, Spanish, Swedish, Thai, Turkish, Vietnamese, and Yiddish) and has been used as a measure for rating depression in studies reported in over 300 publications. McNair reviewed self-evaluations used in antidepressant clinical drug trials conducted from 1955 to 1972 [15]. He reported that the Zung SDS was second only to the MMPI as the most often used scale out of 123 published studies chosen for review and more than twice as many statistical comparisons of treatments have been made with the Zung SDS than with any other scale. In addition, more data and experience with the SDS are available than for any other scale, and on most counts no other widely used self-rating scale has been shown to be superior to it.

Table 21.6. Comparison of Self-Rating Depression Scale indices from patients with depressive disorders in various countries

Country	N	SDS index Mean (SD)
Australia	135	56.4 (16.0)
Canada	136	59.0 (14.0)
Czechoslovakia	360	61.5 (12.5)
England	105	61.8 (10.5)
Germany	79	65.1 (10.8)
India	430	69.8 (12.8)
Italy	82	62.2 (6.6)
Japan	50	59.7 (7.3)
Korea	96	70.0 (24.4)
Netherlands	95	66.1 (11.7)
United States	360	64.0 (12.0)

SDS Results in Nonpsychiatric Settings

The SDS has been used as a screening diagnostic tool to detect depression in patients treated for medical and surgical problems. When the SDS was administered in a general medical screening clinic of a university teaching hospital, to which patients usually came complaining of a physical medical problem, 35% of these patients scored in the morbidity range of the SDS, which is an index of 50 or above [18]. In a recent study where the SDS was given to over 1000 patients seen in a family medicine centre, 13% of these patients had scored 55 or above and had depression corresponding to DSM-III diagnostic criteria for a major affective disorder [33]. When the SDS was given to over 1000 elderly male hypertensive outpatients, 43% of the subjects scored in the morbid range of the SDS [8]. In another study, 50 patients who had sustained acute trauma to the spinal and paraspinal structures were given the SDS. Seventy percent of these patients had indices of 50 or higher [6]. A number of studies on patients with chronic pain have been reported. Patients with severe or disabling migraine headaches demonstrated the presence of depressive symptoms [4, 5]. Also in patients with chronic stable back pain due to a demonstrable organic cause, the SDS showed that this patient population had significantly higher SDS indices than did normal control subjects [16]. In studies of the relationship between depression and alcoholism, results indicated that depressive symptomatology is very high in alcoholic patients [20].

The Depression Status Inventory (DSI)

Goals of the DSI

In the recording of patient symptomatology for clinical or research purposes, studies that rate only the interviewer's impressions or record only self-evaluations from the patient are less useful than when both methods are used and particularly if the instruments employed identical operational definitions for the disorder. In order to obtain an interviewer rating, we could use a global rating system or an existing scale such as the Hamilton Rating Scale for Depression. However, to compare the SDS results with the Hamilton or any other scale is difficult inasmuch as they do not measure exactly the same thing. For example, the Hamilton Rating Scale for Depression includes ratings for anxiety that would confound a measure of depression in the total score. Thus, the disadvantage of each instrument of looking only in one direction is not necessarily corrected by the addition of the other.

After the development of a patient self-rating scale for the measurement of depressive symptomatology in the form of the SDS, I constructed an inventory that would record the results of a clinical interview [27]. The goals were: to provide an interviewer-rated scale that corresponded to the SDS with respect to the diagnostic criteria used, to have a standardized method of recording the patient's clinical status using a semistructured inventory and to record responses in a quantitative manner rather than as yes or no.

Table 21.7. The Zung Depression Status Inventory (DSI)

	Interview guide for DSI	Severity of observed or reported responses:			
		None	Mild	Moderate	Severe
1. Depressed mood	Have you been feeling sad or depressed lately?	1	2	3	4
2. Diurnal variation	Is there any part of the day when you feel worst? How do you feel most mornings?	1	2	3	4
3. Crying spells	Do you have crying spells or feel like it?	1	2	3	4
4. Sleep disturbance	How have you been sleeping?	1	2	3	4
5. Decreased appetite	How is your appetite?	1	2	3	4
6. Weight loss	Have you lost any weight?	1	2	3	4
7. Decreased libido	Has there been any recent change in your interest in sex? Do you enjoy looking, talking, or being with attractive women/men?	1	2	3	4
8. Constipation	Do you have trouble with constipation?	1	2	3	4
9. Tachycardia	Have you had times when your heart was beating faster than usual	1	2	3	4
10. Fatigue	How easily do you get tired?	1	2	3	4
11. Psychomotor retardation	Do you feel slowed down in doing the things you usually do?	1	2	3	4
12. Confusion	Do you ever feel confused and have trouble thinking?	1	2	3	4
13. Psychomotor agitation	Do you find yourself restless and can't sit still?	1	2	3	4
14. Irritability	How easily do you get irritated?	1	2	3	4
15. Indecisiveness	How are you at making decisions?	1	2	3	4
16. Hopelessness	How hopeful do you feel about the future?	1	2	3	4
17. Personal devaluation	Do you ever feel useless and not wanted?	1	2	3	4
18. Emptiness	Do you feel life is empty for you?	1	2	3	4
19. Dissatisfaction	Do you still enjoy the things you used to?	1	2	3	4
20. Suicidal ruminations	Do you feel others would be better off if you were dead?	1	2	3	4

Copyright © W. Zung, 1972. All rights reserved.

Table 21.8. Statistical analyses comparing mean DSI and SDS scores of various diagnostic groups tested

Diagnosis	N	Mean DSI score	Mean SDS index
Depressive disorders	96	61	65
Schizophrenia	25	48	51
Anxiety disorder	22	50	53
Personality disorder	54	52	56
Transient situational disturbance	12	44	48
		$P<0.01$	$P<0.01$

Construction of the DSI

The procedure for the development of the DSI was: deciding what is to be measured in terms of explicitly defined units, formulating instructions on how to observe and elicit behavior and information to complete the DSI, and using the DSI to obtain a data base for purposes of studying the psychometric properties of the scale. The constructed DSI is shown in Table 21.7.

The DSI and SDS were simultaneously administered to 225 patients and the results are shown in Table 21.8. Analysis of variance and t-tests showed that the mean scores of patients with a diagnosis of depression were significantly higher than scores obtained from the other five diagnostic groups ($P<0.01$). Similarly, the SDS scores of the various diagnostic groups showed that patients with depression scored significantly higher than those with other diagnoses ($P<0.01$).

The correlation between the DSI and the SDS was 0.87 (Pearson's r). Split-half correlation for the ten even-numbered and the ten odd-numbered DSI items was 0.81 ($P<0.01$), indicating a high reliability and internal consistency. Simultaneous ratings using the DSI were performed by two raters and the interrater reliability as calculated by product moment correlation was significant ($P<0.01$), with an r value of 0.91.

Both the DSI and SDS were used in several investigations including a clinical trial to evaluate Gerovital H3 as an antidepressant drug by comparing it with imipramine and placebo [32], and in an investigation of longitudinal changes occurring in patients with depression only, dementia only, depression and dementia, and normal healthy elderly controls [29].

References

1. American Psychiatric Association. 1980. Diagnostic and Statistical Manual of Mental Disorders, 3rd Ed. American Psychiatric Association, Washington DC.
2. Brown, G. L., and Zung, W. W. K. 1972. Depression scales: Self- or physician-rating? Compr. Psychiatry 13: 361–367.
3. Byrne, D. 1980. The prevalence of symptoms of depression in an Australian general population. Aus. N. Z. J. Psychiatry 14: 65–71.
4. Couch, J., Ziegler, D., and Hassanein, R. 1976. Evaluation of the relationship between migraine headache and depression. Headache 15: 41–50.

5. Couch, J., Ziegler, D., and Hassanein, R. 1976b. Amitriptyline in the prophylaxis of migraine. Neurology 26: 121-127.
6. Crobsy, A. 1969. The use of the SDS after traumatic injury. J. Am. Osteopath. Assoc. 69: 269-270.
7. FDA guidelines for psychotropic drugs. 1974. Psychopharmacol. Bull. 10: 70-91.
8. Friedman, M., and Bennet, P. 1977. Depression and hypertension. Psychosom. Med. 39: 134-142.
9. Fukuda, K., and Kobayashi, S. 1973. A study on a self-rating depression scale. Psychiatrica et Neurologia Japonica 75: 673-679.
10. Hamilton, M. 1960. A rating scale for depression. J. Neurol. Neurosurg. Psychiatry 23: 56-62.
11. Hinchlif, M., Lancashi, M., and Roberts, F. 1971. Study of eye-contact changes in depressed and recovered psychiatric patients. Br. J. Psychiatry 119: 213-215.
12. Humphrey, M. 1967. Functional impairment in psychiatric out-patients. Br. J. Psychiatry 113: 1141-1151.
13. Marone, J., and Lubin, B. 1968. Relationship between set 2 of the depression adjective checklists (DACL) and Zung Self-rating Depression Scale (SDS). Psychol. Rep. 22: 333-334.
14. Master, R., and Zung, W.W.K. 1977. Depressive symptoms in patients and normal subjects in India. Arch. Gen. Psychiatry 34: 972-974.
15. McNair, D. 1974. Self-evaluations of antidepressants. Psychopharmacologia 37: 281-302.
16. Mendelson, G., Kranz, H., and Kidson, M. 1977. Acupuncture for chronic pain. Clin. Exp. Neurol. 14: 154-161.
17. Prange, A. 1969. Enhancement of imipramine antidepressant activity by thyroid hormone. Am. J. Psychiatry 126: 39-51.
18. Raft, D., Spencer, R., Toomey, T., and Brogan, D. 1977. Depression in medical out-patients. Diseases of the Nervous System 38: 999-1004.
19. Rhee, J., and Shin, S. 1978. An ophthalmologic and psychiatric study on the headache: chiefly on the depression, anxiety, deviations and refractive errors. Chungnam Medical Journal 5: 57-66.
20. Shaw, J., Donley, P., Morgan, D., and Robinson, A. 1975. Treatment of depression in alcoholics. Am. J. Psychiatry 132: 641-644.
21. Stumphauzer, J., and Cantor, J. 1968. Depression and responses to humour. Veterans Administration Psychology Newsletter, February.
22. Zung, W.W.K. 1965. A self-rating depression scale. Arch. Gen. Psychiatry 12: 63-70.
23. Zung, W.W.K. 1967. Factors influencing the Self-Rating Depression Scale. Arch. Gen. Psychiatry 16: 543-547.
24. Zung, W.W.K. 1969. A cross-cultural survey of symptoms in depression. Am. J. Psychiatry 126: 116-121.
25. Zung, W.W.K. 1969. Effect of antidepressant drugs on sleeping and dreaming: III. On the depressed patient. Biol. Psychiatry 1: 283-287.
26. Zung, W.W.K. 1972. How normal is depression? Psychosomatics 13: 174-178.
27. Zung, W.W.K. 1972. The Depression Status Inventory: An adjunct to the Self-rating Depression Scale. J. Clin. Psychol. 28: 539-543.
28. Zung, W.W.K. 1973. From art to science: The diagnosis and treatment of depression. Arch. Gen. Psychiatry 29: 328-337.
29. Zung, W.W.K. 1982. The puzzle of depression diagnoses: A binomial solution. In: J. Cavenar and H. Brodie (eds.), Critical Problems in Psychiatry. Lippencott, Philadelphia.
30. Zung, W.W.K., Richards, C., and Short, M. 1965. Self-rating depression scale in an out-patient clinic. Arch. Gen. Psychiatry 13: 508-515.
31. Zung, W.W.K., van Praag, J., Dijkstra, P., and van Winzum, P. 1975. Cross-cultural survey of symptoms in depressed and normal adults. In: T. Itil (ed.), Transcultural Neuropsychopharmacology. Bozak, Istanbul.
32. Zung, W.W.K., Gianturco, D., Pfeiffer, E., Wang, H.S., Whanger, A., Bridge, T., and Potkin, S. 1974. Pharmacology of depression in the aged: Evaluation of Gerovital H3 as an antidepressant drug. Psychosomatics 15: 127-131.
33. Zung, W.W.K., Magill, M. Moore, J., and George, D. 1983. Recognition and treatment of depression in a family medicine practice. J. Clin. Psychiatry 44: 3-6.

Chapter 22 Depression Scales Derived from the Hopkins Symptom Checklist

R. S. LIPMAN

The Hopkins Symptom Checklist (HSCL) is a patient self-report symptom inventory derived from the Cornell Medical Index. The HSCL was developed initially to measure the more common psychoneurotic complaints of outpatients [18]. An early version of the instrument, the "Discomfort Scale," was used by Parloff et al. [26] and by Frank et al. [11] as an improvement measure in their studies of psychotherapy. Frank et al. [11], for example, employed a 41-item version of the HSCL in a series of psychotherapy studies.

History

Since 1960, the major development of the HSCL was supported by grants from the Psychopharmacology Research Branch, National Institute of Mental Health to the Johns Hopkins University (MH-04732, MH-15720, MH-24354, MH-26101); to the University of Pennsylvania (MH-04732, MH-08958); and to the University of Chicago (HSM-42-69-59). This development, which included several versions of the HSCL, varying in length from 35 items to 58 items to 90 items, grew out of the collaboration among Ronald S. Lipman and Seymour Fisher (NIMH); Lee C. Park, Lino Covi, and Leonard R. Derogatis (Johns Hopkins University); Karl Rickels and Robert W. Downing (University of Pennsylvania; and E. H. Uhlenhuth (Johns Hopkins University and University of Chicago) [3, 4, 7, 8, 17, 19, 20, 21, 32, 36, 38, 42].

While the major psychometric development of the HSCL has focused on a 58-item version, a 35-item version of the HSCL was included in the Early Clinical Drug Evaluation Unit (ECDEU) battery of the Psychopharmacology Research Branch [12].

The HSCL-58 has been extensively reviewed in two recent publications [7, 8]. Repeated factor analyses of the HSCL-58 have revealed the presence of five primary dimensions of symptomatology which have been labeled interpersonal sensitivity, somatization, anxiety, depression, and cognitive-performance difficulty or obsessive-compulsive. These dimensions have shown adequate reliability, good construct validity, reasonable factorial invariance, and differential sensitivity to change in controlled studies of psychotropic drugs and psychotherapy.

The factor analysis of a 72-item version of the HSCL based on the pretreatment scores of a depressed nonpsychotic outpatients who participated in a NIMH-PRB

Drug-Group Psychotherapy trial initiated in 1969 [3, 4, 17] revealed the presence of an anger-hostility, phobic-anxiety, and sleep difficulty factor.

The most recent version of the HSCL is a 90-item scale evolved from prior versions of the HSCL to provide a more complete representation of phobic-anxiety and anger-hostility and to develop two additional dimensions reflective of more seriously disturbed symptomatology, i.e., psychoticism and paranoid ideation[1] [22] (Appendix A). A factor analysis of the HSCL-90 performed on the pretreatment self-ratings of more than 300 nonpsychotic outpatients with symptoms of depression and anxiety revealed the presence of 8 clinically meaningful factors. These orthogonal factors each contained at least five items and were labeled somatization, phobic-anxiety, retarded depression, agitated depression, obsessive-compulsive, interpersonal sensitivity, anger-hostility, and psychoticism.

Depression Subscales (35- and 58-item HSCL)

Since this book focuses on the evaluation of depressive states, the various factors derived from the HSCL that measure depression are presented in Tables 22.1–22.7. Table 22.1 presents the depression dimension contained in the 35-item HSCL. The nine items subsumed under the depression dimension reflect the basic mood dysphoria and many of the associated somatic complaints experienced by depressed patients, i.e., "difficulty in falling asleep or staying asleep" and "poor appetite." The cognitive content of the depression measure is also reflective of Beck's formulation (1) in that it contains the item "feeling hopeless about the future" and "blaming yourself for things." These two items are reflective of a negative view of oneself and one's future. Feelings of anhedonia are reflected in the item "loss of sexual interest or pleasure."

Since the 35-item HSCL is no longer very often used in clinical trials, a more detailed explication of the depression dimension will be presented with regard to that dimension as it is defined by the 11 items shown in Table 22.2.

Table 22.1. Depression factors from the 35-item HSCL

No.	Item
9.	Blaming yourself for things
18.	Crying easily
22.	Loss of sexual interest or pleasure
24.	Poor appetite
26.	Difficulty in falling asleep or staying asleep
27.	Feeling hopeless about the future
28.	Feeling blue
29.	Feeling lonely
35.	Thoughts of ending your life

---

[1] A copy of the HSCL-90 can be obtained by writing to Dr. Ron Lipman, Friends Hospital, Dept. of Research, Roosevelt Boulevard at Adams Avenue, Philadelphia, PA 19124

Table 22.2. HSCL depression (test-retest reliability coefficient)

Items	(r11)
Feeling low in energy or slowed down	
Thoughts of ending your life	
Poor appetite	
Feeling blue	
Feeling no interest in things	
Feeling hopeless about the future	
Blaming yourself for things	
Loss of sexual interest or pleasure	
Crying easily	
Feeling lonely	
Constipation	(0.81)

Basically, this 11-item depression dimension was developed on the basis of clinical consensus. Historically, the HSCL was scored for "psychic" and "somatic" symptoms, for target symptoms (symptoms independently checked as bothersome by the patient and the patient's treating doctor), and for total score. In this regard, each item of the HSCL was rated by the patient in terms of how much the item bothered him/her during the past week on a four-point intensity scale (1, not at all; 2, a little bit; 3, quite a bit; 4, extremely). To the clinician, it seemed obvious that the 58-item HSCL contained a number of different dimensions of "neuroticism" [20]. Working independently, Rickels and Uhlenhuth both employed experienced psychiatrists and clinical psychologists to subdivide the HSCL items into more homogeneous symptom clusters. Since these independent efforts produced excellent clinical concordance, only one grouping and its development will be described. The following four a priori clusters were specified: (1) anxiety, (2) depression, (3) anger-hostility, and (4) obsessive-compulsive phobia. At two rating sessions, 2 weeks apart, 20 experienced clinicians independently categorized the items of the HSCL using the clusters indicated above. Only those items allocated to each cluster that were agreed upon by at least 75% of the raters at both sessions were retained as defining the cluster. In fact, the first six of the items, as shown in Table 22.2, were designated as defining depression by all 20 raters at both rating sessions.

A depression factor was also found statistically when the 58-item HSCL ratings of a very large sample ($N=1115$) of anxious neurotic outpatients was factor analyzed. This factor contained only four items: (1) "poor appetite," (2) "crying easily," (3) "loss of sexual interest or pleasure," and (4) "feeling no interest in things." An earlier factor analysis by Mattson et al. [24] had found the items "feeling low in energy or slowed down" and "constipation" to be significantly loaded on a depression factor. The results of this early work have been summarized by Williams et al. [42]. Despite the larger number of items contained in the depression cluster, as contrasted with the depression factor (e.g., 11 items vs 4 items), the correlation of patient scores on these depression measures was found to be very high, $r=0.86$ [20]. A considerable amount of psychometric work has been done with the 58-item HSCL. This research has been summarized by Derogatis et al. [7].

In this regard, the depression cluster, as presented in Table 22.2, has demonstrated adequate reliability. The degree of internal consistency, as defined by coefficient alpha, was 0.86. Test-retest reliability, based on a sample of over 400 anxious neurotic outpatients tested 1 week apart, was 0.81. Normative data are also available for the 58-item version of the HSCL. The individuals comprising the normative sample were 735 noninstitutionalized adults living in Oakland, California. The HSCL was administered to each respondent by a trained interviewer as part of a 60- to 90-min interview session which focused on the health of the person. This group represents a true probability sample of households in the Oakland area. The mean depression cluster score in this normative group ($X=1.14$, $SD=0.28$) was found to be substantially lower than the mean depression score ($X=2.04$, $SD=0.63$) of a large sample ($N=1435$) of anxious neurotic outpatients, which, in turn, was significantly lower than the mean depression score ($X=2.62$, $SD=0.63$) of a sample ($N=367$) of nonpsychotic depressed outpatients. This logically expected rank ordering of the severity of depression in these samples is a good example of the criterion-related validity of the HSCL. Along these same lines, Prusoff and Klerman [27] utilized a discriminant function approach to see whether or not the HSCL, in terms of the 58 items and in terms of the 5 HSCL dimensions, was capable of differentiating between patient samples diagnosed as having depressive disorders or anxiety states. The 364 patients in the anxious and depressed groups were matched for age, sex, social class, and race. The depressed cohort scored significantly higher on the depression dimension of the HSCL-58 than on the anxiety dimension, whereas the opposite pattern characterized the anxious group. The 68% discrimination of the anxious and depressed cohorts found in this study on the basis of HSCL scores was significantly better than chance.

In addition to factor-analytic studies using patient self-ratings on the HSCL-58, the ratings of psychiatrists have also been subject to factor analysis. Lipman et al. [21] reported psychiatric ratings of 837 anxious outpatients. The doctor form of the HSCL contained the same four-point scale as the patient version which describes the degree of distress that each symptom caused the patient during the previous week. The doctor also used a "not elicited" category. The 7 items with significant factor loadings on the factor labeled depression were all contained among the 11 items of the depression cluster (Table 22.2). The items with statistically significant factor loadings above 0.45 were: (1) "thoughts of ending your life," (2) "feeling blue," (3) "loss of sexual interest or pleasure," (4) "feeling hopeless about the future," (5) "poor appetite," (6) "feeling lonely," and (7) "constipation." Clearly, this correspondence among the items comprising the depression factor and the depression cluster buttresses our confidence in the validity of these constructs.

In addition to its reliability, criterion validity, and construct validity, the depression cluster of the HSCL-58 has proven sensitive to the differential effects of tricyclic antidepressants versus placebos and tranquilizers (cf., for example, 3, 17, 28). Kellner has referred to this ability of scales to differentiate the effects of "active medication" from placebo as "chemical validation" [15].

Another application of depression cluster scores has involved using a minimum cutoff score on the depression cluster as a prerequisite for the selection of depressed patients for drug trials [5, 23].

In our experience this procedure has worked very well, particularly in the selection of "symptomatic volunteers" for drug trials. We have employed a mean score of 1.70 as a minimal criterion, which corresponds to a score 2 standard deviations higher than the mean score of 1.14 obtained by our normative sample on the depression cluster. In the context of a drug trial with depressed outpatients using this minimal criterion [17], actual mean pretreatment depression cluster symptom levels were found to be roughly four standard deviations (SDs) higher than the normative mean. After 16 weeks of treatment, imipramine patients, on average, were found to be only 1.5 SDs above the normative mean for depression, while placebo patients were 3 SDs above the mean and diazepam patients were about 3.75 SDs above the mean. Treatment effect analyses in this study [17] strongly favored the efficacy of imipramine over the other medications.

Depression Subscales (HSCL-90)

While other versions of the HSCL have also been developed to meet the needs of specific studies, the 90-item version of the HSCL represents a major milestone in the development of the instrument [22]. The 90-item version of the HSCL contains the core items that defined the five basic dimensions of outpatient psychopathology from the HSCL-58. Items were also added to measure some dimensions better, and an attempt was made to measure two newly postulated dimensions of more severe psychopathology, i.e., paranoid ideation and psychoticism. The HSCL-90 has been incorporated by the National Institute of Mental Health into the basic ECDEU battery [11] and has been recommended, by the Clinical Research Branch in its publication on rating scales, for use as a psychotherapy change measure. It is currently included as an outcome measure in the ongoing Psychotherapy of Depression project being supported by the NIMH. The HSCL-90 and all other versions of the HSCL are in the public domain.

The postulated composition of the depression scale of the HSCL-90 is presented in Table 22.3. The depression cluster contains 13 items, 9 of which were also contained in the depression cluster of the HSCL-58. Two items were deleted: "poor appetite" and "constipation." In this regard, many depressed patients tend to over-

Table 22.3. HSCL-90: postulated depression factor

No.	Item
5.	Loss of sexual interest or pleasure
14.	Feeling low in energy or slowed down
15.	Thoughts of ending your life
20.	Crying easily
22.	Feeling of being trapped or caught
26.	Blaming yourself for things
29.	Feeling lonely
30.	Feeling blue
31.	Worrying too much about things
32.	Feeling no interest in things
54.	Feeling hopeless about the future
71.	Feeling everything is an effort
79.	Feelings of worthlessness

eat and constipation is a frequent side-effect of the antidepressant medications, and it seemed desirable to avoid confounding therapeutic effects with adverse treatment emergent symptoms. Four items were added: (1) "feeling everything is an effort," (2) "feelings of worthlessness," (3) "feeling of being trapped or caught," and (4) "worrying too much about things." These items either had borderline factor loadings on depression dimensions in prior factor analyses or were new items (e.g., items 1 and 2 above) which were frequently used as descriptions of depression in the literature.

The basic validity of this depression dimension has already been established in the prior research done with the very similar dimension contained in the 58-item version of the HSCL. A recent concurrent validation study with the HSCL-90 [9] compared the dimensions of the HSCL-90 with the standard clinical scales of the Minnesota Multiphasic Personality Inventory (MMPI) using a sample of 209 "symptomatic volunteers" as subjects. The HSCL 90 depression cluster scale was found to be most highly correlated with the content Depression Scale (0.75) and the cluster Depression Scale (0.68) of the MMPI. The authors conclude that the various depression scales were measuring "analogue constructs."

The dimensional structure of the HSCL-90 has also been subjected to a confirmatory empirical test with a sample of 1002 heterogeneous outpatients [6]. A modified factor-analytic method, a "Procrustes solution," was used to compare the hypothesized nine clinical clusters of the HSCL-90 with the factor analytic structure of the instrument as determined empirically. The hypothetical depression cluster (see Table 22.3) proved to be an excellent match to the empirical factor. Only one item, "loss of sexual interest or pleasure," was missing in the Varimax procedure while all 13 items had substantial loadings in the Procrustes procedure. An extra item, "feeling lonely even when you are with people," also loaded in the empirical solutions. It will be recalled that this item also appeared in the retarded depression factor found by Lipman et al. [22] in their orthogonal factor analysis. These confirmations of hypothesized and observed depression dimensions clearly contribute to the construct validity of the HSCL-90 depression scales.

A factor analysis of the 90-item version of the HSCL was performed on the pretreatment ratings of 320 outpatients with symptoms of depression and anxiety [22]. Eight clinically meaningful orthogonal factors were found, including the presence of two depression factors. The larger depression factor, called retarded depression, is presented in Table 22.4.

This factor rather closely resembles previous depression clusters and a depression factor found in the factor analysis of a 72-item HSCL that was used in a medication and group psychotherapy study with nonpsychotic, depressed outpatients [17]. In fact, eight of the ten items that were contained in the orthogonal depression factor of the 72-item HSCL were also present in the retarded depression factor as shown in Table 22.4. The correspondence between the retarded depression factor and the a priori postulated depression cluster (Table 22.3) was also quite good. The factor contained 9 of the 13 items postulated to form an orthogonal depression dimension.

The second depression factor that emerged from the factor analysis of the HSCL-90 was interpreted as representing agitated or anxious depression. This nine-item factor is presented in Table 22.5.

Table 22.4. HSCL-90 9 factor solution

Item No.	Factor loading	Factor 3: depression (retarded)
14.	0.49	Feeling low in energy or slowed down
15.	0.67	Thoughts of ending your life
23.[a]	0.42	Suddenly scared for no reason (2)
28.	0.58	Feeling blocked in getting things done
29.	0.65	Feeling lonely
30.	0.63	Feeling blue
31.	0.41	Worrying too much about things
32.	0.61	Feeling no interest in things
33.[a]	0.47	Feeling fearful (2)
46.[a]	0.41	Difficulty making decisions (6)
54.	0.67	Feeling hopeless about the future
59.	0.52	Thoughts of death or dying
71.[a]	0.53	Feeling everything is an effort
77.	0.60	Feeling lonely even when you are with people
79.	0.60	Feelings of worthlessness
88.	0.51	Never feeling close to another person

Note: This factor explains 8.56% of the variance in the rotated matrix
[a] Split loading; if higher on another factor, the number of the other factor is given in parentheses

Table 22.5. HSCL-90 9 factor solution

Item No.	Factor loading	Factor 7: agitated depression
2.	0.60	Nervousness or shakiness inside
17.	0.41	Trembling
19.	0.51	Poor appetite
20.	0.48	Crying easily
44.	0.57	Trouble falling asleep
57.	0.43	Feeling tense or keyed up
64.	0.66	Awakening in the early morning
66.	0.63	Sleep that is restless or disturbed
75.	0.43	Feeling nervous when you are left alone

Note: This factor explains 5.45% of the variance in the rotated matrix

The "crying easily" item is reflective of dysphoric mood. "Poor appetite" and the three sleep difficulty items are congruent with their counterpart's items in the Research Diagnostic Criteria (RDC) for major depressive disorders [34]. Anxiety and/or agitation is represented by "nervousness or shakiness inside," "trembling," "feeling tense or keyed up," and "feeling nervous when you are left alone." Although the agitated depression factor was not postulated on an a priori basis, in hindsight it seems relevant to the anxious or agitated subtype of depressed patient identified by Overall and his associates [14, 25]. In a similar vein, Rickels et al. [30] performed a factor analysis on the Zung Self-Rating Depression Scale and found that the 20-item scale also contained two orthogonal depression factors. Factor 1, which they called "retarded depression," contained such items as "hopeless about the future," "feel useless," "life is empty," and "don't enjoy things." The second depression factor, which they labeled "anxious depression," contained the items "crying spells," "trouble sleeping," "restless," and others. The similarity between these factors from the Zung Self-Rated Depression Scale and the retarded and agitated/anxious depression factors from the HSCL-90 is quite evident.

As with the depression cluster and factor of the HSCL-58, the depression cluster and depression factors of the HSCL-90 have demonstrated very substantial internal consistency and test-retest reliability (Pearson's rs vary from 0.82 to 0.90).

Unfortunately, a true probability sample of normal households is not available to establish normative data for the HSCL-90, which employed a five-point item-rating scale: 1 = not at all, 2 = a little bit, 3 = moderately, 4 = quite a bit, and 5 = extremely. It will be recalled that the HSCL-58 contained a four-point item-rating scale in which the anchor point "moderately" was not included. It is clear, however, that patient populations score significantly higher on the depression scales of the HSCL-90 than do nonpatients. In this regard, Ravaris et al. [29], for example, report pretreatment mean depression cluster scores of 3.36 in a sample of 100 depressed outpatients diagnosed by RDC criteria as primarily having nonpsychotic major depressive disorders. In a sample of mixed depressed and anxious outpatients Lipman et al. [22] found a slightly lower but comparable mean depression cluster severity level of 2.98 and a mean severity level of 2.97 for retarded depression and 2.64 for agitated/anxious depression. By contrast, a sample of nonpatient "normals" ($N = 974$) was referred to by Ravaris et al. [29] as having a substantially lower mean depression cluster score of 1.36. The sample of patients in the Ravaris et al. [29] study were about 4 standard deviations higher on the depression cluster of the HSCL-90 than were the nonpatient normals (SD for normals = 0.44). Using an 80-item version of the HSCL which contained all the anxiety and depression items of the HSCL-90 and most of the other items with the exception of psychoticism items, Lipman [16] contrasted the cluster scores of a carefully diagnosed sample of 385 depressed outpatients with 220 anxious outpatients. The diagnostic procedures employed in this study are detailed by Downing et al. [10], but the main point is that the independent diagnostic classification of patients proved quite reliable (kappa of 0.62). Downing et al. [10] demonstrated, using the five a priori clusters of the HSCL-58, that the depressed group scored significantly higher on the depression cluster ($P < .001$) whereas the anxious group scored significantly higher on the anxiety cluster ($P < .025$). Lipman extended these analyses to the comparable clusters of the HSCL-90 with the same results. Of even more interest, however, were the results of a comparison of the specific symptoms, which were rated higher by anxious than by depressed patients and vice versa. Items rated highest by anxious patients, relative to depressed patients, are given in Table 22.6.

The items shown in Table 22.6 are clinically meaningful and in DSM-III terminology they are associated with a diagnosis of agoraphobia with panic attacks. A similar analysis of items rated higher by depressed than by anxious patients was cut off after nine items, since the depressed sample was relatively more distressed on all the items of the HSCL-90 with the exception of those nine items listed in Table 22.6. The nine items rated relatively highest by the depressed cohort are presented in Table 22.7.

Again, these items form a clinically meaningful cluster of symptoms which are clearly reflective of depression. The depressive syndrome includes symptoms of

Table 22.6. HSCL symptoms relatively highest in anxious outpatients

1. Feeling afraid you will faint in public
2. Numbness or tingling in parts of your body
3. Heart pounding or racing
4. Trouble getting your breath
5. Having to avoid certain things, places, or activities because they frighten you
6. Spells of terror or panic
7. Feeling uneasy in crowds such as shopping or at a movie
8. Hot or cold spells
9. A lump in your throat

Table 22.7. HSCL symptoms relatively highest in depressed outpatients

1. Feeling hopeless about the future
2. Feeling all the pleasure and joy has gone out of your life
3. Feeling no interest in things
4. Thoughts of ending your life
5. Not getting any fun out of life
6. Crying easily
7. Sleep that is restless or disturbed
8. Feeling you may never enjoy yourself again
9. Feelings of worthlessness

dysphoric affect, withdrawal of interest, anhedonia, feelings of futility and hopelessness, as well as suicidal ideation and some somatic components of depression, e.g., sleep difficulty. It is suggested that future clinical trials might include this item definition of depression to determine its sensitivity to pharmacotherapy and psychotherapy effects. In this regard, the depression cluster of the HSCL-90 has been shown sensitive to differences of drug effects in depressed populations [29, 34, 39].

In a preliminary analysis of the clinical improvement of 70 patients diagnosed as having a primary major depressive disorder by RDC criteria, both the agitated depression factor and the retarded depression factor of the HSCL-90 showed a statistically reliable advantage for group cognitive-behavior therapy, alone and in combination with imipramine, as contrasted with traditional group therapy. The study lasted 4 months and the data was analyzed 1, 2, 3, and 4 months after treatment. The statistical advantages mentioned above were found 2, 3, and 4 months after treatment. Beck Depression Inventory [2] scores, by contrast, only revealed significant differences among the treatments at 3 and 4 months, not at the earlier 2-month period. The Hamilton Depression Scale [13], as completed by a "blind" independent clinical evaluator at these same time periods, showed statistically significant but generally less sensitive discriminations among treatment conditions than did the HSCL-90 depression cluster.

Of the various factors and clusters of depression derived from the Hopkins Symptom Checklist, those presented in Tables 22.2 and 22.3 have been most widely employed in outcome trials and should, therefore, be considered the best validated. The retarded (Table 22.4) and agitated (Table 22.5) depression factors have been reported first in 1979 [22] and are not yet in common use although the author has found them sensitive to psychotherapy and antidepressant drug effects in at least one study. The set of nine HSCL symptoms that were found most distressing to depressed outpatients (Table 22.7) were reported in 1982 [16] and have not yet been studied in the context of a treatment outcome trial.

While the depression factors and cluster, as reported in Tables 22.4 and 22.5 and Table 22.7, respectively, have a high level of face validity, they should be still considered as requiring additional study and validation.

There have been few, if any, studies in which the factors or clusters of the HSCL-90 have been used as free-standing scales, i.e., independent of the entire 90-item scale. In principle, such usage would be comparable to the Zung Self-Rating Depression Scale [43], which has demonstrated adequate validity.

In summary, the various clinical clusters of depression as derived from the HSCL as well as the depression factors of agitated/anxious depression and retarded depression derived from the HSCL-90 have, to greater or lesser extents, proved reliable, valid, and sensitive to differential effects of pharmacotherapy, psychotherapy, and the combination of these modalities. The use of minimal cutoff severity scores on depression as an intake inclusion criterion also seems likely to enhance the sensitivity of clinical trials. While observer-rated measures of depression are an important aspect of treatment assessment research, ultimately, as Uhlenhuth, Lipman, Chassan, Hines, and McNair [37] have stressed, "... it is the patient's opinion with all its biases that is most relevant for the initiation and maintenance of treatment."

Appendix A The HSCL-90

MH 9-53   National Institute of Mental Health
5-73
                                    SCL-90

Instructions: Below is a list of problems and complaints that people sometimes have. Please read each one carefully. After you have done so, please fill in one of the numbered spaces to the right that best describes HOW MUCH THAT PROBLEM HAS BOTHERED OR DISTRESSED YOU DURING THE PAST WEEK INCLUDING TODAY. Mark only one numbered space for each problem and do not skip any items. Make your marks carefully using a No. 2 pencil. DO NOT USE A BALLPOINT PEN. If you change your mind, erase your first mark carefully. Please do not make any extra marks on the sheet. Please read the example below before beginning.

Example:

How Much Were You Bothered by:	Not at All	A Little Bit	Moderately	Quite a Bit	Extremely
1. Backaches					

How Much Were You Bothered by:		Not at All	A Little Bit	Moderately	Quite a Bit	Extremely
1. Headaches	1.	0	1	2	3	4
2. Nervousness or shakiness inside	2.	0	1	2	3	4
3. Unwanted thoughts, words, or ideas that won't leave your mind	3.	0	1	2	3	4
4. Faintness or dizziness	4.	0	1	2	3	4
5. Loss of sexual interest or pleasure	5.	0	1	2	3	4
6. Feeling critical of others	6.	0	1	2	3	4
7. The idea that someone else can control your thoughts	7.	0	1	2	3	4
8. Feeling others are to blame for most of your troubles	8.	0	1	2	3	4
9. Trouble remembering things	9.	0	1	2	3	4
10. Worried about sloppiness or carelessness	10.	0	1	2	3	4
11. Feeling easily annoyed or irritated	11.	0	1	2	3	4
12. Pains in heart or chest	12.	0	1	2	3	4
13. Feeling afraid in open spaces or on the streets	13.	0	1	2	3	4
14. Feeling low in energy or slowed down	14.	0	1	2	3	4
15. Thoughts of ending your life	15.	0	1	2	3	4
16. Hearing voices that other people do not hear	16.	0	1	2	3	4
17. Trembling	17.	0	1	2	3	4
18. Feeling that most people cannot be trusted	18.	0	1	2	3	4
19. Poor appetite	19.	0	1	2	3	4
20. Crying easily	20.	0	1	2	3	4
21. Feeling shy or uneasy with the opposite sex	21.	0	1	2	3	4
22. Feeling of being trapped or caught	22.	0	1	2	3	4
23. Suddenly scared for no reason	23.	0	1	2	3	4
24. Temper outbursts that you could not control	24.	0	1	2	3	4

Depression Scales Derived from the Hopkins Symptom Checklist

How Much Were You Bothered by:	Not at All	A Little Bit	Moderately	Quite a Bit	Extremely
25. Feeling afraid to go out of your house alone .... 25.	0	1	2	3	4
26. Blaming yourself for things ...... 26.	0	1	2	3	4
27. Pains in lower back .... 27.	0	1	2	3	4
28. Feeling blocked in getting things done .... 28.	0	1	2	3	4
29. Feeling lonely .... 29.	0	1	2	3	4
30. Feeling blue .... 30.	0	1	2	3	4
31. Worrying too much about things . 31.	0	1	2	3	4
32. Feeling no interest in things ...... 32.	0	1	2	3	4
33. Feeling fearful .... 33.	0	1	2	3	4
34. Your feelings being easily hurt ... 34.	0	1	2	3	4
35. Other people being aware of your private thoughts .... 35.	0	1	2	3	4
36. Feeling others do not understand you or are unsympathetic .... 36.	0	1	2	3	4
37. Feeling that people are unfriendly or dislike you .... 37.	0	1	2	3	4
38. Having to do things very slowly to insure correctness .... 38.	0	1	2	3	4
39. Heart pounding or racing .... 39.	0	1	2	3	4
40. Nausea or upset stomach .... 40.	0	1	2	3	4
41. Feeling inferior to others .... 41.	0	1	2	3	4
42. Soreness of your muscles .... 42.	0	1	2	3	4
43. Feeling that you are watched or talked about by others .... 43.	0	1	2	3	4
44. Trouble falling asleep .... 44.	0	1	2	3	4
45. Having to check and double-check what you do .... 45.	0	1	2	3	4
46. Difficulty making decisions ..... 46.	0	1	2	3	4
47. Feeling afraid to travel on buses, subways, or trains .... 47.	0	1	2	3	4
48. Trouble getting your breath ...... 48.	0	1	2	3	4
49. Hot or cold spells .... 49.	0	1	2	3	4

How Much Were You Bothered by:	Not at All	A Little Bit	Moder- Ately	Quite a Bit	Ex- treme- ly
50. Having to avoid certain things, places, or activities because they frighten you .... 50.	0	1	2	3	4
51. Your mind going blank .... 51.	0	1	2	3	4
52. Numbness or tingling in parts of your body .... 52.	0	1	2	3	4
53. A lump in your throat .... 53.	0	1	2	3	4
54. Feeling hopeless about the future .... 54.	0	1	2	3	4
55. Trouble concentrating .... 55.	0	1	2	3	4
56. Feeling weak in parts of your body .... 56.	0	1	2	3	4
57. Feeling tense or keyed up ...... 57.	0	1	2	3	4
58. Heavy feelings in your arms or legs .... 58.	0	1	2	3	4
59. Thoughts of death or dying ..... 59.	0	1	2	3	4
60. Overeating .... 60.	0	1	2	3	4
61. Feeling uneasy when people are watching or talking about you .... 61.	0	1	2	3	4
62. Having thoughts that are not your own .... 62.	0	1	2	3	4
63. Having urges to beat, injure, or harm someone .... 63.	0	1	2	3	4
64. Awakening in the early morning .... 64.	0	1	2	3	4
65. Having to repeat the same actions such as touching, counting, washing .... 65.	0	1	2	3	4
66. Sleep that is restless or disturbed .... 66.	0	1	2	3	4
67. Having urges to break or smash things .... 67.	0	1	2	3	4
68. Having ideas or beliefs that others do not share .... 68.	0	1	2	3	4

Depression Scales Derived from the Hopkins Symptom Checklist

How Much Were You Bothered by:	Not at All	A Little Bit	Moderately	Quite a Bit	Extremely
69. Feeling very self-conscious with others .... 69.	0	1	2	3	4
70. Feeling uneasy in crowds, such as shopping or at a movie ... 70	0	1	2	3	4
71. Feeling everything is an effort .... 71.	0	1	2	3	4
72. Spells of terror or panic .... 72.	0	1	2	3	4
73. Feeling uncomfortable about eating or drinking in public ...... 73.	0	1	2	3	4
74. Getting into frequent arguments .. 74.	0	1	2	3	4
75. Feeling nervous when you are left alone .... 75.	0	1	2	3	4
76. Others not giving you proper credit for your achievements ..... 76.	0	1	2	3	4
77. Feeling lonely even when you are with people .... 77.	0	1	2	3	4
78. Feeling so restless you couldn't sit still .... 78.	0	1	2	3	4
79. Feelings of worthlessness .... 79.	0	1	2	3	4
80. Feeling that familiar things are strange or unreal .... 80.	0	1	2	3	4
81. Shouting or throwing things ..... 81.	0	1	2	3	4
82. Feeling afraid you will faint in public .... 82.	0	1	2	3	4
83. Feeling that people will take advantage of you if you let them .... 83.	0	1	2	3	4
84. Having thoughts about sex that bother you a lot .... 84.	0	1	2	3	4
85. The idea that you should be punished for your sins .... 85.	0	1	2	3	4
86. Feeling pushed to get things done....................... 86.	0	1	2	3	4
87. The idea that something serious is wrong with your body....................... 87.	0	1	2	3	4

How Much Were You Bothered by:	Not at All	A Little Bit	Moder- Ately	Quite a Bit	Ex- treme- ly
88. Never feeling close to another person .... 88.	0	1	2	3	4
89. Feelings of guilt .... 89.	0	1	2	3	4
90. The idea that something is wrong with your mind .... 90.	0	1	2	3	4

References

1. Beck, A. T. 1976. Cognitive Therapy and the Emotional Disorders. Universities Press, New York.
2. Beck, A. T., Ward, C. H., Mendelson, M., Mock., and Erbough, J. 1961. Inventory for measuring depression. Arch. Gen. Psychiatry 4: 561-571.
3. Covi, L., Lipman, R. S., Derogatis, L. R., Smith, J. E., and Pattison, J. H. 1974. Drugs and group psychotherapy in neurotic depression. Am. J. Psychiatry 131: 191-198.
4. Covi, L., Lipman, R. S., Alarcon, R. D., and Smith, V. K. 1976. Psychotherapy interaction in depression. Am. J. Psychiatry 133: 502-508.
5. Covi, L., Lipman, R. S., McNair, D., and Czwelinsky, T. 1979. Symptomatic volunteers in multicenter trials. Prog. Neuropsychopharmacol. 3: 521-533.
6. Derogatis, L. R., and Cleary, P. A. 1977. Confirmation of the dimensional structure of the SCL-90: A study in construct validation. J. Clin. Psychol. 33: 981-989.
7. Derogatis, L. R., Lipman, R. S., Rickels, K., Uhlenhuth, E. H., and Covi, L. 1974. The Hopkins Symptom Checklist (HSCL) - A Measure of Primary Symptom Dimensions. In: P. Pichot (ed.), Psychological Measurements in Psychopharmacology - Modern Problems in Pharmacopsychiatry, pp. 79-110. Karger, Basel.
8. Derogatis, L. R., Lipman, R. S., Rickels, K., Uhlenhuth, E. H., and Covi, L. 1974. The Hopkins Symptoms Checklist - a self-report symptom inventory. Behav. Sci. 19: 1-15.
9. Derogatis, L. R., Rickels, K., and Rock, A. F. 1976. The SCL-90 and the MMPI: A step in the validation of a new self-report scale. Br. J. Psychiatry 128: 280-289.
10. Downing, R. W., Rickels, K., McNair, D., Lipman, R. S., Kahn, R. J., Fisher, S., Covi, L., and Smith, V. K. 1981. Description of sample, comparison of anxious and depressed groups, attrition rates. Psychopharmacol. Bull. 17: 94-97.
11. Frank, J. R., Gliedman, L. E., Imber, S. D., Nash, E. H., and Stone, A. R., 1957. Why patients leave psychotherapy. Archives of Neurological Psychiatry 77: 283-299.
12. Guy, W. C. 1976. ECDEU Assessment Manual for Psychopharmacology Revised, DHEW Publication No. (ADM) 76-338, U. S. Government Printing Office, Washington, D. C.
13. Hamilton, M. A. 1960. A rating scale for depression. J. Neurol. Neurosurg. Psychiatry 23: 56-62.
14. Hollister, L. E., Overall, J. E., Shelton, J., Pennington, V., Kimbell, I., and Johnson, M. 1967. Amitryptiline, perphenazine, and amitryptiline - perphenazine combination in different depressive syndromes. Arch. Gen. Psychiatry 17: 486-493.
15. Kellner, R., Sheffield, B. F., and Simpson, G. M. 1978. The value of self-rating scales in drug trials with nonpsychotic patients. Prog. Neuropsychopharmacol. 2: 197-205.
16. Lipman, R. S. 1982. Differentiating anxiety and depression in anxiety disorders: Use of rating scales. Psychopharmacol. Bull. 18: 69-77.
17. Lipman, R. S., and Covi, L. 1976. Outpatient treatment of neurotic depression-medication and group psychotherapy. In: R. L. Spitzer and J. Zubin (eds.), Evaluation of Psychological Therapies, pp. 178-218. Johns Hopkins University Press, Baltimore MD.

18. Lipman, R.S., Cole, J.O., Park, L.C., and Rickels, K. 1965. Sensitivity of symptom and non-symptom-focused criteria of outpatient drug efficacy. Am. J. Psychiatry 122 (1): 24-27.
19. Lipman, R.S., Park, L.C., and Rickels, K. 1966. Paradoxical influence of a therapeutic side-effect interpretation. Arch. Gen. Psychiatry 15: 462-474.
20. Lipman, R.S., Covi, L., Rickels, K., Uhlenhuth, E.H., and Lazar, R. 1968. Selected measures of change in outpatient drug evaluation: Psychopharmacology - a review of progress. 1957-1967. (PHS Publication No. 1836), U.S. Government Printing Office, Washington, D.C.
21. Lipman, R.S., Rickels, K., Covi, L., Derogatis, L.R., and Uhlenhuth, E.H. 1968. Factors of symptom distress - Doctor ratings of anxious neurotic patients. Arch. Gen. Psychiatry 21: 328-338.
22. Lipman, R.S., Covi, L., and Shapiro, A.K. 1979. The Hopkins Symptom Checklist (HSCL): Factors derived from the HSCL-90. J. Affective Disord. 1: 9-24.
23. Lipman, R.S., Covi, L., Downing, R.W., Fisher, S., Kahn, R.J., McNair, D.M., Rickels, K., and Smith, V.K. 1981. Pharmacotherapy of anxiety and depression: rationale and study design. Psychopharmacol. Bull. 3: 91-94.
24. Mattsson, N.B., Williams, H.V., Rickels, K., Lipman, R.S., and Uhlenhuth, E.H. 1969. Dimensions of symptom distress in anxious neurotic outpatients. Psychopharmacol. Bull. 5: 19-32.
25. Overall, J.E., Hollister, L.E., Johnson, M., and Pennington, U. 1966. Nosology of depression and differential response to drugs. J. Am. Med. Assoc. 195: 946-948.
26. Parloff, M.D., Kelman, H.C., and Frank, J.D., 1954. Comfort, effectiveness and self-awareness as criteria of improvement in psychotherapy. Am. J. Psychiatry 5: 343-351.
27. Prusoff, B., and Klerman, G.L. 1954. Differentiating depressed from anxious neurotic outpatient: Use of discriminant function analysis for separation of neurotic affective states. Arch. Gen. Psychiatry 30: 302-309.
28. Raskin, A., Schulterbrandt, J.G., Reating, N., and McKeon, J.J. 1970. Differential response to chlorpromazine, imipramine, and a placebo among subgroups of hospitalized depressed patients. Arch. Gen. Psychiatry 23: 164-173.
29. Ravaris, C.L., Robinson, D.S., Ives, J.O., Nies, A., and Bartlett, D. 1980. Phenelzine and amitriptyline in the treatment of depression: a comparison of present and past studies. Arch. Gen. Psychiatry 37: 1075-1080.
30. Rickels, K., Lipman, R.S., Park, L.C., Covi, L., Uhlenhuth, E.H., and Mock, J.E. 1971. Drugs, doctor warmth, and clinic setting in the symptomatic response to minor tranquilizers. Psychopharmacologia (Berlin) 20: 128-152
31. Rickels, K., Downing, R.W., Lipman, R.S., Fisher, E., and Randall, A.M. 1973. The Self-Rating Depression Scale (SDS) as a measure of psychotropic drug response. Dis. Nerv. Syst. 34: 98-104.
32. Rickels, K., Garcia, C.R., Lipman, R.S., Derogatis, L.R., and Fisher, E.L. 1976. The Hopkins Symptom Checklist - Assessing emotional distress in obstetric-gynecologic practice. Primary Care 3: 751-764.
33. Robinson, D.S., Nies, A., Ravaris, L., Ives, J.O., and Bartlett, D. 1978. Clinical pharmacology of phenelzine. Arch. Gen. Psychiatry 35: 629-635.
34. Robinson, D.S., Nies, A., Concella, J., and Cooper, T.B. 1981. Phenelzine plasma levels, pharmacokinetics and clinical outcome. Psychopharmacol. Bull. 17: 154-157.
35. Spitzer, R.L., Endicott, J., and Robins, E. 1978. Research diagnostic criteria: rationale and reliability. Arch. Gen. Psychiatry 35: 773-782.
36. Uhlenhuth, E.H., Rickels, K., Fisher, S., Park, L.C., Lipman, R.S., and Mock, J. 1966. Drug, doctor's verbal attitude and clinic setting in the symptomatic response to pharmacotherapy. Psychopharmacologia (Berlin) 9: 392-418.
37. Uhlenhuth, E.H., Lipman, R.S., Chassan, J.B., Hines, L.R., and McNair, D.M. 1970. Methodological issues in evaluating the effectiveness of agents for treating anxious patients. In: J. Levine, B., Schiele, and L. Bouthilet (eds.), Principles and Problems in Establishing the Efficacy of Psychotropic Agents. U.S. Public Health Service, Chevy Chase, MD.
38. Uhlenhuth, E.H., Lipman, R.S., Balter, M.B., and Stern, M. 1974. Symptom intensity and life stress in the city. Arch. Gen. Psychiatry 31: 759-764.
39. Uhlenhuth, E.H., Glass, R.M., and Fishman, M.W. 1979. Multiple crossover design with an anti-anxiety agent and an antidepressant. Psychopharmacol. Bull. 15: 37-40.

40. Waskow, I. E., and Parloff, M. B. (eds.). 1975. Psychotherapy Change Measures. National Institute of Mental Health, Rockville, MD.
41. Weissman, M. M., Pottenger, M., Kleber, H., Ruben, H., and Williams, D. 1977. Symptom patterns in primary and secondary depression. Arch. Gen. Psychiatry 34: 854–862.
42. Williams, H. V., Lipman, R. S., Uhlenhuth, E. H., and Rickels, K. 1968. Replication of symptom distress factors in anxious neurotic outpatients. Multivariate Behavior Research 3: 199–212.
43. Zung, W. W. K. 1965. A self-rating depression scale. Arch. Gen. Psychiatry 12: 63–70.

Chapter 23 The Wittenborn Psychiatric Rating Scale

J. R. WITTENBORN

The Development of a Set of Observer-Rating Scales

The Wittenborn Psychiatric Rating Scale (WPRS) is an observer-rating scale [10, 12]. The distinction offered by the term "observer" may be more apparent than real, however. In a given situation observers may share the same sensory experience, but the observations generated by the sensory input can vary widely from observer to observer. The observational response of one rater to a sensory experience may be instantaneous, unitary, unambiguous, and reliable. For another rater the same observation based on the same sensory input may be a complex judgment that accrued from a process involving both inference and deduction. Whether a given rating should be considered an observation or a judgment depends, in part, upon the background, current responsibility, and training of the rater.

The WPRS was conceived shortly after World War II. During the forties there was a great diagnostic emphasis in psychiatry. Experience with various clinics, Veteran's Administration (VA) installations, and private practitioners led to the inescapable conclusion that the implications of diagnostic designations and the frequency with which they were used could vary substantially from clinic to clinic. Clinical investigators, in particular, were handicapped by the lack of suitable standard assessments of psychopathological behavior.

The desired standardization required an emphasis on observed behavioral manifestations and insofar as possible minimized the involvement of interpretative judgments. The first task was to identify those manifestations which were considered by psychiatrists to have a pertinence for functional, as contrasted with organic, psychopathology. The psychiatrists of the Yale Department of Psychiatry, as well as other southern New England psychiatrists, were asked to assist in developing a symptom-rating procedure that would be comprehensive in its coverage of symptoms of functional disorders and would generate symptomatic descriptions that would not vary from rater to rater. In an interview situation, each psychiatrist was asked to describe a behavioral manifestation of a particular diagnostic syndrome and to describe behavior that he or she would consider as indication of a maximal degree of the behavioral manifestation and also to describe a minimal indication. Each of the resulting large number of descriptive statements was edited so that the meaning was unambiguous. These statements were then placed in graded sequences of four statements each so that each set of four statements formed a scale implying increasing psychopathology.

These graded sequences of edited descriptive statements were processed through several pretesting stages so that the emerging set of rating scales was accepted by the psychiatrists without further revision and could be offered as a comprehensive sampling of observable manifestations of psychopathology. Care was taken to ensure that the arrangement of the items on the continuum always reflected increasing severity.

Thus, the scales of the WPRS were generated in a pragmatic manner. They did not reflect any particular point of view and were not deduced from any recognized theory or theories. Their only claim to pertinence lay in the fact that they were generated by the responses of United States psychiatrists when asked what they observed in their patients as evidence of psychopathology.

There are many ways in which descriptive continua may be developed. The duration of an observable manifestation, the frequency with which the manifestation occurs, the burden the manifestation places upon the patient or on those who share his life, and the number of different aspects of the patient's life distorted or burdened by these manifestations may all be used as a basis for distinguishing between behaviors. The rating continua of the WPRS were judged to reflect the seriousness of the psychopathological gravity of the observed behavior.

The scales offered the particular advantage of reviewing the entire spectrum of pathological behavioral manifestations of a given patient, regardless of how relevant or irrelevant to a patient's illness a particular rater regarded some of the behaviors. Thus, the scales could claim a standard descriptive significance not limited to the patient's presenting problems or to the therapist's prejudgments. The set of scales that survived pretesting described 55 distinguishable symptoms, far too many for economical description.

A Scoring Rationale

Descriptive terms and designations often have overlapping implications, and their intercorrelations usually suggest the possibility of conceptual, as well as descriptive, economy. Such possibilities can be efficiently explored by multiple-factor analysis of the intercorrelations among the set of descriptive items [8]. This method was used to display the pattern of interrelationships among the 55 scales of the WPRS (eventually reduced to 52).

The first factor analysis was based on the symptom ratings for a heterogeneous unselected sample of 140 male chronic patients at the Veterans Administration Hospital at Northampton, Massachussetts [11]. The scales fell into seven groups, six of which could be associated with classical diagnostic entities, i.e., hebephrenic deterioration, conversion hysteria, catatonic excitement, anxiety, paranoid schizophrenia, and paranoid condition. In the present context, the seventh constellation is most interesting. It comprised symptoms descriptive of both a manic state and a depressed state, but the correlations between the factor and these classes of symptoms bore opposite signs, with the manic symptoms bearing a positive sign and the depressive symptoms bearing a negative sign. Thus, the factor could be described as bipolar, but it was considered descriptively useful to treat the manic symptoms as comprising one of the symptom constellations appropriate for scoring and the depressive symptoms as another inversely related scoring constellation.

In order to examine the descriptive generality of the symptom constellations inherent in this comprehensive set of symptom-rating scales, psychiatrists prepared ratings for 1000 consecutive admissions to the Connecticut State Hospital at Middletown [21]. A sample of 240 of these new admissions was selected on the basis of two criteria: age under 60 years and a functional illness uncomplicated by brain damage or toxic conditions, including addiction. When the symptom ratings for this sample of patients were intercorrelated and factor analyzed, seven factors emerged, six of which were readily identified with six of the factors found in the Northampton sample [11]. The seventh factor in the acute sample described an obsessive-compulsive-phobic condition. The hebephrenic-deteriorated factor found in the chronic Northampton sample was not found in the acutely ill, newly admitted patients at Middletown. In this sample, as in the Northampton sample, items describing a manic state and the items describing a depressed state formed a bipolar factor. This consistency in the symptom constellations found in two quite different samples of patients suggested that mental hospital patients may be described in terms of a standard set of symptom constellations.

The emphasis on observation and the fact that the rating scales were presented unlabeled and in random order suggest that the symptom constellations were objective summaries of the patient's observable behavior. Nevertheless, there was a possibility that these symptom constellations were an artifact of the training and perceptual predispositions of the psychiatrists, and a study was undertaken to examine this possibility.

Two psychiatrists who differed in age, sex, cultural background, theoretical bias, and training were on the staff of the Middletown Hospital during this period. Both psychiatrists were rating patients who were generally quite similar. Accordingly, it was possible to factor analyze symptom ratings for a sample of 79 patients rated by Dr A and independently to analyze the same set of rating scales for 119 patients rated by Dr B [30]. Because of the modest size of these samples, the analysis was limited to a common set of 20 selected symptoms representative of the major symptom constellations identified in the large Northampton and Middletown samples. These two factor analyses were conducted by different statistical analysts using the same method, and the resulting factor loadings were compared. The factors generated by these two sets of data differed very little and resembled factors identified in the analyses of two prior samples. For example, the symptom-rating scale describing feelings of impending doom correlated 0.606 with the depressive factor defined by Dr A's data and 0.689 with the depressive factor based on Dr B's data. These findings suggest that the symptom constellations found among these rating scales may be relatively independent of the bias and orientation of the rater.

When raters represent professional disciplines which differ with respect to the content and goals of their training, the roles they assume, and their opportunities for observation, some difference in symptom ratings may emerge. Psychiatrists, clinical psychologists, and nurses rated the same sample of depressed female patients, and the ratings generated by the psychiatrists and psychologists were quite similar [31]. Psychiatrists and psychologists generated symptom ratings that differed substantially from those provided by nurses. When ratings by psychiatrists and psychologists were compared with ratings by nurses, the nurses underrated the severity of the patient's manifestations, underestimated the subjective aspects of the patient's illness, and overgeneralized. Much of this difference may be due to the fact that the nurses assume a direct day-to-day responsibility for the physical status of the patient, whereas the psychiatrist and the psychologist have the responsibility for being aware of the nature and status of the patient's mental illness.

Although symptom patterns found in a heterogeneous sample of patients with functional disorders may not vary greatly among well-motivated raters who know the content and procedures of the WPRS and have opportunity to observe all relevant aspects of the patient's illness, the pattern of symptoms can vary according to restrictions in the composition of the sample. This was illustrated by two analyses: one based on the ratings of the 20 representative symptoms in a sample of organic patients of advanced age [28] and the other based on funtional patients under 30 years of age [29]. Among the old patients, the anxiety constellation and the paranoid symptom complex were clearly distinguishable. A broad constellation of excited manic behavior was also well defined. Other symptomatic constellations found in the prior analyses, including the depressive constellation, were no longer distinguishable. In the young sample, the constellations of anxiety, manic state, depression, paranoia, and conversion hysteria were all discrete and clearly identified. There was some tendency, however, for mania and schizophrenic excitement symptoms to form a single constellation in the young sample, a noticeable contrast with the distinction between mania and schizophrenic excitement in the large samples which were heterogeneous with respect to age.

Symptoms, Groupings, and Diagnoses

Although at one time the rating scales were described as a quantified multiple diagnostic procedure, no formal diagnostic use was intended for the WPRS which was to provide a summary description of behavioral manifestations observable within some arbitrarily predetermined period.

The correspondence between a formal psychiatric diagnosis and descriptions based on the WPRS was examined for a group of patients bearing a simple diagnosis based on the consensus of a traditional case conference. A group of patients with a diagnosis of manic-depressive psychosis (manic state) was selected for this purpose. The symptomatic similarity of the patients was examined by factor analysis [25]. The correlations between pairs of patients were based on the similarity or dissimilarity with which they were rated on the set of 55 symptom-rating scales. The interrater consistency for these ratings had been found to be sufficient for this purpose [30]. To minimize artifacts each scale was standardized before the interpatient correlations were computed. If this sample of 20 patients had been symptomatically homogeneous, the patients would have been rated in essentially the same way. They would have borne high positive correlations with each other, and only one factor would have emerged. Within this small group of patients with the simple manic diagnosis, there were six factors, indicating that six subgroups could be identified on the basis of symptom ratings. Regardless of the group in which they fell, all patients had high scores on the manic state cluster, but they varied widely with respect to other symptom clusters, particularly paranoid condition and paranoid schizophrenia. A similar analysis showed symptomatic heterogeneity among 20 patients with the diagnosis involutional psychosis [24]. Scores on the symptom constellations showed the expected relationships with various external considerations, such as the background of the patient's illness [22] and his or her behavior in occupational therapy situations [23].

The Scores of the WPRS as Criteria

The WPRS has been shown to provide a sufficiently sensitive assessment of depressed states to reflect the action of antidepressant medication. In one of the first applications for this purpose, the score for the depression constellation provided a statistically significant discrimination between depressed women who had been treated with iproniazid and depressed women who had received an indistinguishable placebo [32].

In a subsequent study, both the anxiety and the depression scores on the WPRS provided a significant distinction between depressed female patients treated with imipramine and those treated with placebo [33]. Patients who were involutional, who had had a schizophrenic disorder, or who had had a manic-depressive diagnosis responded to imipramine with increased restlessness and fear of impending doom. In contrast, the patients who were reactive or neurotic responded favorably to imipramine in these symptomatic respects [18].

In a particularly comprehensive analysis of responses to placebo, iproniazid, imipramine, and ECT, changes associated with the treatment were distinguished from changes associated with various nontreatment factors which were potential predictors of individual differences in therapeutic response [15, 17]. The depression, phobic, and anxiety scores of the WPRS were significantly related to the use of iproniazid as constrasted with placebo ($P<.05$) when the variance of many nontreatment factors had been statistically eliminated. In this analysis, it was found also that the phobic score had a significant association with imipramine as contrasted with placebo ($P<.05$) and that both the depression score and the anxiety score of the WPRS had a significant association with ECT ($P<.05$).

There are several reports where the scores of the original WPRS have been used as dependent variables in clinical investigations. A good example is provided by a study of the responses of alcoholic and nonalcoholic patients during a prolonged period of experimental drinking [7]. Seven of the nine WPRS scores showed significant changes during the course of drinking, and the magnitude of these changes was, in part, an effect of whether the subject had a history of alcoholism.

The Revised WPRS

In the mid-fifties, the WPRS was revised and enlarged to include chronic manifestations of the major psychoses. A revised set of 98 scales was prepared. One hundred and fifty male patients at the Veterans Administration Hospital at Lyons, New Jersey, were rated [13], and a comparative group of 135 female patients at the New Jersey State Hospital at Marlboro were rated [26]. Each patient was observed and rated independently by two qualified raters, and the ratings submitted to analysis were a composite of these two ratings. Centroid analyses of the symptom-rating scale intercorrelations were conducted for the male and for the female patients by an independent statistician who, in the interest of objectivity, was unaware of some of the most critical features of the data. The male sample [13] yielded ten factors, including six of those generated in the Connecticut data [21]. The data for the female sample generated 12 factors, including two different aspects of depressive retardation [26].

When these intercorrelations were submitted to a principal component analysis [4, 5], the number of interpretable factors was increased for both the male and the female samples, with the females responsible for more interpretable factors than the males, including four aspects of depression [14]. In order to produce a practicable rating procedure that could yield scores for the most important symptom constellations, some compromises were necessary. Twelve major factors plus 11 secondary factors provide the final scoring spectrum for the revised WPRS. Only 72 of the 98 items involved in the analytical explorations were retained for practical application. The revised WPRS, like the original form, minimized the use of judgments and interpretations and continued to prefer observations as the basis for ratings.

A comparison of schizophrenic and depressed samples illustrates the descriptive potential of the 12 scores generated by the revised WPRS (Table 23.1). The samples were drawn from the inpatients of the New Jersey State Hospital at Marlboro [26] and were limited to depressed females and schizophrenic males. All cluster scores contributed to the differentiation, and no one target symptom complex was sufficient to provide a symptomatic assessment for these two diagnostic entities. In view of the present interest in depression, it is useful to note that the symptomatic manifestation of a depressed sample can be examined in terms of four subcategories of the depressive symptom complex.

A 24-month study of changes in a sample of 75 schizophrenic men provided the opportunity to examine the sensitivity of the depressive retardation score when the patient is in the process of active change and the stability of this score when the patient's condition has stabilized [20]. The greatest portion of the reduction in depressive retardation score occurred by the end of 6 months, and changes thereafter were relatively modest. The correlation between the pretreatment depressive retardation score and the depressive retardation score at the end of 6 months was only 0.29. The correlation between the score at 6 months and the score at 12 months was 0.51. The correlation between the 12th month and the 18th month was 0.78 and between the 18th month and the 24th month was 0.80. The increasing correlation between successive ratings during the course of treatment corresponds to the reduction in the depressive retardation score during the first 6 months of treatment and the modest change thereafter.

Table 23.1. Mean standard scores[a] for symptom clusters

Symptom clusters		Depressed women x̄ (n = 157)	Schizophrenic men x̄ (n = 86)
I	Anxiety	6	7
II	Hysterical conversion	1	3
III	Manic state	2	4
IV	Depressive total	6	7
	(a) Obstructive	(1)	
	(b) Apathy	(5)	
	(c) Withdrawal	(7)	
	(d) Affective flatness	(3)	
V	Schizophrenic excitement total	3	6
VI	Psychotic belligerence total	2	6
VII	Paranoid	1	6
VIII	Hebephrenic total	4	5
IX	Compulsive-obsessive	5	6
X	Intellectual impairment	1	4
XI	Homosexual dominance	2	4
XII	Ideas of grandeur	1	3

[a] Raw scores based on the sum of ratings for scales comprising a cluster were transformed to standard scores, which ranged from 1 to 10

The revised WPRS, like the original 52-item scale, has been used in predictive studies, and numerous significant correlations may be found between changes in WPRS scores, e.g., anxiety and depression, and various predictor items [34]. The WPRS has been applied also as a criterion for the definitions of samples [1, 27] and as a standard by which samples may be compared [9].

In response to the need for a shortened observer symptom-rating scale procedure that would lend itself to the assessment of outpatients and to situations where numerous repeated assessments were anticipated, scales representing the principal symptom groups were selected from the long revised form and combined as an abbreviated form [19]. This form has found some use in studies of the efficacy of psychotropic substances [6]. Unfortunately, there has been some tendency to combine all the scales in the short form into a total score, despite the fact that in most situations the scores for each of the symptom constellations represented by small groups of scales will prove more discriminating than the total score.

Some Comments on Symptom Clusters

In a culturally and linguistically homogeneous community, analyses of independent samples can generate essentially the same constellations of symptoms, but it does not necessarily follow that culturally diverse samples will generate the same constellations of symptoms. The degree to which symptom constellations, in the perceptions of the rater, are a consequence of characteristics of the society in which his patients have lived and developed their psychopathologies, or are in some way intrinsic to the structure and physiologic function of man, has not been explored.

Because of the common elements in the training of all psychiatrists, scales that invite the rater to rate his judgment of the patient may be unsuitable for the purpose of intercultural comparisons. For such an exploration, meticulously discrete statements of generally observable behavior should be defined and used as the standard units of observation.

Some tentative explorations based on the WPRS may be brought to the reader's attention. To some extent, at least, sex has been a major cultural distinction in most parts of the world, including the United States. Privileges, responsibilities, role models, standards of conduct, and acceptable modes of expression have all combined to create two pervasive subcultures. It is not surprising, therefore, to have found contrasts between men and women in the constellations of psychiatric symptoms they develop [14].

The WPRS has been translated into various languages. Among these are Czech, French, German, Italian, Japanese, Korean, Portuguese, and Swedish.

When symptom constellations generated by newly admitted mental hospital patients in the State of New Jersey were compared with the symptom constellations generated by a sample of newly admitted patients from southern Italy, several differences emerged [35]. These differences have been interpreted as consistent with contrasts between the highly mobile consumer-oriented American community and the expressive, socially stable, ethnically homogeneous Italian community with its family orientation. Symptoms corresponding to the American description of anxiety states were intercorrelated in the American sample, but this pattern of intercorrelations was modified, if not obscured, in the Italian sample. In addition, some schizophrenic symptoms were correlated with some of the symptoms comprising the depressive retardation pattern found in the American sample. In contrast, many of the symptoms associated with schizophrenic excitement in the American data were not a part of the comparable Italian constellation.

The WPRS was applied to both male and female samples in Korea. Depressive retardation involved more items in the Korean data than in the American data [16]. A pervasive factor of psychotic belligerence was much more clearly defined among the Korean women than among the Korean men. Other contrasts have been described, including differences between the symptom constellations of American and Puerto Rican samples [3], of American and Czechoslovakian patients [35], and of European and "Oriental" Jews [2].

Serious attempts to relate these differences in symptom constellations with national or regional cultures are obviously premature. If these contrasts or some features of them can be confirmed in other samples drawn from the same population, they might help document a cultural significance for some manifestations of psychopathology.

Acknowledgment. The preparation of this manuscript was supported in part by a grant from the Cape Branch Foundation, Dayton, New Jersey.

References

1. Baugher, D., and Wittenborn, J.R. 1980. Some dimensions of dysphorias and their assessment. J. Nerv. Ment. Dis. 168: 75-83.
2. Goldman, I.M. 1971. Psychopathology of European and 'Oriental' Jews. Unpublished doctoral dissertation, Rutgers The State University, New Brunswick, New Jersey.
3. Gonzalez-Pabon, J.F. 1971. Patterns of psychopathology: Correspondences and distinctions between samples of American and Puerto Rican mental hospital patients. Unpublished doctoral dissertation, Rutgers The State University, New Brunswick, New Jersey.
4. Hotelling, H. 1933. Analysis of a complex of statistical variables into principal components. Journal of Educational Psychology 24: 417-441, 498-520.
5. Kaiser, H.F. 1952. Varimax solution for primary mental abilities. Psychometr. Monogr. no. 6. University of Chicago Press, Chicago.
6. Lapierre, Y.D., Tremblay, A., Gagnon, A., Monpremier, P., Berliss, H., and Cyewumi, L.K. 1982. A therapeutic and discontinuation study of clobazam and diazepam in anxiety neurosis. J. Clin. Psychiatr. 43: 372-374.
7. Nathan, P.E. and O'Brien, J.S. 1971. An experimental analysis of the behaviour of alcoholics and nonalcoholics during prolonged experimental drinking: A necesssary precursor of behaviour therapy? Behaviour Therapy 2: 455-476.
8. Thurstone, L.L. 1947. Multiple Factor Analysis. University of Chicago Press, Chicago.
9. Tonowski, R.R. 1978. Depressed alcoholic women: Personality characteristics and life events. Unpublished doctoral dissertation, Rutgers The State University, New Brunswick, New Jersey.
10. Wittenborn, J.R. 1950. A new procedure for evaluating mental hospital patients. J. Consult. Psychol. 14: 500-501.
11. Wittenborn, J.R. 1951. Symptom patterns in a group of mental hospital patients. J. Consult. Psychol. 15: 290-302.
12. Wittenborn, J.R. 1955. Wittenborn Psychiatric Rating Scales Manual. Psychological Corporation, New York.
13. Wittenborn, J.R. 1962. The dimensions of psychosis. J. Nerv. Ment. Dis. 134: 117-128.
14. Wittenborn, J.R. 1964. Psychotic dimensions in male and female hospital patients: A principal component analysis. J. Nerv. Ment. Dis. 138: 460-467.
15. Wittenborn, J.R. 1966. The assessment of clinical change. In: J.O.Cole and J.R.Wittenborn (eds.), Pharmacotherapy of Depression, pp. 67-90. Charles Thomas Publisher, Springfield.
16. Wittenborn, J.R. 1966. Psychiatric syndromes as a cultural phenomenon. In: Proceedings of the Vth International Congress of the Collegium Internationale Neuropsychopharmacologicum, pp. 521-524. Exerpta Medica International Congress Series No. 129. Excerpta Medica, Amsterdam.
17. Wittenborn, J.R. 1966. Factors which qualify the response to iproniazid and to imipramine. In: J.R. Wittenborn and P.R.A. May (eds.), Prediction of Response to Pharmacotherapy, pp. 125-146. Charles Thomas Publisher, Springfield.
18. Wittenborn, J.R. 1969. Diagnostic classification and response to imipramine. In: P.R.A. May and J.R. Wittenborn (eds.), Psychotropic Drug Response. Charles Thomas Publisher, Springfield.
19. Wittenborn, J.R. 1976. Wittenborn Psychiatric Rating Scale. In: W.Guy (ed.), ECDEU Assessment Manual for Psychopharmacology, Revised 1976. U.D. DHEW, PHS, National Institute of Mental Health, Washington D.C.
20. Wittenborn, J.R. 1977. Stability of symptom ratings for schizophrenic men. Arch. Gen. Psychiatry 34: 437-440.
21. Wittenborn, R.R., and Holzberg, J.D. 1951. The generality of psychiatric syndromes. J. Consult. Psychol. 15: 372-380.
22. Wittenborn, J.R., and Lesser, G.S. 1951. Biographical factors and psychiatric symptoms. J. Clin. Psychol. 7: 317-322.
23. Wittenborn, J.R., and Mettler, F.A. 1951. Practical correlates of psychiatric symptoms. J. Consult. Psychol. 15: 505-510.
24. Wittenborn, J.R., and Bailey, C. 1952. The symptoms of involutional psychosis. J. Consult. Psychol. 16: 13-17.

25. Wittenborn, J. F., and Weiss, W. 1952. Patients diagnosed manic depressive psychosis – manic state. J. Consult. Psychol. 16: 193–198.
26. Wittenborn, J. R., and Smith, J. B. K. 1964. A comparison of psychotic dimensions in male and female hospital patients. J. Nerv. Ment. Dis. 138: 375–382.
27. Wittenborn, J. R., and Buhler, R. 1979. Somatic discomforts among depressed women. Arch. Gen. Psychiatry 36: 465–471.
28. Wittenborn, J. R., Bell, E. G., and Lesser, G. S. 1951. Symptom patterns among organic patients of advanced age. J. Clin. Psychol. 7: 328–331.
29. Wittenborn, J. R., Mandler, G., and Waterhouse, I. K. 1951. Symptom patterns in youthful mental hospital patients. J. Clin. Psychol. 7: 323–327.
30. Wittenborn, J. R., Herz, M. I., Kurtz, K. H., Mandell, W., and Tatz, S. 1952. The effect of rater differences on symptom rating scale clusters. J. Consult. Psychol. 16: 107–109.
31. Wittenborn, J. R., Plante, M., and Burgess, F. 1961. A comparison of physicians' and nurses' symptom ratings. J. Nerv. Ment. Dis. 133: 515–518.
32. Wittenborn, J. R., Plante, M., Burgess, F., and Livermore, N. 1961. The efficacy of electroconvulsive therapy, iproniazid and placebo in the treatment of young depressed women. J. Nerv. Ment. Dis. 133: 316–332.
33. Wittenborn, J. R., Plante, M., Burgess, F., and Maurer, H. 1962. A comparison of imipramine, electroconvulsive therapy and placebo in the treatment of depressions. J. Nerv. Ment. Dis. 135: 131–137.
34. Wittenborn, J. R., Kiremitci, N., and Weber, E. S. P. 1973. The choice of alternative antidepressants. J. Nerv. Ment. Dis. 156: 97–108.
35. Wittenborn, J. R., Vinar, O., and Monteleone, I. V. 1975. Cultural factors in psychopathological manifestations. In: T. M. Itil and E. Itil (eds.), Transcultural Neuropsychopharmacology, pp. 111–128. Bosak Publishing Co., Istanbul, Turkey.

Chapter 24 The Melancholia Scale: Development, Consistency, Validity, and Utility

P. BECH and O. J. RAFAELSEN

Introduction

The Melancholia scale (MES) was designed to be an observer-rating scale quantifying the severity of depressive states in all types of patients and serving to identify depressed patients or to assess the response to antidepressive therapy.

Rating scales can be defined as a clinical assessment procedure measuring one or more aspects (dimensions or axes) of psychopathology. Within depressive disorder [3] it has been found necessary to describe patients on two dimensions: (a) first to recognize a depressive case (the quantitative aspect of severity, e.g., minor versus major) and (b) if a case has been recognized then to put forward a theory about it (the qualitative aspect of depression, e.g., endogenous versus nonendogenous depression).

The original work, upon which the MES was based, endeavored to elucidate which features distinguish depressed patients quantitatively on the dimension of severity [3]. The MES is derived from a subgroup of six items of the Hamilton Depression Scale (HAM-D) [15, 16] that we found to represent a one-dimensional measure of depressive states. The sum of these items, the total score, was an acceptable reduction of the detailed information covered by the individual items [7]. The remaining HDS items might, hereafter, be conceived as more qualitative than quantitative, i.e., describing those clinical features that distinguish depressed patients qualitatively on an axis of diagnosis, which has recently been emphasized by Roth and co-workers [21]. Hence, the HAM-D seems to contain a heterogeneous sample of items while the MES is exclusively a quantitative scale sensitive to changes in the severity of depressive states. The MES is thus a melancholia *state* scale, e.g., categorizing patients in no depression, minor, or major depression.

Development of the MES

Each of the MES items is operationally defined on a five-point scale similar to the nine most weighted items of the HAM-D. By having an even number of positive ratings (mild, moderate, severe, extreme) the "error of central tendency" is reduced. Since the first 17-item version of the HAM-D was published in 1960 [15], it has repeatedly been demonstrated that the quantitative aspect of depression can be adequately assessed by the application of approximately ten items [3]. The MES encompasses eleven items (see Appendix A). As discussed elsewhere [5] and mentioned above, the MES has been developed on the basis of the following six HAM-D items which we found to constitute a one-dimensional measurement of depressive states: "depressed mood," "guilt," "work and interest," "retardation," "psychic anxiety," and "general somatic symptoms." As "retardation" refers to various aspects of depressive states we have included motor, verbal, emotional, and intellectual items of retardation. By this subdivision of "retardation" we have endeavored to balance items of depressive signs (observed during the interview) with items of depressive symptoms (as reported by the patient). The MES is an observer scale which can be administered by psychiatrists, psychologists, or other skilled observers. It is recommended to make use of a semistructured interview following the ordinary clinical tradition as far as possible. The criterion or rule for the item combination of MES is the total score of the 11 items. No other algorithm is recommended, as the scale has been constructed as a one-dimensional scale for the severity of depression.

Our analysis of the MES is so far limited to patients observed by psychiatrists. For use in general practice research we have designed a more simple MES version [4] by redefining the MES items on a two-point scale (0 = absent and 1 = present). Using an eight-item version of the HAM-D (an item sample covered by the MES), Fisch et al. [11] have only found small differences between psychiatrists and general physicians in evaluating the severity of depression. However, further studies with the MES in general practice research are certainly needed.

Consistency of the MES

There are three major sets of criteria for using the summed total score to ascertain the degree of depression [3]:
1. *Homogeneity* refers to the structure by which the items mutually agree, often equal to internal consistency. A rating scale is homogeneous if the measure is independent of the part of the scale (or the subgroup of items) that has been used to obtain the rating score.
2. *Reliability* refers to the extent (a) to which it may be expected that different observers obtain the same score on the same rating occasion or (b) to which it may be expected that the same observer (or patient) obtains the same score on different rating occasions. Usually (a) is called interrater reliability and (b) is called the test-retest reliability.
3. *Applicability* or transferability refers to the extent to which the scale scores can be applied to various groups of patients (e.g., diagnosis, age, sex, culture) or to the same group of patients examined repeatedly during a treatment period. This means that the rating scale is expected to be a stable "yardstick" – e.g., not measuring "anxiety" when applied to females and "depression" when applied to males.

Any conclusion based on the MES will be in accordance with what has been found consistent for the six-item HAM-D subscale. Hence, the applicability and homogeneity of the MES, evaluated by use of Rasch statistics [3, 4, 7] across such variables as plasma levels of imipramine, age, sex, weekly rating occasions, and diagnosis, are determined and have recently been confirmed by Maier and Philipp [18].

Factor analysis has often been used to measure the convergent or internal consistency. However, when a single "common factor" is expected, there is no need for factor analysis. In this sense, therefore, the homogeneity of the MES has been tested by comparing each of the 11 items with the total score of the remaining items as originally suggested by Wherry [24]. The essential aim of this method is to use the total score of the MES as a criterion of internal consistency. Items that correlate most strongly with the corresponding total score of the remaining items are then considered to be homogeneous. The results obtained by this method supported the contention that the MES is a homogeneous scale (Table 24.1). The generally higher correlation coefficients found in our first study [5] may be due to the fact that the patients in this study were tested both when depressed and again when recovering, while in the other studies ratings were obtained only when the patients were depressed.

Table 24.1. The Melancholia Scale: evaluation of homogeneity

No.	Item	Bech and Rafaelsen [5] ($n=44$)	Gjerris et al. [13] ($n=24$)	Bech et al. [8] ($n=35$)
1.	Retardation (motor)	0.71	0.62	0.62
2.	Retardation (verbal)	0.73	0.50	0.41
3.	Retardation (intellectual)	0.88	0.51	0.61
4.	Anxiety (psychic)	0.62	0.47	0.24
5.	Suicidal impulses	0.58	0.75	0.60
6.	Lowered mood	0.77	0.80	0.73
7.	Self-depreciation	0.58	0.44	0.51
8.	Retardation (emotional)	0.72	0.75	0.61
9.	Sleep disturbances	0.61	0.13	0.44
10.	Tiredness and pains	0.52	0.01	0.32
11.	Work and interests	0.73	0.65	0.37

Each of the scale items compared with the corresponding total score of the remaining items.

It is often held that there is a lower limit for the number of items on a rating scale beyond which the inter-observer reliability is adversely affected. However, when the 11-item MES was compared with the 17-item HAM-D or the 14-item Hamilton Anxiety Scale (HAM-A) it was found (Table 24.2) that the three scales all had an adequate reliability. When testing the reliability of a large group of raters, situations will often emerge where there is not the same number of raters per patient throughout the study. As shown in Table 24.2, we have in such situations used the Spearman test by comparing each rater with the average assessments for the remaining group of raters. All the Spearman coefficients are of statistical significance ($P<0.01$). Using another nonparametric test, the Kendell coefficient of concordance (W), which gives the average intercorrelation when all four raters participated, we found that the three scales were of acceptable reliability: The Kendell W was 0.79 ($P<0.01$), for the HAM-D [19]; 0.90 ($P<0.01$), for the HAM-A [13]; and 0.81 ($P<0.01$), for the MES [13]. Within the frame of parametric statistics, Bartko and Carpenter [2] have developed an intraclass correlation coefficient (ICC) which does not require the same number of raters per patient. Using the most conservative, unbiased version of the ICC(U) in a study with 35 patients and 9 observers we found this coefficient to be 0.82 ($F=32.1$, $P<0.001$) [8].

Table 24.2. Interrater reliability: A comparison of scales for affective disorders. Correlation of each rater with the average value for the remaining group of raters by Spearman coefficients r_s

Raters	Hamilton Depression Scale [19] 17 items	Hamilton Anxiety Scale [13] 14 items	Melancholia Scale [13] 11 items	Melancholia Scale [18] 11 items
A	0.79	0.79	0.93	0.87
B	0.93	0.86	0.92	0.92
C	0.83	0.81	0.91	0.86
D	0.84	0.80	0.80	0.82

$P<0.01$ for all r_s

The Validity of the MES

We have evaluated the concurrent validity of the MES by determining how it correlated (Spearman r_s) with other scales. In a population of depressed patients, the MES correlated significantly both with the 17-item HAM-D ($r_s=0.97$, $P<0.001$) and the 6-item HAM-D subscale ($r_s=0.96$, $P<0.001$). In this connection it should be emphasized that in another study on the plasma level of clomipramine and antidepressive effect we found the 6-item HAM-D (and thereby the MES) more sensitive than the 17-item HAM-D [20], resulting in a significant correlation of -0.53 ($P<0.05$) for posttreatment 6-item HDS scores and in an insignificant correlation of -0.34 for posttreatment 17-item HDS when related to the plasma levels of clomipramine. Moreover, for patients classified as endogenously depressed an r_s of 0.73 was obtained ($P<0.01$) whereas for patients classified as nonendogenously depressed an r_s of 0.30 ($P>0.05$) was obtained, when MES and HAM-A were correlated [13]. Hence, within the group of nonendogenous or neurotic depressives anxiety (HAM-A) and depression (HAM-D) are quantitatively two independent dimensions.

In principle, the dimensions of depressive states (MES) and the dimension of diagnosis (endogenous versus nonendogenous) have been considered mutually independent. In our first study [19] we found a positive, but insignificant, correlation between MES and the diagnostic index of depression, $r_s=0.46$, $P>0.05$, $n=13$. In our next study [8] we found a weak but significant correlation between the MES and the Newcastle diagnostic indices, $r_s = 0.41$ and $r_s = 0.35$, respectively ($P < 0.05$, $n = 35$). It has repeatedly been shown that the HAM-D, in contrast to the Newcastle diagnostic indices, has no diagnostic or prognostic validity in predicting response to antidepressant treatment [3], and our preliminary results with the MES seem, thus, to indicate that it is an outcome scale, not a diagnostic scale. As discussed elsewhere [3], we have *not* followed the tradition of measuring the construct validity by factor analysis. From a clinical point of view it is of importance that the MES contains items for the rating of the three elements which have been shown to be the cornerstones of melancholic states, namely (1) lowered mood, including self-depreciation and suicidal impulses, (2) worrying and tension, and (3) psychomotor retardation including work and interests [9, 14, 17]. Moreover, when attempting to measure the essentials of the melancholic state we have found it useful to look at its clinical opposite – the manic state – and the MES has been constructed to counterbalance our mania scale [3, 6], thus covering the whole affective spectrum of manic-melancholic states.

Utility of the MES

In scientific investigations the MES has been found easy and uncomplicated to use. As pretreatment definition of the target symptomatology of depressive states we have previously published the following standardized MES values: 0–5, no depression; 6–14, mild depression; 15–25, moderate depression; 26–44, severe depression [5]. In a subsequent study [8] we have compared the MES values with the Feighner criteria [10] and with the DSM-III criteria [1] for major depressive episodes (Table 24.3). As can be seen from this table, a score of 15 or more on the MES seems to be an adequate cutoff value for major depressive episodes.

Table 24.3. Comparison of the MES values with the Feighner criteria and the DSM-III criteria

Classification system	Depressive episode	Melancholia Scale median (25 percentiles)	Number of patients
DSM-III [1]	Major	19 (15–24)	26
	Minor	13 (11–17)	9
Feighner [10]	Definite	20 (17–25)	20
	Nondefinite	14 (11–17)	15

Using weekly ratings during a therapeutic trial, the MES can measure treatment effects. We recommend using a score between 0 and 5 for full remission, and 6 to 14 for partial response to treatment.

Apart from the original Scandinavian version an English [3] and a German version [12] have been released. French, Italian, Japanese, and Spanish versions are in preparation [23]. These MES versions have to be tested locally for their interrater reliability and applicability before they can be used in scientific studies.

Conclusion

The MES is primarily a research tool for measuring treatment effects. It is a melancholic state scale which has been developed from the Hamilton Depression Scale to measure more strictly the quantitative aspect of depression. Analyses of the consistency of the MES have justified that the criterion for item combinations of its 11 items is the total score. As research criteria of treatment effects we have recommended an MES score of between 0 and 5 for full remission and an MES score of between 6 and 14 for partial response.

Appendix A Melancholia Rating Scale: Scoring Instructions

Introduction

The melancholia scale consists of 11 items. The interviewer should judge the patient's condition at the time of the interview when assessing the presence and degree of the individual items. Some items are, however, less suitable for a "here-and-now" evaluation, e.g., sleep disturbances. It is necessary here to judge the condition during the 3 days prior to the interview. When in doubt the interviewer should solicit information from ward personnel or relatives.

The duration of the interview should be no less than 15 min and no more than 30 min. In principle the interview technique is not different from clinical tradition. Pressure should not be exerted on patients, who as far as possible should be allowed to explain their situations in their own words. The interviewer should remain unaffected by spontaneous intermissions as these represent an integral part of the observation.

The rating should always take place at a fixed hour, e.g., between 8:00 and 9:30 a.m., to avoid the influence of diurnal variation. The scale is basically quantitative; it has been constructed for the sole purpose of rating the actual clinical picture, and it is not to be considered a diagnostic tool. When the scale is applied in repeated (weekly) ratings, each assessment should be independent. The rater should therefore avoid taking a look at or recalling former interviews and likewise should not ask for changes that might have taken place from the last interview; instead he or she should elucidate the patient's condition during the preceding 3 days.

For the various items it is assumed that each scale step contains the lower steps, e.g., scale step 3 includes the statements of scale steps 2 and 1. Normal function is always rated as 0.

The following glossary represents guidelines for ratings:

1. Activity (motor)
0: Normal motor activity, adequate facial expression
1: Slightly decreased motor activity, facial expression slightly rigid (retarded)
2: More pronounced motor retardation (e.g., reduced gestures, slow pace)

The Melancholia Scale

3: All movements very slow
4: Motor retardation approaching or including stupor

2. *Activity (verbal)*

This item includes changes in flow of speech and the capacity to verbalize thoughts and emotions
0: Normal verbal activity
1: Slightly reduced verbal expression or inertia in conversation
2: More pronounced inertia in conversation, e. g., a trend to longer intermissions
3: When the interview is clearly prolonged due to long pauses and brief responses
4: When the interview can only be completed with marked difficulty

3. *Retardation (intellectual)*

0: Normal intellectual activity
1: The patient has to make an effort to concentrate on his or her work
2: Even with a major effort it is difficult for the patient to concentrate on his or her work. Less initiative than usual. The patient easily experiences "brain fatigue"
3: Marked difficulties with concentration, initiative, and decision-making. For example, can hardly read a newspaper or watch television. Score 3 as long as the retardation has not clearly influenced the interview
4: When the patient during the interview has shown marked difficulty in following normal conversation

4. *Anxiety (psychic)*

This item includes tension, irritability, worry, insecurity, fear, and apprehension approaching panic. It may often be difficult to distinguish between the patient's experience of anxiety ("psychic" or "central" anxiety phenomena) and the physiological ("peripheral") anxiety manifestations which can be observed, e. g., hand tremor and sweating. Most important is the patient's report on worry, insecurity, uncertainty, experiences of fear and panic, i. e., the psychic ("central") anxiety
0: When the patient is neither more nor less anxious or insecure or tense than usual
1: When the patient is somewhat more anxious, tense, or insecure than usual
2: When the patient clearly expresses a state of anxiety, insecurity, worry, and tension which he or she finds difficult to control and which therefore may interfere with his or her daily work
3: When the anxiety or insecurity from time to time is very marked and experienced as panic, i. e., when anxiety gets out of control
4: When the patient more constantly is in a state of panic. It is difficult to distract the patient from his or her feeling of panic and this interferes with the interview

5. *Suicidal impulses*

0: No suicidal impulses
1: The patient feels that life is not worthwhile, but expresses no wish to die
2: The patient wishes to die, but has no plans to end his or her own life
3: It is probable that the patient contemplates committing suicide

4: If the patient in the days prior to the interview has tried to commit suicide, or if the patient in the ward is under special observation due to suicidal risk

6. *Lowered mood*

This item covers both the verbal and the nonverbal communication of sadness, depression, despondency, helplessness, and hopelessness
0: Neutral mood
1: The patient vaguely indicates that he or she is more despondent and depressed than usual
2: When the patient, more clearly, is disturbed by unpleasant experiences, although he or she is without helplessness or hopelessness
3: The patient shows clear nonverbal signs of depression, e.g., repeated weeping, face pale and grayish, frowning, and unsteady voice
4: The patient's remarks or non-verbal signs of despondency and helplessness, from which he cannot be distracted, dominate the interview

7. *Self-depreciation and guilt feeling*

This item covers lowered self-esteem
0: No self-depreciation or guilt feeling
1: Vague self-depreciation; the patient feels that he or she has not lived up to expectations, that he or she may have failed
2: Self-depreciation or guilt feeling is more clearly present. Patient may feel he has been a burden to his family or that his work capacity has been reduced during the actual episode of illness. It is important to note whether the patient unreasonably reproaches him- or herself for small omissions or failures, such as not to have done his or her duty or to have harmed others. Such self-accusations are often focused on incidents in the past, prior to the actual episode
3: The patient suffers from severe guilt feeling and will often express the feeling that the actual suffering is some sort of a punishment. Score 3 as long as the patient intellectually can see that his or her view is unfounded
4: The guilt feeling is firmly maintained and resists any counterargument, thereby becoming a paranoid idea

8. *Emotional retardation*

This item covers the reduced interest and emotional contact with other human beings. The wish or ability to communicate one's own feelings and opinions and to share joy and sorrow is experienced by the patient as being alien and painful
0: Normal interest and emotional contact with others
1: Less wish or ability to be together with new or distant acquaintances
2: The patient isolates him- or herself to a certain degree and has no need or ability to establish closer contact with people met away from home (workmates, fellow patients, ward personnel)
3: The patient isolates him- or herself also in relation to family members and feels emotionally indifferent even to near friends and family

4: Totally isolated. Is unable to feel any human contact. Considers him- or herself dead emotionally

9. *Sleep disturbances*

This item covers only the patient's subjective experience of the duration of sleep (hours of sleep per 24-h period) and sleep depth (superficial and interrupted sleep versus deep and steady sleep). The rating is based on three preceding nights, irrespective of administration of hypnotics or sedatives
0: Usual sleep duration and sleep depth
1: Sleep duration is slightly reduced (e. g., due to difficulties in falling asleep), but no change in sleep depth
2: Sleep depth is now also reduced, sleep being more superficial. Sleep as a whole somewhat disturbed
3: Sleep duration as well as sleep depth is markedly changed. The broken sleep periods total only a few hours per 24-h period
4: It is difficult here to ascertain sleep duration as sleep depth is so shallow that the patient speaks of short periods of slumber or dosing, but no real sleep

10. *Tiredness and pains*

This item includes weakness, faintness, tiredness, fullness, and soreness merging into real pains more or less diffusely located to muscles or inner organs. Muscle fatigue is normally located in the extremities. The patient may give this as the reason for difficulties in his or her work as he or she has a feeling of tiredness or heaviness in arms and legs. Muscle pains are often located in the back, neck, or shoulders perceived as tensions or headache. The feeling of fullness and heaviness increasing to real sensations of pain is often broadly located as "chest discomfort" (different from heart pains), abdominal pains, and head pains (different from simple headache). It is often difficult to discern between "psychic" and "physical" pains. Special notice should be taken of vague "psychic" pains
0: The patient is neither more nor less tired or troubled by bodily discomfort than usual
1: Vague feelings of muscular fatigue or other somatic discomfort
2: Feelings of muscular fatigue or somatic discomfort are more pronounced. Painful sensations sometimes occur
3: Muscular fatigue or diffuse pain is clearly present, which interferes with the patient's daily work
4: Muscular fatigue and diffuse pains are constantly causing the patient severe distress

11. *Work and interests*

This item includes both motivation and work actually carried out. Especially for housewives it may be difficult to assess this item, as such patients are less prone to remark that they have difficulties with their daily housework. They will often use statements such as "I have been less hard-working or conscientious lately"

A. At first rating of the patient
0: Normal work activity
1: The patient expresses problems due to lack of motivation, and/or trouble in carrying out the usual workload, which the patient, however, manages to do without reduction
2: More pronounced deficiency due to lack of motivation and/or trouble in carrying out the usual work. Here the patient has reduced work capacity, cannot maintain normal speed, copes with less on the job or at home; the patient may stay home some days or tries to leave early
3: The patient has been sick-listed; or the patient has been hospitalized (as a day-patient or with full hospitalization) but can participate for some hours per day in the ward activities
4: The patient is fully hospitalized and generally unoccupied without participation in the ward activities

B. At weekly ratings
0: a) The patient has resumed work at his or her normal activity level
   b) The patient will have no trouble resuming normal work
1: a) The patient is working, but at a reduced activity level, either due to lack of motivation or due to difficulties in the accomplishment of his or her normal work
   b) The patient is not working, and it is still doubtful that normal work can be resumed without difficulty
2: a) The patient is working, but at a clearly reduced level, either due to episodes of nonattendance or due to reduced work time
   b) The patient is still hospitalized or sick-listed, participates more than 3-4 h/day in ward (or home) activities, but is only capable of resuming normal work at a reduced level. If hospitalized the patient is able to change from full-stay to day-patient status
3: The patient is unable to undertake normal work, but participates for 3-4 h/day in ward activities. It may be considered desirable to change the patient's hospitalization to day-patient status, but discharge is not recommended
4: The patient is still fully hospitalized and on the whole unable to participate in ward activities

References

1. American Psychiatric Association. 1980. Diagnostic and Statistical Manual of Mental Disorders. 3rd Ed. (DSM-III). American Psychiatric Association, Washington DC.
2. Bartko, J.J., and Carpenter, W.T. 1976. On the methods and theory of reliability. J. Nerv. Ment. Dis. 163: 307-317.
3. Bech, P. 1981. Rating scales for affective disorders: Their validity and consistency. Acta Psychiatr. Scand. 64 (suppl. 295): 1-101.
4. Bech, P. 1985. The use of rating scales for affective disorders. In: T. Helgason (ed.), Methodology in evaluation of psychiatric treatment. European Medical Research Council. Cambridge University Press, Cambridge.

5. Bech, P., and Rafaelsen, O.J. 1980. The use of rating scales exemplified by a comparison of the Hamilton and the Bech-Rafaelsen Melancholia Scale. Acta Psychiatr. Scand. 62 (suppl. 285): 128-131.
6. Bech, P., Bolwig, T.G., Kramp, P., and Rafaelsen, O.J. 1979. The Bech-Rafaelsen Mania Scale and the Hamilton Depression Scale. Acta Psychiatr. Scand. 59: 420-430.
7. Bech, P., Allerup, P., Gram, L.F., Reisby, N., Rosenberg, R., Jacobsen, O., and Nagy, A. 1981. The Hamilton Depression Scale. Evaluation of objectivity using logistic models. Acta Psychiatr. Scand. 63: 290-299.
8. Bech, P., Gjerris, A., Andersen, J., Bøjholm, S., Kramp, P., Bolwig, T.G., Kastrup, M., Clemmesen, L., and Rafaelsen, O.J. 1985. The Melancholia Scale and the Newcastle Scales: Item-combinations and inter-observer reliability. Br. J. Psychiatry 143: 58-63.
9. Beck, A.T. 1967. Depression: Clinical, Experimental, and Theoretical Aspects. University of Pennsylvania Press, Philadelphia.
10. Feighner, J.P., Robins, E., Guze, S.B., Woddruff, Jr., R.A., Winokur, G., and Munoz, R. 1972. Diagnostic criteria for use in psychiatric research. Arch. Gen. Psychiatr. 26: 57-63.
11. Fisch, H.U., Hammond, K.R., and Joyce, C.R.B. 1982. On evaluating the severity of depression: An experimental study of psychiatrists. Br. J. Psychiat. 140: 378-383.
12. Gastpar, G., and Gastpar, M. 1982. Unpublished, Basel.
13. Gjerris, A., Bech, P., Bøjholm, S., Bolwig, T.G., Kramp, P., Andersen, J., and Rafaelsen, O.J. 1983. The Hamilton Anxiety Scale: Evaluation of homogeneity and interobserver reliability in patients with depressive disorders. J. Affective Disord. 5: 163-170.
14. Goldberg, D. 1972. The Detection of Psychiatric Illness by Questionnaire. Maudsley Monograph No. 21. Oxford University, Press, London.
15. Hamilton, M. 1960. A rating scale for depression. J. Neurol. Neurosurg. Psychiatry. 23: 56-62.
16. Hamilton, M. 1967. Development of a rating scale for primary depressive illness. Br. J. Soc. Clin. Psychol. 6: 278-296.
17. Kielholz, P., Terzani, S., and Gastpar, M. 1979. Treatment for therapy resistant depression. International Pharmacopsychiatry 14: 94-100.
18. Maier, W., and Philipp, M. 1985. Comparative analysis of observer depression scales. Acta Psychiatr. Scand. In press.
19. Rafaelsen, O.J., Bech, P., Bolwig, T.G., Kramp, P., and Gjerris, A. 1980. The Bech-Rafaelsen combined rating scale for mania and melancholia. In: K. Achte, V. Aalberg, and J. Lönnqvist (eds.), Psychopathology of depression. Psychiatria Fennica (suppl.) 327-331.
20. Reisby, N., Gram, L.F., Bech, P., Sihm, F., Krautwald, O., Elly, J., Ortman, J., and Christiansen, J. 1979. Clomipramine: plasma levels and clinical effects. Commun. Psychopharmacol. 3: 341-351.
21. Roth, M., Mountjoy, D.O., and Caetano, D. 1982. Further investigations into the relationship between depressive disorders and anxiety states. Pharmacopsychiatria 15: 135-141.
22. Spitzer, R.J., Endicott, J.E., and Robins, E. 1978. Research Diagnostic Criteria. Arch. Gen. Psychiatry 35: 773-782.
23. Unpublished Melancholia Scales: Ballus, C., Cassano, G.B., Takahashi, R., and Zarifian, E. have prepared the Spanish, Italian, Japanese, and French versions, respectively.
24. Wherry, R.J., Campbell, J.T., and Perloff, R. 1951. An empirical verification of the Wherry Gaylood iterative factor analysis procedure. Psychometrika 16: 67-74.

Chapter 25 Clinical Self-Rating Scales (CSRS) of the Munich Psychiatric Information System (PSYCHIS München)

D. VON ZERSSEN

Introduction

In order to assess the present mental state of patients at admission to and discharge from a psychiatric hospital and to record changes in their general mood state during hospitalization or within special research projects, a series of self-rating scales [5, 29, 30] were constructed as a supplement to clinical-rating scales (such as the inpatient multidimensional psychiatric scale [IMPS] according to Lorr and Klett [15]). All these scales, together with additional scales for the evaluation of premorbid personality traits and the respective scoring procedures, constitute a subsystem of the Munich psychiatric information system (PSYCHIS München [1]) developed at the Max Planck Institute of Psychiatry (MPIP). At present the data bank of this system contains questionnaire data on more than 3500 psychiatric inpatients, well over 700 medical patients, and approximately 4000 subjects from the general population investigated in epidemiological studies [8, 26, 29 a] by means of these scales or a subset of them. The scales have also been applied in various other clinical and outpatient settings, pharmacological laboratories, etc., within and outside the Federal Republic of Germany.

The Clinical Self-Rating Scales (CSRSs; in German, *Klinische Selbstbeurteilungs-Skalen,* KSb-S) have been translated into English (see Appendix A), French [3, 11], Italian, Japanese, Russian, and Spanish, and one of them, an adjective mood scale, also into Lithuanian, Slovakian, Czech, Danish, and Swedish. The scales exist in two parallel versions, for each of which normative values from the adult general population of the Federal Republic of Germany and reference values from various psychiatric samples have been provided. A detailed description is given in the test manuals [29 a-d] according to the *Standards for Educational and Psychological Tests and Manuals* (see [4], pp. 1479-1508).

The CSRSs have proven particularly useful in the investigation of affective disorders, above all the various types of depression [28]. This area will be the focus of the following report on the construction and application of the scales.

Construction of the Scales

The CSRSs are composed of items that were selected from the psychiatric literature, existing symptom scales, and psychiatric case records, all reflecting disturbances of a patient's affective or cognitive functioning at the subjective level of symptoms (see Table 25.1). They comprise three questionnaires with parallel versions and two additional questionnaires (CL° and AS$_{10}$; see below):

1. The Adjective Mood Scale (AMS and its parallel version AMS'; in German, *Befindlichkeits-Skala*, Bf-S/Bf-S', with 28 items each) for the assessment of fluctuations in well-being (or rather its reduction) such as diurnal variations in mood or mood changes during drug treatment of a depressive disorder [6, 33].

Table 25.1. Survey of scales described in this article

Questionnaire (system)	Abbreviation and references	Area of disturbance	No. of items	Comment
Clinical self-rating scales of the Munich Psychiatric Information System (PSYCHIS, München)	CSRS [29a, 30]	Present state of subjective disturbances		Parallel forms (S') for the scales (S) (1) through (3) with normative values of the average population (for probands with an IQ ≥ 80)
1. Adjective Mood Scale (two parallel versions S/S')	AMS/AMS' [29a, d, 30, 32]	Actual reduction of well-being	28/28	Designed for the assessment of short-term mood changes by repeated measurements
2. Complaint List (two parallel versions L/L' with one supplementary list L°)	CL/CL'/CL° [29b, 30, 31]	Somatic and general complaints	24/24/17	Items of CL° (not scored!) only serving as additional information on specific complaints
3. Paranoid Depression Scale (two parallel versions S/S')	PDS/PDS' [29c, 30, 34]	Paranoid tendencies (P/P') and depressive tendencies (D/D'); furthermore a tendency toward denial of illness (DI/DI')	43/43	Beyond DI/DI' further control measures regarding motivation (M) and discrepancy (DC) between identical or similar items of the two parallel versions
Depression Scale (two parallel versions S/S')	DS/DS' [29c]	As above (D/D')	16/16	Subscale of PDS/PDS' (without control items and scales)
4. Anxiety Scale$_{10}$	AS$_{10}$	State anxiety	10	Composed of a factorially homogeneous subset of items from the SAS [36] and the SDS [35]

2. The Complaint List (CL and its parallel version CL'; in German, *Beschwerden-Liste*, B-L/B-L', with 24 items each, as well as one supplementary list, CL°, or, in German, B-L°, with 17 items, not used for calculating a scale value but serving as an additional source of information about a patient's symptoms) contains items describing either somatic or general complaints as reported by the majority of medical and, in particular, psychiatric patients (see [21, 31]), in the latter partially expressing the degree of somatization of the underlying emotional disorder, e.g., depression.
3. The multidimensional Paranoid Depression Scale (PDS; in German, *Paranoid-Depressivitäts-Skala*, and its parallel version PDS' with 43 items each) comprised of two clinical scales for depressive (DS/DS') and paranoid symptoms (PS/PS'), respectively (16 items each separately for both the parallel versions), one control scale for the ascertainment of a tendency to the denial of illness (DIS/DIS': eight items, identical in both parallel versions), and three items regarding the patient's motivation (M) to cooperate in the test situation (all three identical in both parallel versions). If the two parallel versions are applied to the same individual within short intervals (a few hours or around 24 h), a discrepancy (DC) score can be calculated from the item scores of the eight items of the control scale, which are identical in both questionnaires, and four items of the Depression Scale, which are very similar in content in both questionnaires and correlate highly with each other. A high value of DC (as the sum of differences between item scores of identical or similar items in the two parallel forms) points to inconsistencies of the responses and may thus reveal that the test results are meaningless.

In studying subjects with nonpsychotic depression where marked paranoid tendencies cannot be expected, the subscale for assessing symptoms of depression (DS and/or DS' with 16 items each) may be applied separately. The aforementioned control measures are, however, only included in the complete questionnaire (PDS and PDS').
4. In addition to the questionnaires described in the manuals [29a-d], a ten-item version of Zung's Self-Rating Anxiety Scale (SAS; [36]) has been used experimentally since 1977. This „Anxiety Scale₁₀" (AS_{10}) contains those items (eight from the SAS and two - item Nos. 9 and 10 - from the SDS; [35]) that, according to a principal component analysis of data from a sample of 314 subjects (185 psychiatric inpatients and 129 healthy controls), constitute a homogeneous factor not represented in our symptom scales CL and DS and may, therefore, reflect a somewhat different aspect of a patient's emotional state than these scales (and their parallel forms) do. It should be pointed out, however, that during the construction of our scales a clear differentiation between anxiety and depression at the level of symptom factors could not be achieved [29a], which is in accord with other studies of self-rating scales reported in the literature [17]. Moreover, the original 20-item version of Zung's SAS has proven inferior to the CL and DS, not only with respect to internal consistency but also to clinical validity in the comparison of psychiatric patients and controls (see Table 25.10) as well as the same patients' mental state at admission and discharge [27].

The CSRSs were developed step by step, starting from a rather large item pool which was then condensed on the basis of intermediate statistical data analyses (following tenets of the classical test theory; see [13]) until highly consistent scales with likewise highly correlating parallel versions had been developed. Although the different scales measure different aspects of a patient's subjective state, the scale values do not vary independently of one another but do show some intercorrelations. A principal component analysis with orthogonal rotation of five vectors (Table 25.2) reveals largely independent dimensions (3 and 4, respectively) for the Denial of Illness Scale (DIS/DIS') and the Paranoid Scale (PS/PS'), one dimension (5) for the Anxiety Scale$_{10}$ (AS$_{10}$), one dimension (2) for the Complaint List (CL/CL') but with additional loadings of DS and AS$_{10}$, and one – most prominent – dimension (1) for both the Depression Scale (DS/DS') and the Adjective Mood Scale (AMS/AMS'), with additional loadings of CL'. It can be assumed on the basis of this analysis that the first principal component represents the most typical features of depression at a subjective level whereas the other dimensions are related to aspects of subjective disturbances which play a more peripheral role in depression, such as physical discomfort (2), a general feeling of sickness (the reverse of the denial of illness: (3), see below under „Application of the Scales"), delusional thinking (4), and anxiety (5).

The relationship of DS/DS', AMS/AMS', and CL/CL' to depressive symptomatology becomes obvious mainly in the analysis of changes in psychopathology during treatment. This is demonstrated by the result of a principal component analysis of differences between scale values obtained at admission and discharge from the same patients by means of the CSRS and the IMPS. As shown in Table 25.3, changes in self-ratings concord fairly well with changes in the corresponding clinical ratings. Clearly, the first dimension represents changes in depressive symptomatology whereas the fourth dimension indicates changes in delusional thinking. The other dimensions reflect either changes in self-description (2: general distress) or in

Table 25.2. Factorial structure of the CSRS of psychiatric inpatients on admission ($n = 420$) according to a principal component analysis with orthogonal rotation on the first five vectors

Scale	Abbreviation	1	2	3	4	5	h^2
Complaint List	CL	0.32	**−0.85**	0.17	0.15	0.21	**0.93**
Parallel Form	CL'	**0.46**	**−0.81**	0.20	0.08	0.15	0.94
Paranoid Scale	PS	−0.02	−0.25	0.15	**0.91**	−0.02	0.91
Parallel Form	PS'	0.07	0.03	0.14	**0.93**	0.16	0.91
Depression Scale	DS	**0.74**	**−0.46**	0.26	0.20	−0.01	0.86
Parallel Form	DS'	**0.78**	−0.31	0.24	0.13	0.34	0.89
Denial of Illness Scale	DIS	−0.18	0.26	**−0.89**	−0.17	0.02	0.92
Parallel Form	DIS'	−0.19	0.08	**−0.89**	−0.16	−0.24	0.92
Adjective Mood Scale	AMS	**0.86**	−0.32	0.12	−0.07	−0.02	0.86
Parallel Form	AMS'	**0.91**	−0.10	0.09	−0.01	0.17	0.89
Anxiety Scale$_{10}$	AS$_{10}$	0.29	**−0.49**	0.25	0.19	**0.72**	0.94
% Total variance		29.03	19.82	17.44	16.96	7.35	

Factor loadings ≧ 0.40 in boldface

clinically assessed psychopathology (3: psychotic excitement; 5: paranoid-hallucinatory and, amazingly, obsessional features; 6: organic features). It can be inferred from the result of this analysis that some of the CSRSs are rather sensitive measures of change in depressive symptomatology: above all, the Adjective Mood Scale (AMS/AMS'), but also the Depression Scale (DS/DS') and, to a certain extent, the Complaint List (CL/CL'). This rather high degree of concordance between self-ratings and clinical ratings is not found in the analysis of cross-sectional measures of psychopathology (see [33], Table 25.4), which means that self-ratings of psychopathology yield clinically more valid results in longitudinal investigations.

Some of the statistical scale characteristics derived from the test manuals [29 b-d], or recent data analyses are presented in Tables 25.4-25.9. The test statistics indicate a rather high factorial homogeneity and, consequently, a high reliability in the sense of internal consistency of all the scales. The parallel test reliability is also

Table 25.3. Factorial structure of the difference between scale values obtained at admission and discharge by means of the CSRS and the IMPS[a] from the same patients as in Table 25.2 ($n = 420$) with orthogonal rotation of the first six vectors

Scale	Abbreviation	1	2	3	4	5	6	h^2
CSRS (Self-rating)								
Complaint List	CL	**0.42**	**0.65**	−0.11	0.19	−0.04	0.02	0.64
Parallel Form	CL'	**0.51**	**0.67**	−0.06	0.13	0.02	0.03	0.73
Paranoid Scale	PS	0.01	0.34	−0.15	**0.80**	−0.07	−0.06	0.78
Parallel Form	PS'	0.10	0.23	−0.16	**0.83**	−0.09	−0.02	0.79
Depression Scale	DS	**0.61**	**0.56**	0.09	0.25	0.02	0.02	0.75
Parallel Form	DS'	**0.65**	**0.48**	0.06	0.22	0.05	0.10	0.72
Denial of Illness Scale	DIS	0.01	**−0.78**	−0.04	−0.08	0.05	0.11	0.62
Parallel Form	DIS'	−0.03	**−0.72**	0.02	−0.09	0.05	0.12	0.54
Adjective Mood Scale	AMS	**0.71**	0.38	0.00	−0.09	0.03	0.03	0.65
Parallel Form	AMS'	**0.76**	0.25	−0.02	0.01	0.02	−0.04	0.64
Anxiety Scale$_{10}$	AS$_{10}$	0.35	**0.54**	−0.09	0.27	−0.05	0.09	0.51
IMPS[a] (clinician's rating)								
Excitement	EXC	−0.18	0.16	**−0.78**	−0.03	0.03	0.10	0.68
Hostile belligerence	HOS	0.01	−0.03	**−0.77**	0.13	−0.07	0.08	0.62
Conceptual disorganization	CNP	−0.09	0.01	**−0.61**	0.06	−0.08	**−0.43**	0.58
Motor disturbances	MTR	0.10	0.10	**−0.59**	−0.04	−0.24	**−0.48**	0.65
Grandiose Expansiveness	GRN	−0.12	−0.06	**−0.63**	0.22	−0.04	0.06	0.46
Paranoid projection	PAR	−0.07	−0.07	**−0.41**	**0.44**	**−0.56**	−0.05	0.69
Perceptual distortions	PCP	−0.06	0.04	−0.14	0.12	**−0.79**	−0.14	0.69
Anxious depression	ANX	**0.69**	0.01	0.19	0.00	−0.24	0.10	0.57
Retardation and apathy	RTD	**0.51**	−0.21	0.01	0.16	0.03	**−0.58**	0.67
Impaired functioning	IMP	**0.66**	−0.04	0.18	−0.03	0.09	−0.10	0.49
Obsessional-phobic	OBS	0.09	0.08	0.03	−0.04	**−0.76**	0.16	0.61
Disorientation	DIS	−0.12	0.19	0.07	−0.01	0.07	**−0.75**	0.63
% Total variance		16.03	14.50	11.57	8.19	7.32	6.34	

[a] According to Lorr [14]
Factor loadings ≥ 0.40 in boldface

high with the exception of PDS/PDS' in the general population sample (probably due to the very low scores on this particular scale in normals). The parallel test correlation in patients can be assumed to be somewhat underestimated since the two forms were administered on two consecutive days shortly after admission to the hospital; thus the value involves the retest reliability, which is necessarily limited in change-sensitive scales within a time span during which marked changes in the patient's mental state may occur, e.g., shortly after hospital admission.

The differences in the distribution of test scores between patients and healthy subjects point to a high discriminating power of the clinical scales and a particularly high sensitivity of the Depression Scale and the Adjective Mood Scale to the symptomatology of depression, which is in concordance with the results presented in Tables 25.2 and 25.3.

Application of the Scales

The scales described in this article have been applied separately or in combination with one another and/or with other self-rating as well as observers' rating scales in various settings (see „Introduction"). It is recommended to use the CSRSs predominantly as adjuncts to clinical ratings and to check the patients' intelligence by means

Table 25.4. Test statistics of the *Complaint List (CL/CL')* from the general population (A) and psychiatric (B) and, in particular, depressive (C)[a] inpatients (males and females, aged 20-64 years)

	A General population		B Psychiatric inpatients		C[a] Depressive inpatients	
	CL	CL'	CL	CL'	CL	CL'
	$n=n'=1761$		$n=n'=420$		$n=n'=104$	
Parallel test correlation	0.85		0.90		0.90	
Odd-even reliability upgraded according to Spearman-Brown	0.90	0.90	0.92	0.92	0.87	0.88
% total variance of 1st unrotated component[b]	28.36	29.15	35.08	37.11	27.89	27.64
1st quartile (Q_1)	5.50	5.50	15.93	15.79	19.83	25.10
2nd quartile (Q_2=median)	11.50	11.50	26.32	29.30	28.90	35.17
3rd quartile (Q_3)	20.50	20.50	38.30	39.75	37.17	42.00
Mean value ($\bar{x}$)	14.26	14.26	26.75	28.19	29.18	33.76
Standard deviation (s)	10.75	10.74	14.81	15.35	12.46	12.22
Skewness	0.82	0.84	0.14	−0.01	0.24	−0.22
Excess	0.33	0.48	−0.73	−0.77	−0.41	−0.34

No. of items per parallel test: 24
Item scores (in key direction): 0-1-2-3
Normal range: 0-23
[a] Subsample of B
[b] From a principal component analysis of the 24 test items

Table 25.5. Test statistics of the *Paranoid Scale (PS/PS')* from the general population (A) and psychiatric (B) and, in particular, depressive (C)[a] inpatients (males and females, aged 20–64 years)

	A General population		B Psychiatric inpatients		C[a] Depressive inpatients	
	PS	PS'	PS	PS'	PS	PS'
	$n = 1693$,	$n' = 1700$	$n = n' = 420$		$n = n' = 104$	
Parallel test correlation	0.58		0.77		0.74	
Odd-even reliability, upgraded according to Spearman-Brown	0.74	0.75	0.86	0.90	0.73	0.88
% total variance of 1st unrotated component[b]	21.20	23.83	34.11	36.01	29.26	29.87
1st quartile (Q_1)	0.00	0.00	2.14	1.52	1.75	0.94
2nd quartile (Q_2 = median)	0.50	0.50	5.50	4.47	4.09	2.94
3rd quartile (Q_3)	2.50	2.50	11.27	10.28	8.90	8.17
Mean value ($\bar{x}$)	2.08	2.53	7.89	7.07	6.25	5.09
Standard deviation (s)	2.92	3.39	7.81	7.65	6.07	5.53
Skewness	2.53	2.91	1.65	1.66	1.29	1.25
Excess	9.39	13.69	3.28	2.77	1.12	0.74

No. of items per parallel test: 16
Item scores (in key direction): 0–1–2–3
Normal range: 0–4
[a] Subsample of B
[b] From a principal component analysis of the 16 test items

Table 25.6. Test statistics of the *Depression Scale (DS/DS')* from the general population (A) and psychiatric (B) and, in particular, depressive (C)[a] inpatients (males and females, aged 20–64 years)

	A General population		B Psychiatric inpatients		C[a] Depressive inpatients	
	DS	DS'	DS	DS'	DS	DS'
	$n = 1693$,	$n' = 1700$	$n = n' = 420$		$n = n' = 104$	
Parallel test correlation	0.76		0.83		0.79	
Odd-even reliability, upgraded according to Spearman-Brown	0.80	0.81	0.91	0.91	0.90	0.86
% total variance of 1st unrotated component[b]	27.93	30.90	42.24	41.21	39.94	33.89
1st quartile (Q_1)	1.50	2.50	9.14	10.92	16.86	18.17
2nd quartile (Q_2 = median)	3.50	5.50	17.43	19.56	23.50	24.25
3rd quartile (Q_3)	6.50	8.50	27.50	28.27	32.50	32.25
Mean value ($\bar{x}$)	5.46	7.09	18.65	19.71	23.88	24.39
Standard deviation (s)	4.74	5.47	11.23	11.10	10.42	9.65
Skewness	1.85	1.65	0.21	0.13	−0.20	−0.25
Excess	5.20	4.03	−0.99	−0.88	−0.75	−0.58

No. of items per parallel test: 16
Item scores (in key direction): 0–1–2–3
Normal range: 0–10
[a] Subsample of B
[b] From a principal component analysis of the 16 test items

Table 25.7. Test statistics of the *Denial of Illness Scale (DIS/DIS')* from the general population (A) and psychiatric (B) and, in particular, depressive (C)[a] inpatients (males and females, aged 20-64 years)

	A General population		B Psychiatric inpatients		C[a] Depressive inpatients	
	DIS	DIS'	DIS	DIS'	DIS	DIS'
	$n=1693$,	$n'=1700$	$n=n'=420$		$n=n'=104$	
Parallel test correlation	0.79		0.79		0.82	
Odd-even reliability, upgraded according to Spearman-Brown	0.82	0.84	0.77	0.82	0.63	0.73
% total variance of 1st unrotated component[b]	44.35	43.93	40.54	44.94	33.57	38.77
1st quartile (Q_1)	12.50	12.50	6.38	5.88	7.36	7.25
2nd quartile (Q_2 = median)	15.50	15.50	9.69	10.55	10.17	10.59
3rd quartile (Q_3)	17.50	16.50	13.79	14.24	13.00	13.61
Mean value ($\bar{x}$)	15.19	14.76	9.95	10.17	10.16	10.29
Standard deviation (s)	4.12	4.27	5.11	5.34	4.37	4.68
Skewness	−1.03	−0.94	0.21	0.05	−0.01	0.03
Excess	1.49	1.14	−0.37	−0.72	−0.22	−0.45

No. of items per parallel test: 8
Item scores (in key direction): 0-1-2-3
Normal range: 12-18
[a] Subsample of B
[b] From a principal component analysis of the eight test items

Table 25.8. Test statistics of the *Adjective Mood Scale (AMS/AMS')* from the general population (A) and psychiatric (B) and, in particular, depressive (C)[a] inpatients (males and females, aged 20-64 years)

	A General population		B Psychiatric inpatients		C[a] Depressive inpatients	
	AMS	AMS'	AMS	AMS'	AMS	AMS'
	$n=n'=1761$		$n=n'=420$		$n=n'=104$	
Parallel test correlation	0.86		0.78		0.70	
Odd-even reliability, upgraded according to Spearman-Brown	0.93	0.91	0.96	0.96	0.94	0.93
% total variance of 1st unrotated component[b]	33.22	32.60	47.44	49.51	37.89	39.52
1st quartile (Q_1)	3.50	4.50	18.50	15.62	31.83	27.50
2nd quartile (Q_2 = median)	9.50	9.50	34.04	31.17	40.83	40.00
3rd quartile (Q_3)	16.50	17.50	43.77	43.75	46.17	46.30
Mean value ($\bar{x}$)	11.86	12.46	30.97	29.41	37.60	36.61
Standard deviation (s)	9.75	9.62	15.54	15.99	12.65	12.79
Skewness	1.15	1.18	−0.43	−0.18	−0.99	−0.88
Excess	1.30	1.59	−0.98	−1.21	0.49	−0.01

No. of items per parallel test: 28
Item scores (in key direction): 0-1-2
Normal range: 0-21
[a] Subsample of B
[b] From a principal component analysis of the 28 test items

Table 25.9. Test statistics of the *Anxiety Scale₁₀ (AS₁₀)* from the general population (A) and psychiatric (B) and, in particular, depressive (C)[a] inpatients (males and females, aged 20-64 years)

	A General population	B Psychiatric inpatients	C[a] Depressive inpatients
	AS_{10} $n = 104$	AS_{10} $n = 420$	AS_{10} $n = 104$
Odd-even reliability, upgraded according to Spearman-Brown	0.71	0.86	0.82
% total variance of 1st unrotated component[b]	26.79	41.84	36.77
1st quartile (Q_1)	2.58	3.18	4.36
2nd quartile (Q_2 = median)	4.57	6.86	8.10
3rd quartile (Q_3)	6.59	11.45	12.50
Mean value ($\bar{x}$)	5.03	7.94	8.70
Standard deviation (s)	3.45	6.05	5.43
Skewness	1.16	0.82	0.38
Excess	1.72	0.25	−0.67

No. of items: 10
Item scores (in key direction): 0-1-2-3
Normal range: 0-8
[a] Subsample of B
[b] From a principal component analysis of the ten test items

of a short verbal intelligence test, e.g., the subtest „information" of the Bellevue Scale of Wechsler [24] – setting an estimated verbal IQ < 80 as an exclusion criterion for further investigation. For the exclusion of subjects whose self-ratings may be strongly influenced by a tendency to the denial of illness, a score of 19 or above on the DIS (eight items each in PDS and PDS') can be recommended. A low score on this scale (≤ 11) may indicate a tendency "to claim undesirable symptoms in personality inventories" [7]. In patients, it seems to indicate mainly a high sensitivity to physical or emotional discomfort (above all, in depressives) or a tendency to complain (predominant in all types of neurotics). Therefore, the scale can serve also as an inverse (!) measure of a tendency to express feelings of sickness and not only as a control measure for the clinical scales.

The normal ranges of test scores in Tables 25.4–25.9 refer to a convention suggested in the general part of the test manuals ([29a] Fig. 4). The ranges are based on the frequency distribution of test scores in the general population. Furthermore, the tables with more detailed information on these distributions (presented in the appendices to the test manuals [29b-d]) may be explored for a clinically and statistically meaningful classification of scores. Thus, stannine values of 7 or above on the Depression Scale (DS/DS') are suspect of a clinically relevant disturbance in the emotional sphere whereas such values on the Complaint List (CL/CL') or on the Adjective Mood Scale (AMS/AMS') may reflect somatic disorders as well (see [20]), and the respective value on the Paranoid Scale (PS/PS') is related to emotional disturbances mainly in the case of psychotic depression but, above all, points more or less directly to a disturbance in the cognitive sphere of reality testing.

The clinical relevance of high stannine values on the Anxiety Scale$_{10}$ (AS$_{10}$) has not yet been elucidated. The original (20-item) scale (SAS) did not discriminate as well as our CSRSs between a diagnostically heterogeneous group of 94 psychiatric inpatients and 91 healthy controls of similar sex and age distribution ([27]; see [30] and Table 25.10); only Zung's Self-Rating Depression Scale (SDS [35]) achieved a higher ranking of discriminating power than some of our CSRSs although it did not reach the DS in that respect. The Psychoticism Scale [9], although discriminating between psychiatric patients in general and normals to the same extent as the Paranoid Scale (PS), turned out to be almost totally nonspecific for psychotic disorders which were most specifically differentiated by the PS from normality and other disorders. The Self-Rating Anxiety Scale (SAS [36]) was comparatively the least-sensitive indicator of mental abnormality in general and was, moreover, nonspecific for neurotic disorders where it could have been expected to reach higher values than in psychotic disorders.

The Adjective Mood Scale was not included in Wittmann's study since it had been constructed particularly for longitudinal and not for cross-sectional investigations. However, in a recent cross-sectional comparison including AMS/AMS' (see Table 25.11), this scale, too, discriminated very well between depressives and controls. The data presented in Table 25.11 confirm the high clinical validity of the CSRS, especially of AMS/AMS' and DS/DS', but also of CL/CL', as measuring instruments of depression.

The normative values for the CSRSs refer to the age range of 20-64 years. Judging from preliminary data analyses of protocols from the population survey and from clinical investigations, the age ranges of 15-19 and 65-79 years are also covered by the norms for the narrower age range of 20-64 years. As an example, Fig. 25.1 presents the comparison of scale values of the Complaint List (CL/CL') between psychiatric inpatients with the diagnosis of either a depressive ($n=18$/group) or a paranoid syndrome ($n=4$/group) of the age ranges of 65-79 and 50-64 years, matched by sex and diagnosis, and two groups of the same age distribution from a general population sample investigated by Dilling et al. [8]. The scale values of CL and CL' are very similar for both age groups in the patient sam-

Table 25.10. Rate of misclassifications[a] and the *phi* coefficient (r_{phi})[a] from a comparison of psychiatric inpatients ($n=94$) and healthy controls ($n=91$) regarding various self-rating scales[b]

Scale	Abbreviation	% misclassified	r_{phi}
Complaint List	CL	33.5	0.35
Paranoid Scale	PS	36.2	0.33
Depression Scale	DS	19.5	0.61
Self-Rating Anxiety Scale	SAS[c]	39.5	0.21
Self-Rating Depression Scale	SDS[c]	27.0	0.50
Psychoticism Scale	P[d]	35.1	0.30

[a] Based on the median of the total sample ($n=185$) and not the cutoff point providing a minimum of misclassifications as reported elsewhere; von Zerssen ([32], Table 25.4)
[b] According to Wittmann [27]
[c] According to Zung [37]
[d] According to Eysenck and Eysenck ([9], see 2)

Table 25.11. Rate of misclassifications,[a] the *phi* coefficient (r_{phi}),[a] and the (more appropriate) tetrachoric correlation coefficient (r_{tet})[a] from a comparison of depressive inpatients (46 with endogenous and 58 with neurotic depression) and sex- and age-matched controls ($n = 104$) from the general population sample ($n = 1952$)[b] regarding the CSRS (without the control scale DIS/DIS')

Scale	Abbreviation	% misclassified	r_{phi}	r_{tet}
Complaint List	CL	26.9	0.46	0.66
Parallel Form	CL'	19.2	0.62	0.82
Paranoid Scale	PS	30.7	0.38	0.57
Parallel Form	PS'	38.0	0.24	0.37
Depression Scale	DS	11.5	0.77	0.94
Parallel Form	DS'	11.1	0.78	0.94
Adjective Mood Scale	AMS	12.0	0.76	0.93
Parallel Form	AMS'	15.4	0.69	0.89
Anxiety Scale$_{10}$[c]	AS$_{10}$	35.8	0.28	0.43

[a] Based on the median of the total sample ($n = 208$)
[b] See von Zerssen ([29a], Table 25.7)
[c] $n = 162$, equal number of patients (subsample of $n = 104$) and matched controls, from Wittmann [27]

ple on admission and also in the population sample. The reduction in the patients' scores from admission to discharge is somewhat more pronounced in the older group but not significantly so. The similarity between the age groups at admission and discharge was also found with respect to the scores of both parallel versions of the other CSRSs (PS/PS', DS/DS', AMS/AMS'). Compared with considerably younger age groups (e.g., 20-34 years), the values of the CSRSs are somewhat higher in the elderly, but this is also true of the age range of 50-64 years and reflects, most probably, a slight increase in physical and emotional discomfort with age.

Sex is another source of variance in values of the CSRSs. Here, too, the differences can be assumed to indicate real differences in the phenomena to be measured by the scales. This is demonstrated by the comparison of "cases" of both sexes defined operationally in a population survey ($n = 1743$) by means of scale values of the Depression and/or Paranoid Scale, with the expectancy values for the sex ratio derived from a sample of the same age distribution [34]. The stannine values had been calculated for the total sample irrespective of sex differences in the distribution of the scores. It turned out that females scored in the upper range significantly more often than males only on the Depression Scale but not on the Paranoid Scale, where males were even overrepresented in the upper range of scores, considering the age distribution of both sexes in the total sample. Consequently, the female preponderance in elevated depression scores cannot be sufficiently explained by a higher tendency on the part of women to acknowledge symptoms since such a tendency should also show up in the values of the Paranoid Scale. Women, at least in

Fig. 25.1. Test statistics of two groups of psychiatric inpatients of the MPIP with either depression or paranoid psychosis and from the general population, regarding the complaint List, CL/CL'

Clinical Self-Rating Scales

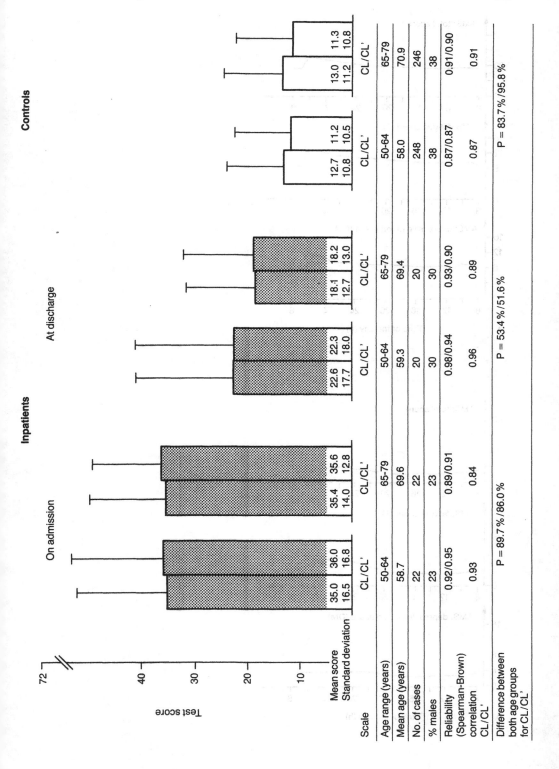

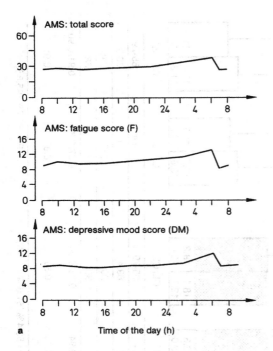

a

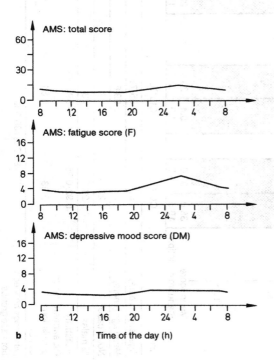

b

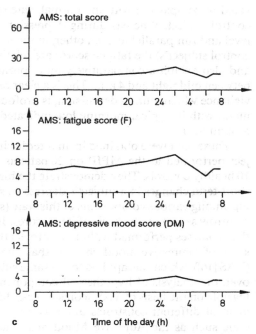

Fig. 25.2 a–c. Diurnal variation in the general mood state, the degree of fatigue, and, more specifically, depressive mood according to the Adjective Mood Scale (AMS) in an elderly woman. **a** During an episode of endogenous depression; **b** after complete remission; **c** in a control subject of the same sex and similar age

industrialized cultures, show more depressive symptoms than men (see [25, 34]).

It becomes evident from this analysis that the CSRS scores are influenced mainly by a subject's clinical condition. Changes in this condition are, at least with respect to its subjective components, rather sensitively reflected by changes in repetitively recorded scores. This is clearly shown by the changes in scale values of the Complaint List from admission to discharge, as exemplified in Fig. 25.1.

The Adjective Mood Scale AMS/AMS' is particularly sensitive even to rather subtle changes in well-being assessed within short intervals of time (see also [12]). In Figs. 25.2 a–c diurnal variations in mood are illustrated as the educed waveform of the AM scores obtained every 3 h during the day (from 7 a.m. to 10 p.m.) and once at night (at around 2:30 a.m.) over a 2-week period without medication in an elderly woman during an episode of endogenous depression and, several months later, in a fully recovered state (again free of medication) and, for comparison, in a healthy control subject of the same sex and similar age. In addition to the total score, two subscores (based on eight items each) arrived at hypothetically are plotted in the same manner, one of them reflecting the degree of fatigue (F; see Appendix A, AMS) and the other one that of specifically depressive mood (DM; see Appendix A, AMS). During depression, the total score and the two subscores are clearly elevated in comparison with the normal state of the same individual and that of the control subject. Whereas during depression both subscores reach about the same level and run parallel to each other, in the normal state (the patient's as well as the control subject's) the fatigue scores are relatively higher than the depression scores and also exhibit a comparatively more pronounced diurnal variation with a peak between midnight and 4 a.m. This is a clear reflection of the circadian fluctuation of vigilance which, during depression, is profoundly modified by the patient's state of mood with its typical morning low indicated by a phase shift of the peak value to around 6 a.m.

These data were obtained in an interdisciplinary chronobiological research project performed at the MPIP on 20 patients with major depressive disorders and 10 healthy controls. They demonstrate the high sensitivity of the AM values even to short-term changes in a subject's depressive state and the possibility of differentiating among various components of this state (such as fatigue and depressive mood in a narrow sense) on the basis of item scores. It can be concluded from the statistical data analyses performed within this project that the AM scores are more valid measures of depressive mood changes than the scores of the Visual Analogue Scale (VAS [16]), which was applied to the same subjects at the same points in time. Moreover, the analysis of hypothetical components of fluctuations in well-being is not feasible on the basis of VAS scores (unless different VASs are used for the measurement of different constructs under consideration). An advantage of a multi-item scale such as the Adjective Mood Scale lies in the possibility to form different scores from subsets of items according to hypothetical constructs or to the results of multivariate statistical analyses even retrospectively, i.e., after the data collection has been completed.

Examples of the application of AMS/AMS' in therapeutic trials which are the domain of this particular scale were given in a paper on self-rating scales in the evaluation of psychiatric treatment ([32]; see also [3, 6]). Another indication for the application of AMS/AMS' is the long-term observation of patients, e.g., during hospital treatment. Here, repetitive measurements at 2-day intervals (as routinely performed at the Psychiatric Department of the MPIP; see [1, 18]) provide the data base for visual [19] or purely statistical analyses [22, 23] of mood changes in relation to diagnosis, treatment interventions [10], etc. The description of these methods, however, goes beyond the scope of this presentation.

Appendix A

Questionnaires with scoring key (see abbreviations of scales in text)

CL
C..........................
Clinic: .... Ward: .... Date: .... Time: ....
Day of Week: .... Test Duration: ....
ID No: .... ICD No.: .... V-IQ: ....

To be filled in by the patient:
Last Name: .... Maiden Name: ....
First Name: .... Date of Birth: .... Age: ....
Occupation: .... Sex: ....

Please complete this list of complaints carefully. Check one of the four columns according to the degree of your agreement or disagreement. Please answer all the questions.

I am suffering from the following:	Severely	Moderately	Scarcely	Not at all
1. A feeling of choking, a lump or tightness in the throat	3	2	1	0
2. Shortness of breath	3	2	1	0
3. A feeling of weakness	3	2	1	0
4. Difficulty in swallowing	3	2	1	0
5. Stabbing chest pains or twinges	3	2	1	0
6. A sensation of pressure or fullness in the stomach	3	2	1	0
7. Fatigue	3	2	1	0
8. Nausea	3	2	1	0
9. Heartburn or burping due to stomach acidity	3	2	1	0
10. Irritability	3	2	1	0
11. Brooding	3	2	1	0
12. Heavy perspiration	3	2	1	0
13. Lumbago or back pain	3	2	1	0
14. Inner restlessness	3	2	1	0

	Severely	Moderately	Scarcely	Not at all
15. A sensation of heaviness or fatigue in the legs	3	2	1	0
16. Restless feeling in the legs	3	2	1	0
17. Extreme sensitivity to heat	3	2	1	0
18. Extreme sensitivity to cold	3	2	1	0
19. Excessive need of sleep	3	2	1	0
20. Insomnia	3	2	1	0
21. A feeling of dizziness or light-headedness	3	2	1	0
22. Trembling	3	2	1	0
23. Neck or shoulder pain	3	2	1	0
24. Weight loss	3	2	1	0

CL'

C' ....
Clinic: .... Ward: .... Date: .... Time: ....
Day of Week: .... Test Duration: ....
ID No.: .... ICD No.: .... V-IQ: ....

To be filled in by the patient:
Last Name: .... Maiden Name: ....
First Name: .... Date of Birth: .... Age: ....
Occupation: .... Sex: ....

Please complete this list of complaints carefully. Check one of the four columns according to the degree of your agreement or disagreement. Please answer all the questions.

I am suffering from the following:	Severely	Moderately	Scarcely	Not at all
1. Headaches, head pressure, or face pains	3	2	1	0
2. Fatigue	3	2	1	0
3. Loss of balance	3	2	1	0
4. Attacks of breathlessness	3	2	1	0
5. A feeling of suffocation	3	2	1	0
6. A tendency to cry	3	2	1	0
7. A lack of appetite	3	2	1	0
8. Hiccups	3	2	1	0
9. Palpitations or irregular heartbeats	3	2	1	0
10. A tendency to become quickly exhausted	3	2	1	0
11. Feelings of anxiety	3	2	1	0
12. Stomachaches or abdominal pains	3	2	1	0
13. Constipation	3	2	1	0
14. A lack of energy	3	2	1	0
15. Pains in joints or limbs	3	2	1	0
16. Diminished ability to concentrate	3	2	1	0
17. Cold feet	3	2	1	0
18. A lack of sexual response	3	2	1	0
19. Blushing easily	3	2	1	0
20. Feeling cold	3	2	1	0

	Severely	Moderately	Scarcely	Not at all
21. Hot flashes	3	2	1	0
22. Gloomy thoughts	3	2	1	0
23. Inner tension	3	2	1	0
24. A sensation of numbness, burning, or itching in hands and/or feet	3	2	1	0

Clinical Self-Rating Scales

CL°
           C° ....
Clinic: .... Ward: .... Date: .... Time: ....
Day of Week: .... Test Duration: ....
ID No.: .... ICD No.: .... V-IQ: ....

To be filled in by the patient:
Last Name: .... Maiden Name: ....
First Name: .... Date of Birth: .... Age: ....
Occupation: .... Sex: ....

Please complete this list of complaints carefully. Check one of the four columns according to the degree of your agreement or disagreement. Please answer all the questions.

I am suffering from the following:	Severely	Moderately	Scarcely	Not at all
1. A chronic cough...................				
2. Diarrhea				
3. Difficulty urinating				
4. Itching				
5. Swollen feet				
6. Blood in the stool				
7. Inability to eat certain foods				
8. Tiredness of living				
9. Visual disturbances				
10. Skin changes				
11. An enormous appetite				
12. Great thirst				
13. Forgetfulness				
14. Vomiting				
15. Fainting spells or other attacks of unconsciousness				
16. Problems at home or at work				
17. (Women:) Menstrual problems				

In addition I have the following problems:
....
....
....

PDS

P .... D .... DI ...... DC .....
Clinic: .... Ward: .... Date: .... Time: ....
Day of Week: .... Test Duration: ....
ID No.: .... ICD No.: .... V-IQ: ....

To be filled in by the patient:
Last Name: .... Maiden Name: ....
First Name: .... Date of Birth: .... Age: ....
Occupation: .... Sex: .....

Please read the following. Decide whether or not each statement applies to you. Check *one of the four columns* to the right according to the degree of your agreement or disagreement. Please complete all the questions carefully, with a minimum of hesitation, and *on your own*.

	Completely true	Mostly true	Partly true	Not true	
1. I understand the instructions	3	2	1	0	M
2. I am willing to answer each question as truthfully as possible	3	2	1	0	M
3. I enjoy all sorts of games and pastimes	0	1	2	3	D
4. I am more sensitive to criticism than I used to be	3	2	1	0	D
5. Lately I have been very anxious and easily startled	3	2	1	0	D
6. I have a cold now and then	0	1	2	3	DI
7. I am being influenced by others against my will	3	2	1	0	P
8. I cry easily	3	2	1	0	D
9. I have had the feeling that the world was coming to an end	3	2	1	0	P
10. Occasionally I feel tired	0	1	2	3	DI
11. People are wrong to think I am ill	3	2	1	0	P
12. Sometimes my body moves by itself	3	2	1	0	P
13. I am afraid of losing my mind	3	2	1	0	D
14. I feel down and depressed	3	2	1	0	D
15. Someone wants to destroy my mind	3	2	1	0	P
16. I cannot understand what I read as well a I used to	3	2	1	0	D
17. I would like most of all to take my own life	3	2	1	0	D

Clinical Self-Rating Scales

	Completely true	Mostly true	Partly true	Not true	
18. At times I have been so worked up that I could hardly fall asleep	0	1	2	3	DI
19. Some days I cannot concentrate as well as on others	0	1	2	3	DI
20. I am constantly being watched and controlled by others	3	2	1	0	P
21. In the morning I feel particularly bad	3	2	1	0	D
22. I suffer from peculiar physical changes	3	2	1	0	P
23. There are people who try to steal my thoughts and ideas	3	2	1	0	P
24. I no longer have any relationship with others .	3	2	1	0	D
25. There are comments being made about all my thoughts and actions	3	2	1	0	P
26. I am frightened sometimes	0	1	2	3	DI
27. People are envious of my knowledge, discoveries, and special experiences	3	2	1	0	P
28. I have peculiar experiences such as visions, inspirations, and the like	3	2	1	0	P
29. From time to time I am in a bad mood	0	1	2	3	DI
30. Someone wants to kill me	3	2	1	0	P
31. I feel that I am about to go to pieces	3	2	1	0	D
32. I have the feeling that I am being influenced by electric currents, rays, or hypnosis	3	2	1	0	P
33. Occasionally I have an upset stomach	0	1	2	3	DI
34. I am constantly afraid of saying or doing something wrong	3	2	1	0	D
35. Sometimes I feel a superhuman and overwhelming force in me....................	3	2	1	0	P
36. I am much less interested in my love life now than I used to be	3	2	1	0	D
37. The moment I think of something, others already know what I am thinking	3	2	1	0	P
38. For some things I have to create my own words which others do not always understand	3	2	1	0	P

	Completely true	Mostly true	Partly true	Not true	
39. I often feel simply miserable	3	2	1	0	D
40. Sometimes my heart pounds with excitement .	0	1	2	3	DI
41. As hard as I try, I cannot think logically at all .	3	2	1	0	D
42. I no longer have any feelings	3	2	1	0	D
43. I believe I have answered every question truthfully	3	2	1	0	M

Clinical Self-Rating Scales

PDS'

P'.......... D'...... DI'..... DC.....
Clinic:.................. Ward:........ Date:......... Time:........
Day of Week:..................... Test Duration:.....................
ID No.:........................ ICD No.:.............. V-IQ:........

To be filled in by the patient:
Last Name:.................... Maiden Name:........................
First Name:.................... Date of Birth:............... Age:....
Occupation:... Sex:....

Please read the following. Decide whether or not each statement applies to you. Check *one of the four columns* to the right according to the degree of your agreement or disagreement. Please complete all the questions carefully, with a minimum of hesitation, and *on your own*.

	Completely true	Mostly true	Partly true	Not true	
1. I understand the instructions	3	2	1	0	M'
2. I am willing to answer each question as truthfully as possible	3	2	1	0	M'
3. Sometimes I am in a bad mood	0	1	2	3	DI'
4. I must really force myself to do anything	3	2	1	0	D'
5. Someone has been stealing my thoughts	3	2	1	0	P'
6. Lately I always feel like crying	3	2	1	0	D'
7. I see things, animals, or people that others do not see	3	2	1	0	P'
8. Sometimes my heart pounds with excitement	0	1	2	3	DI'
9. My appetite has decreased	3	2	1	0	D'
10. Sometimes I am sure other people can tell what I am thinking	3	2	1	0	P'
11. Sometimes I feel so restless that I cannot sit still for a minute	3	2	1	0	D'
12. I have had very strange and unusual experiences	3	2	1	0	P'
13. Sometimes I am frightened	0	1	2	3	DI'
14. People have been spying on me	3	2	1	0	P'
15. I do not sleep well at night	3	2	1	0	D'
16. I wish people would just leave me alone	3	2	1	0	P'
17. I feel empty inside	3	2	1	0	D'
18. I like to occupy myself with mysterious things	3	2	1	0	P'

	Completely true	Mostly true	Partly true	Not true	
19. I am looking into the future full of hope	0	1	2	3	D'
20. Some days I cannot concentrate as well as on others.................................	0	1	2	3	DI'
21. I feel tense and in knots	3	2	1	0	D'
22. I am being tortured and harassed with certain instruments and objects	3	2	1	0	P'
23. Lately every little thing upsets me	3	2	1	0	D'
24. I have changed somehow	3	2	1	0	D'
25. When I think, I often hear my thoughts being spoken out loud	3	2	1	0	P'
26. I often think about suicide.................	3	2	1	0	D'
27. I feel nervous and restless	3	2	1	0	D'
28. Occasionally I have ESP	3	2	1	0	P'
29. I feel lonely even when I am with other people	3	2	1	0	D'
30. Sometimes I feel as though someone makes me do something through hypnosis	3	2	1	0	P'
31. If people had not been against me, I would have been much more successful in life	3	2	1	0	P'
32. Sometimes I am so excited I can hardly fall asleep.................................	0	1	2	3	DI'
33. I can think as clearly as ever	0	1	2	3	D'
34. Now and then I have a cold	0	1	2	3	DI'
35. I suffer from hearing voices that others do not hear	3	2	1	0	P'
36. I no longer feel any contact with others	3	2	1	0	D'
37. I occasionally feel tired	0	1	2	3	DI'
38. Somehow everyone around me has changed..	3	2	1	0	P'
39. I feel as though my ability to think is diminishing.................................	3	2	1	0	D'
40. I think people are conspiring against me	3	2	1	0	P'
41. Occasionally I have an upset stomach	0	1	2	3	DI'
42. Someone has control over my thoughts	3	2	1	0	P'
43. I believe I have answered every question truthfully..............................	3	2	1	0	M'

DS

D..........

Clinic:................... Ward:......... Date:.......... Time:.........
Day of Week: .... Test Duration: ....
ID No.: .... ICD No.: .... V-IQ: ....

To be filled in by the patient:
Last Name: .... Maiden Name: ....
First Name: .... Date of Birth: .... Age: ....
Occupation:... Sex: ....

Please read the following. Decide whether or not each statement applies to you. Check *one of the four columns* to the right according to the degree of your agreement or disagreement. Please complete all the questions carefully, with a minimum of hesitation, and *on your own*.

	Completely true	Mostly true	Partly true	Not true
1. I enjoy all sorts of games and pastimes	0	1	2	3
2. I am more sensitive to criticism than I used to be	3	2	1	0
3. Lately I have been very anxious and easily startled...............................	3	2	1	0
4. I cry easily	3	2	1	0
5. I am afraid of losing my mind	3	2	1	0
6. I feel down and depressed	3	2	1	0
7. I cannot understand what I read as well as I used to	3	2	1	0
8. I would like most of all to take my own life ...	3	2	1	0
9. In the morning I feel particularly bad	3	2	1	0
10. I no longer have any relationship with others .	3	2	1	0
11. I feel that I am about to go to pieces	3	2	1	0
12. I am constantly afraid of saying or doing something wrong	3	2	1	0
13. I am much less interested in my love life now than I used to be	3	2	1	0
14. I often feel simply miserable	3	2	1	0
15. As hard as I try, I cannot think logically at all .	3	2	1	0
16. I no longer have any feelings...............	3	2	1	0

DS'

D' ....

Clinic: .... Ward: .... Date: .... Time: ....
Day of Week: .... Test Duration: ....
ID No.: .... ICD No.: .... V-IQ: ....

To be filled in by the patient:
Last Name: .... Maiden Name: ....
First Name: .... Date of Birth: .... Age: ....
Occupation: .... Sex: ....

Please read the following. Decide whether or not each statement applies to you. Check *one of the four columns* to the right according to the degree of your agreement or disagreement. Please complete all the questions carefully, with a minimum of hesitation, and *on your own*.

	Completely true	Mostly true	Partly true	Not true
1. I must really force myself to do anything	3	2	1	0
2. Lately I always feel like crying	3	2	1	0
3. My appetite has decreased	3	2	1	0
4. Sometimes I feel so restless that I cannot sit still for a minute	3	2	1	0
5. I do not sleep well at night	3	2	1	0
6. I feel empty inside	3	2	1	0
7. I am looking into the future full of hope	0	1	2	3
8. I feel tense and in knots	3	2	1	0
9. Lately every little thing upsets me	3	2	1	0
10. I have changed somehow	3	2	1	0
11. I often think about suicide................	3	2	1	0
12. I feel nervous and restless	3	2	1	0
13. I feel lonely even when I am with other people	3	2	1	0
14. I can think as clearly as ever	0	1	2	3
15. I no longer feel any contact with others	3	2	1	0
16. I feel as though my ability to think is diminishing	3	2	1	0

AMS

AM ....
Clinic: .... Ward: .... Date: .... Time: ....
Day of Week: .... Test Duration: ....
ID No.: .... ICD No.: .... V-IQ: ....

To be filled in by the patient:
Last Name: .... Maiden Name: ....
First Name: .... Date of Birth: .... Age: ....
Occupation: .... Sex: ....

Below you will find pairs of words or expressions. Please decide – without taking too long – which of the two corresponds most closely to the way you feel now. Check the box to the left of this word. Mark "neither-nor" only if you are completely unable to decide between the two.

At the moment, I am feeling:

		More		More			Neither-nor
F	1.	0	Refreshed	2	Listless		1
F	2.	2	Indifferent toward others	0	Interested in others		1
DM	3.	0	Pleased	2	Depressed		1
	4.	0	Successful	2	Unsuccessful		1
	5.	2	Irritable	0	Peaceful		1
F	6.	2	Indecisive	0	Ready to make decisions		1
DM	7.	0	Cheerful	2	Tearful		1
	8.	0	In a good mood	2	In a bad mood		1
F	9.	2	Lacking in appetite	0	With a good appetite		1
	10.	0	Sociable	2	Withdrawn		1
DM	11.	2	Unworthy	0	Worthy		1
	12.	0	Relaxed	2	Tense		1
	13.	0	Happy	2	Unhappy		1
	14.	2	Shy	0	Communicative		1
	15.	2	Sinful and wicked	0	Pure		1
	16.	0	Secure	2	Threatened		1
DM	17.	2	Abandoned	0	Cared for		1
DM	18.	0	Even-tempered	2	Driven		1
DM	19.	0	Confident	2	Insecure		1
	20.	2	Miserable	0	Comfortable		1
	21.	0	Flexible	2	Inflexible		1
F	22.	2	Tired	0	Rested		1

		More		More		Neither-nor
F	23.	2	Hesitant	0	Firm	1
DM	24.	0	Calm	2	Restless	1
F	25.	2	Lacking in energy	0	Energetic	1
	26.	2	Useless	0	Indispensable	1
F	27.	2	Sluggish	0	Lively	1
DM	28.	0	Superior	2	Inferior	1

Clinical Self-Rating Scales

AMS'

AM' ....

Clinic:................... Ward:......... Date:.......... Time:.........
Day of Week:...................... Test Duration:.....................
ID No.:....................... ICD No.:.............. V-IQ:.........

To be filled in by the patient:
Last Name:.................... Maiden Name:........................
First Name:.................... Date of Birth:............... Age:....
Occupation:... Sex:....

Below you will find pairs of words or expressions. Please decide – without taking too long – which of the two corresponds most closely to the way you feel now. Check the box to the left of this word. Mark "neither-nor" only if you are completely unable to decide between the two.

At the moment, I am feeling:

		More		More		Neither-nor
	1.	0	Outgoing	2	Inhibited	1
	2.	0	In good spirits	2	Gloomy	1
F	3.	2	Lacking in drive	0	Motivated	1
	4.	2	Easily ill	0	Healthy	1
	5.	0	Determined	2	Aimless	1
	6.	2	Serious	0	Lighthearted	1
	7.	2	Lacking in ideas	0	Full of ideas	1
DM	8.	2	Sensitive	0	Thick-skinned	1
DM	9.	2	Pessimistic	0	Optimistic	1
DM	10.	0	Carefree	2	Brooding	1
F	11.	2	Worn out	0	Alert	1
	12.	0	Capable of love	2	Incapable of love	1
DM	13.	2	Guilty	0	Innocent	1
F	14.	2	Exhausted	0	Revived	1
	15.	2	Tired of living	0	Enjoying life	1
DM	16.	0	Good-natured	2	Mean	1
	17.	0	Merry	2	Sad	1
DM	18.	0	Loved	2	Unloved	1
F	19.	2	Lazy	0	Active	1
	20.	2	Reserved	0	Responsive	1
F	21.	0	Full of life	2	Lifeless	1
F	22.	0	Spirited	2	Inert	1
F	23.	0	Attentive	2	Absent-minded	1
DM	24.	2	Desperate	0	Hopeful	1

		More		More		Neither-nor
	25.	0	Contented	2	Dissatisfied	1
	26.	2	Timid	0	Bold	1
F	27.	0	Strong	2	Weak	1
DM	28.	0	On an even keel	2	Uneasy	1

AS₁₀

A ....

Clinic:................. Ward:........ Date:......... Time:........
Day of Week: .... Test Duration: ....
ID No.: .... ICD No.:............. V-IQ ....

To be filled in by the patient:
Last Name: .... Maiden Name: ....
First Name: .... Date of Birth:............... Age:....
Occupation:.. Sex:....

Please read the following. Decide whether or not each statement applies to you. Check *one of the four columns* to the right according to the degree of your agreement or disagreement. Please complete all the questions carefully, with a minimum of hesitation, and *on your own*.

	Completely true	Mostly true	Partly true	Not true
1. I get upset easily or feel panicky	3	2	1	0
2. My arms and legs shake and tremble	3	2	1	0
3. I can feel my heart beating fast	3	2	1	0
4. I am bothered by dizzy spells	3	2	1	0
5. I have fainting spells or feel like it	3	2	1	0
6. I get feelings of numbness and tingling in my fingers and toes.........................	3	2	1	0
7. My face gets hot and blushes	3	2	1	0
8. I have nightmares........................	3	2	1	0
9. I am restless and can't keep still	3	2	1	0
10. I am more irritable than usual	3	2	1	0

References

1. Barthelmes, H., and Zerssen, D. von 1978. Das Münchener Psychiatrische Informationssystem (PSYCHIS München). In: P. Reichertz and E. Schwarz (eds.), Informationssysteme in der medizinischen Versorgung. Ökologie der Systeme, pp. 138–145. Schattauer, Stuttgart.
2. Baumann, U., and Dittrich, A. 1975. Konstruktion einer deutschsprachigen Psychotizismus-Skala. Z. Exp. Angew. Psychol. 22: 365–373.
3. Bobon, D.P., Lapierre, Y.D., and Lottin, T. 1981. Validity and sensitivity of the French version of the Zerssen BfS/BfS' self-rating mood scale during treatment with trazodone and amitriptyline. Progr. Neuropsychopharmacol. 5: 519–522.
4. Buros, O.K. (ed.). 1970. Personality Tests and Reviews. Gryphon, Highland Park, N.J.

5. Collegium Internationale Psychiatriae Scalarum (eds.). 1981. CIPS Internationale Skalen für Psychiatrie. Beltz Test, Weinheim.
6. Cording-Tömmel, C., and Zerssen, D. von. 1982. Mianserin and maprotiline as compared to amitriptyline in severe endogenous depression. A new methodological approach to the clinical evaluation of the efficacy of antidepressants. Pharmacopsychiatria 15: 197-204.
7. DeSoto, C.B., and Kuethe, J.L. 1959. The set to claim undesirable symptoms in personality inventories. J. consult. Psychol. 23: 496-500.
8. Dilling, H., Weyerer, S., and Castell, R. 1984. Psychische Erkrankungen in der Bevölkerung. Enke, Stuttgart.
9. Eysenck, S.B.G., and Eysenck, H.J. 1972. The questionnaire measurement of psychoticism. Psychol. Med. 2: 50-55.
10. Gudat, U., and Revenstorff, D. 1976. Interventionseffekte in klinischen Zeitreihen. Arch. Psychol. (Frankf.) 128: 16-44.
11. Heimann, H., Bobon-Schrod, H., Schmocker, A.M., and Bobon, D.P. 1975. Auto-évaluation de l'humeur par une liste d'adjectifs, la "Befindlichkeits-Skala" (BS) de Zerssen. Encéphale n.s. 1: 165-183.
12. Linden, M., and Krautzig, E. 1981. Befindlichkeitsmessung in kurzzeitigen Abständen: ein experimenteller Beitrag zur Validierung der Befindlichkeitsskala (Bf-S) nach v. Zerssen. Pharmacopsychiatria 14: 40-41.
13. Lord, F.M., and Novick, M.R. 1968. Statistical Theories of Mental Test Scores. Addison-Wesley Publishing Company, Reading, MA.
14. Lorr, M. 1974. Assessing psychotic behavior by the IMPS. In: P. Pichot and R. Olivier-Martin (eds.), Psychological Measurements in Psychopharmacology. Modern Problems in Pharmacopsychiatry, pp. 50-63, Vol. 7. Karger, Basel.
15. Lorr, M., and Klett, C.J. 1967. Inpatient Multidimensional Psychiatric Scale (IMPS), revised manual. Consult. Psychologists. Palo Alto, CA.
16. Luria, R.E. 1975. The validity and reliability of the Visual Analogue Mood Scale. J. Psychiatr. Res. 12: 51-57.
17. Mendels, J., Weinstein, N., and Cochrane, C. 1972. The relationship between depression and anxiety. Arch. Gen. Psychiatry 27: 649-653.
18. Möller, H.J., Barthelmes, H., and Zerssen, D. von. 1983. Forschungsmöglichkeiten auf der Grundlage einer routinemäßig durchgeführten psychiatrischen Basis- und Befunddokumentation. Psychiatr. Clin. (Basel) 16: 45-61.
19. Möller, H.-J., and Zerssen, D. von. 1982. Depressive states occurring during the neuroleptic treatment of schizophrenia. Schizophr. Bull. 8: 109-117.
20. Paetz, D., Krüskemper, G., and Gillich, K.H. 1975. Testpsychologische Untersuchungen über die Befindlichkeit von Patientinnen im Klimakterium während stationärer internistischer Behandlung unter besonderer Berücksichtigung von Oestrogen- und Gestagenwirkung. Z. Gerontol. 8: 358-364.
21. Stieglitz, R.-D., Baumann, U., Tobien, H., and Zerssen, D. von. 1980. Zur Stichproben- und Zeitinvarianz von Testkennwerten bei einer Beschwerdenliste. Z. Exp. Angew. Psychol. 27: 631-654.
22. Strian, F., Heger, R., and Klicpera, C. 1981. The course of depression for different types of schizophrenia. Psychiatr. Clin. (Basel) 14: 205-214.
23. Strian, F., Heger, R., and Klicpera, C. 1982. The time structure of depressive mood in schizophrenic patients. Acta Psychiatr. Scand. 65: 66-73.
24. Wechsler, D. 1958. The Measurement and Appraisal of Adult Intelligence. 4th Ed. Williams and Wilkins, Baltimore.
25. Weissman, M.M., and Klerman, G.L. 1977. Sex differences and the epidemiology of depression. Arch. Gen. Psychiatry 34: 98-111.
26. Wittchen, H.-U. 1983. Der Verlauf und Ausgang behandelter und unbehandelter affektiver Störungen unter psychopathologischen, sozialen und psychologischen Aspekten. Psychol. Habilitationsschrift, University of Munich.
27. Wittmann, B. 1978. Untersuchung über die faktorielle und klinisch-diagnostische Differenzierbarkeit der Syndrome Angst und Depression in der klinischen Selbstbeurteilung sowie über die Beziehung zwischen den Fragebogendimensionen "Paranoide Tendenzen" und "Psychotizismus". Doctoral dissertation, University of Munich.

28. Zerssen, D. von. 1973. Beschwerdenskalen bei Depressionen. Therapiewoche 46: 4426-4440.
29. Zerssen, D. von, in collaboration with Koeller, D.-M. 1976 a-d. Klinische Selbstbeurteilungs-Skalen (KSb-S) aus dem Münchener Psychiatrischen Informations-System (PSYCHIS München), Manuale. (a) Allgemeiner Teil; (b) Die Beschwerden-Liste; (c) Paranoid-Depressivitäts-Skala, Depressivitäts-Skala; (d) Die Befindlichkeits-Skala. Beltz Test, Weinheim.
30. Zerssen, D. von. 1979. Klinisch-psychiatrische Selbstbeurteilungs-Fragebögen. In: U. Baumann, H. Berbalk, and G. Seidenstücker (eds.), Klinische Psychologie. Trends in Forschung und Praxis 2, pp. 130-159. Huber, Bern.
31. Zerssen, D. von. 1981. Körperliche und Allgemeinbeschwerden als Ausdruck seelischer Gestörtheit. Therapiewoche 31: 865-876.
32. Zerssen, D. von. 1983. Self-rating scales in the evaluation of psychiatric treatment. In: T. Helgason (ed.), Methodology in Evaluation of Psychiatric Treatment, pp. 183-204. Cambridge University Press, Cambridge.
33. Zerssen, D. von, and Cording, C. 1978. The measurement of change in endogenous affective disorders. Arch. Psychiatr. Nervenkr. 226: 95-112.
34. Zerssen, D. von, and Weyerer, S. 1982. Sex differences in rates of mental disorders. Int. J. Ment. Health 11: 9-45.
35. Zung, W. W. K. 1965. A self-rating depression scale. Arch. Gen. Psychiatry 12: 63-70.
36. Zung, W. W. K. 1971. A rating instrument for anxiety disorders. Psychosomatics 12: 371-379.
37. Zung, W. W. K. 1974. The measurement of affects: Depression and anxiety. In: P. Pichot and R. Olivier-Martin (eds.), Psychological Measurements in Psychopharmacology. Modern Problems in Pharmacopsychiatry, pp. 170-188, Vol. 7. Karger, Basel.

Chapter 26 The Clinical Interview for Depression[1]

E. S. PAYKEL

Development

The Clinical Interview for Depression is a rating scale for assessment of depression by a trained rater at interview. It is suitable for depressive disorders over a wide range of severity and settings, from inpatients who may be very severely and psychotically depressed, to mildly depressed subjects in general practice and in the community. The item pool is sufficiently wide to allow the instrument also to be used in the assessment of mixed neurotic disorders with admixtures of anxiety, phobic, obsessional and depersonalisation symptoms, in addition to depression.

The origins of the scale were in a modification of the Hamilton Rating Scale for Depression [5] undertaken by Klerman and colleagues in the 1960s at the Massachusetts Mental Health Center, Boston. In this modification additional items were added and ratings changed to uniform seven-point scales, not explicitly anchored. This modified Hamilton Scale was used in several reports including factor-analytic studies [41, 42, 43].

Further development and modification was undertaken by the author in collaboration with Klerman at Yale University in 1966. The new scale included additional items, detailed item definitions, anchor points carefully defined for all scales in terms of the specific phenomena rated, and a semistructured interview format with specified questions. Subsequent revision with further expansion of the item pool was undertaken by the author at St. George's Hospital. The Yale version of the scale has previously been described briefly [20].

Rationale and Description

The rationale behind the scale development was to provide an instrument which would comprehensively rate the symptom phenomena of depression in a manner suitable for a variety of purposes, particularly to obtain a full description, classification and measurement of outcome in treatment studies. Existing instruments were lacking in some aspects. The best and most widely used scale, the Hamilton Rating Scale for Depression [5] lacked a number of important qualitative aspects of depres-

---

[1] This chapter is modified from a paper which appeared in the *Journal of Affective Disorders* 1985, 9: 85-96

sion related to classification and the endogenous-reactive distinction (e.g. reactivity of mood, distinct quality of mood differing from normal experience). Its utility was limited in neurotic depressions because items emphasized the somatic disturbances of endogenous depression. The items which might serve as outcome measures for specific effects of drugs could not be used individually because they were rated only on three-point or five-point scales which did not provide sufficient points for parametric analyses, particularly with the tendency of raters to avoid extreme rating points. Reliable use by non-psychiatrists not sharing a frame of reference with psychiatrists was made difficult by absence of a specified interview format and limited definition of rating anchor points.

Other available depression rating scales showed these deficiencies much more markedly. Particular emphasis in this scale was therefore laid on a comprehensive

Table 26.1. Item content of Clinical Interview for Depression

Feelings of depressed mood[a]
Distinct quality of depression
Diurnal variation - symptoms worse in morning
Diurnal variation - symptoms worse in latter half of day
Reactivity to social environment
Guilt, lowered self-esteem, and worthlessness[a]
Pessimism and hopelessness[a]
Suicidal tendencies[a]
Depersonalisation
Obsessional symptoms
Work and interests[a]
Energy and fatigue[a]
Anxiety psychic - generalised[a]
Panic attacks[a]
Phobic anxiety[a]
Avoidance - main phobia[a]
Anxiety somatic[a]
Anorexia[a]
Increased appetite[a]
Weight loss
Weight gain
Irritability[a]
Initial insomnia[a]
Middle insomnia
Delayed insomnia[a]
Increased sleep
Paranoid ideas
Depressive delusions
Self-pity
Overemphasis of symptoms
Hysterical symptoms
Hypochondriasis
Hostility[a]
Retardation[a]
Agitation[a]
Depressed appearance[a]

[a] Included in short form for repeated ratings

item coverage, wider scale range, definition of items and anchor points, and specification of interview procedure.

The full scale contains 36 items listed in Table 26.1. Each item is defined in detail. Items are rated on seven-point scales with full specification of each anchor point based on severity, frequency and/or quality. Although each point is defined for each item there is across all the scales a similar continuum, with points 1-7 being equivalent respectively to absent (1), minimal/very mild (2), mild (3), moderate (4), marked (5), severe (6), extremely severe (7). One item, depressive delusions, is rated on a four-point scale.

In general there are two major types of item. The most common requires retrospective rating of the condition in the last week on the basis of history supplied by the patient. For most of these, if fluctuation has occurred, symptoms are averaged over time, taking into account frequency and severity. For a few, such as suicidal tendencies, a rating is made of the maximal behaviour shown over the week. The second major type of item, comprising fewer of the total, is rated solely on observable behaviour or verbal interaction manifested at interview.

The scale is set out in the form of a semistructured interview, with items to be rated in a specified order, and specified initial questions for each item which should usually be asked but may be modified if circumstances necessitate it. Further probing, the detail of which is left to the judgment of the interviewer, is required where a symptom is present. A few specified questions need not be asked if preceding information indicates that they are irrelevant. The order of the items was chosen to permit comfortable clinical interviewing. At the end are the items which depend solely on rating of observed behaviour at interview without questioning.

The full interview is intended primarily for use on a single occasion as a description of initial clinical state. It takes 30-45 min to administer. Although it can be used for repeated ratings of progress, the most useful items for repeat are available in a shorter form, taking approximately 20 min, also indicated in Table 26.1. In most drug trial applications it has been used in conjunction with the Raskin Three Area Scale [39] and global clinical impressions of severity of illness and of change, which can be completed reliably following administration of the interview. The Hamilton Rating Scale can also be completed on the basis of the same interview, with additional questioning for genital symptoms, constipation and loss of insight, which were dropped from an earlier version of the Clinical Interview because of doubts regarding reliability and validity.

Table 26.2 sets out a specimen page from the interview format, containing two consecutive illustrative ratings. The full scale is obtainable from the author.

Reliability

The Clinical Interview for Depression has been used principally by psychiatrists, but also by psychologists [26, 2, 19], social workers [48], a sociologist [31], research assistants with bachelor level degrees in psychology or social sciences [23] and medical and nursing students [9, 30]. Training has usually involved interviewing approx-

The Clinical Interview for Depression

Table 26.2. Specimen page from Clinical Interview

5. *Reactivity to social environment* This refers to the changes in mood and symptomatology in direction of either improvement or worsening, as a result of environmental circumstances. Assess degree: average if this varies. "Does what is happening around you make a difference to your depression? Or does it not affect it? Do some things bring it on? If you feel bad are there things which will make you feel a lot better? Does it come on without any reason? Does it change much or stay the same?"	*Column: 20* 1 = Absent. Changes due to environment absent or very rare. 2 = Very mild or occasional. 3 = Mild. Non-specific factors, such as having someone to talk to, produce limited improvement. 4 = Moderate. Such factors or certain more specific situations produce greater improvement or worsening. 5 = Marked. Depression varies to a considerable degree according to situational factors. 6 = Severe. Factors frequently completely remove the depression and precipitate it. 7 = Extreme. The source of the depression is entirely dependent on certain specific situations, being regularly precipitated or entirely removed according to them.
6. *Guilt, lowered self-esteem and worthlessness* This refers to patient's verbal expressions which indicate the extent to which his evaluation of himself and his self-esteem are abnormally lowered, and the degree to which he feels to blame for a variety of acts and omissions. Consider intensity and pervasiveness of both guilt and worthlessness. "Have you had a low impression of yourself? Have you blamed yourself for things you have done in the past or recently? Have you felt guilty about things? Have you felt you have let your friends and family down? Have you felt you are to blame for your illness? In what way? A lot? A little?"	*Column: 21* 1 = Absent 2 = Very mild or occasional feelings of self-blame on borderline of normality. 3 = Mild. Lowered opinion of self without self-blame or guilt. May include some guilt over consequences of illness or realistically regrettable past actions. 4 = Moderate. More intense or pervasive feelings of being a failure, or of guilt or self-blame. 5 = Marked. Persistent, exaggerated feelings of self-blame, guilt. Intense feelings of failure without self-blame. 6 = Severe. Pervasive feelings of self-blame, guilt, worthlessness, regarding many areas. Near delusional. Isolated delusional ideas without similar ideas in other content. 7 = Several clear-cut delusions or hallucinations of self-reproach, guilt, worthlessness.

imately ten patients with a trained interviewer, but need not be extensive, since the detailed format of the scale is self-explanatory and facilitates self-training. Some training videotapes have also been developed.

Table 26.3 sets out findings of two formal interrater reliability studies, one by psychiatrists and one by non-psychiatrists. In Study A [2], conducted in the United States, two British-trained psychiatrists alternately interviewed 14 successive depressed patients, with both raters making independent ratings. In Study B [19], conducted in London, a PhD sociologist and psychologist carried out a similar procedure on 15 neurotic patients, predominantly depressive and relatively mildly ill. Agreement on individual items was examined by product moment correlation, and overall agreement by calculation of mean correlations (after z transformation) and by percentage agreement pooling all item pairs.

Agreement was high and was closely similar for psychiatrist and non-psychiatrist raters. Mean correlations were 0.81 and 0.82 respectively. Agreement to within

Table 26.3. Reliability studies: agreement between two raters

	Correlation between two raters	
	Study A[a] $N=14$	Study B[b] $N=15$
Depressed feelings	0.57	0.94
Distinct quality	0.84	-
Diurnal variation - worse a.m.	0.97	-
Diurnal variation - worse p.m.	0.98	-
Reactivity	0.74	-
Guilt	0.85	0.87
Pessimism	0.92	0.92
Suicidal tendencies	0.99	0.99
Depersonalisation	0.86	0.58
Obsessional symptoms	0.77	0.90
Work and interests	0.61	0.66
Energy and fatigue	0.94	0.83
Anxiety psychic	0.76	0.73
Panic attacks	-	-
Phobic anxiety	-	0.90
Anxiety - somatic	0.58	0.72
Anorexia	0.98	0.89
Increased appetite	0.99	0.89
Weight loss	0.98	-
Weight gain	-	-
Irritability	0.93	0.84
Initial insomnia	0.86	-
Middle insomnia	0.94	-
Delayed insomnia	0.93	-
Increased sleep	-	-
Paranoid ideas	0.89	-
Depressive delusions	0.74	-
Self-pity	0.60	0.89
Overemphasis of symptoms	-	0.90
Hysterical symptoms	-	-
Hypochondriasis	0.95	−0.07
Retardation	0.86	−0.07
Agitation	0.38	0.18
Depressed appearance	0.32	0.47
Mean correlation	0.81	0.82
Item agreement - all item pairs		
Agree completely	67.8%	61.7%
Disagree one point	27.2%	35.3%
Greater disagreement	5.0%	3.0%

-, Item not rated
[a] Two psychiatrists
[b] Sociologist and psychologist

one point was considered acceptable on seven-point scales; it was found in 95% of ratings by psychiatrists and 97% of ratings by non-psychiatrists. The relatively low correlations for hypochondriasis, retardation and agitation in Study B were due to relative absence of these phenomena in the sample so that one-point disagreements on a few cases were high in relation to the total variability.

Validity

The validity of the Clinical Interview for Depression has been investigated primarily regarding sensitivity to change, ability to measure drug effects, utility to discriminate in other situations, such as in classification and in relation to other data. Relationship to other depression-rating scales has also been studied and will be reported in a subsequent section. Data have not yet been analysed on ability to discriminate depressives from normals but the sensitivity to improvement in depression makes it clear that the instrument can differentiate depressed from non-depressed subjects. There is also a paucity of formal data contrasting depressives and normals on the Hamilton Scale [4].

Sensitivity to change has been tested in three studies in which the scale was used as a repeated rating outcome measure. In a study [6] over 4 weeks of 172 depressed women treated with amitriptyline, there was a significant linear trend for improve-

Table 26.4. Change over 6 weeks in outpatient depressives

	Initial Mean	Final Mean	Significance of change[a]
Depressed feelings	3.92	2.47	<0.001
Guilt	2.72	1.93	<0.001
Pessimism	3.34	2.40	<0.001
Suicidal tendencies	1.86	1.35	<0.001
Work and interests	3.84	2.47	<0.001
Energy and fatigue	3.86	2.79	<0.001
Anxiety psychic	3.79	2.62	<0.001
Panic attacks	1.54	1.34	<0.05
Phobic anxiety	1.94	1.63	<0.01
Avoidance, main phobia	1.95	1.63	<0.05
Anorexia	2.85	1.86	<0.001
Increased appetite	1.31	1.60	<0.01
Irritability	2.65	1.92	<0.001
Initial insomnia	2.36	1.65	<0.001
Delayed insomnia	2.05	1.76	<0.05
Hostility	1.18	1.16	NS
Retardation	1.66	1.32	<0.001
Agitation	1.47	1.20	<0.001
Depressed appearance	3.04	1.98	<0.001
Total depression score	28.76	18.74	<0.001
Total anxiety score	9.21	7.22	<0.001

[a] Paired t-test ($N=131$)

ment on all 14 ratings used in the analysis. Significant improvement was also found in an open study of phenelzine [29].

Table 26.4 sets out mean scores and significance of change by t-test in another study [44] in which 131 outpatient depressives and mixed anxiety-depressives were treated with amitriptyline, phenelzine or placebo for 6 weeks. As can be seen there was significant change on all items except one, hostility, on which initial ratings were very low. For most items change was significant at the 0.001 level. Table 26.4 also shows two total scores, for anxiety and depression, described more fully in the next section.

A direct test of the power of the scale to discriminate drug effects has been undertaken in two double-blind controlled trials. The total scores and scale items were highly sensitive after 6 weeks of treatment in discriminating differences between effects of amitriptyline or phenelzine and placebo [44]. In an earlier study [26] the instrument did not distinguish maintenance amitriptyline from placebo in patients relapsing after drug withdrawal, unlike global ratings of relapse and self-report ratings. However, patients only displayed mild symptoms, and the scale was useful in describing symptom patterns of the relapses [28].

Scoring Systems and Factorial Structure

Two subscores, the depression and anxiety total scores, derived on an a priori basis and incorporated in the repeated ratings interview have been used as outcome measures in treatment studies [29, 32, 33, 44]. The depression score, described simply as the total score in earlier reports, incorporates high loading items on the general factor obtained in a principal component analysis in a depressed sample [20].

Table 26.5 shows correlations of individual items of the depression and anxiety total scores with the total scores themselves, in three samples; (1) outpatients with depression and mixed anxiety-depression [44]; (2) depressives, predominantly outpatients, from a controlled trial of a new antidepressant; and (3) depressives, spanning outpatients, day patients and inpatients, from a predictor study of outcome on phenelzine [29]. Both scores appear reasonably homogeneous, with the exceptions of low correlations of retardation and agitation with the depression total score. This may partly be due to the relative absence of these two phenomena in the samples studied. Overall, the item to total correlations, are comparable to those which have been reported for the Hamilton Scale [1].

Unrotated factor structure has been examined in two principal component analyses [20, 40], the second of which also incorporated a small number of history items. Both analyses showed a first component of general severity, a second component contrasting endogenous and neurotic symptoms, and a third component contrasting depressive and anxiety symptoms.

Table 26.6 shows rotated factors, from another analysis. A sample of 119 subjects was used, derived in part from several studies. Subjects were predominantly outpatients with depression and mixed anxiety-depression; a small number of inpatients and day patients were included. Principal component analysis gave 13 components with eigenvalues greater than 1. A series of rotations to the Varimax

Table 26.5. Item to total correlations of depression and anxiety total scores

	Correlations		
	Study 1 N=214	Study 2 N=86	Study 3 N=46
Total depression score			
Depressed feelings	0.65***	0.58***	0.51***
Guilt	0.48***	0.37***	0.58***
Pessimism	0.58***	0.70***	0.63***
Suicidal tendencies	0.51***	0.56***	0.44***
Work and interests	0.50***	0.44***	0.54***
Anorexia	0.54***	0.47***	0.53***
Delayed insomnia	0.34***	0.44***	0.40***
Retardation	0.29***	0.03	0.22
Agitation	0.21***	0.09	−0.06
Depressed appearance	0.33***	0.62***	0.58***
Total anxiety score			
Anxiety psychic	0.55***	0.73***	[a]
Panic attacks	0.76***	0.75***	[a]
Phobic anxiety	0.76***	0.56***	[a]
Anxiety – somatic	0.71***	0.60***	[a]

*** $P < 0.001$
[a] Items not included in study

Table 26.6. Six-factor rotation to Varimax criterion[a]

Depression		Anxiety		Appetite change	
Work and interests[b]	0.70	Phobic anxiety[b]	0.85	Weight loss	0.75
Pessimism[b]	0.60	Avoidance – main phobia[b]	0.84	Anorexia[b]	0.71
Energy and fatigue[b]	0.59			Weight gain	−0.75
Distinct quality	0.58	Panic attacks[b]	0.64	Increased appetite[b]	−0.71
Depressed feelings[b]	0.57	Anxiety – somatic[b]	0.49		
Anxiety psychic[b]	0.53				
Guilt[b]	0.45				
Retardation[b]	0.43				
Insomnia		**Self-pity and hostility**		**Agitation**	
Middle insomnia	0.56	Self-pity	0.72	Agitation[b]	0.54
Initial insomnia[b]	0.52	Overemphasis of symptoms	0.66	Irritability[b]	0.52
Delayed insomnia[b]	0.50			Paranoid ideas	0.50
Increased sleep	−0.63	Hostility[b]	0.61	Diurnal variation – worse a.m.	−0.60

[a] Table shows item loadings of 0.43 and above
[b] Item included in short form for repeated rating

criterion was carried out. The clearest and clinically most relevant structure was obtained by rotating six factors. Two factors clearly corresponded to depression and to anxiety, resembling the two total scores derived from the instrument, except that psychic anxiety, in this sample containing many mixed anxiety-depressives, loaded on the depression factor. Two further factors loaded clearly on appetite/weight change and insomnia. The remaining factors corresponded to self-pity/hostility and, less clearly, agitation. These factors incorporated 28 of the 36 items included in the analysis and appeared to provide a useful set of outcome measures for treatment studies. They should be regarded as provisional, in view of the underrepresentation of hospitalised patients in the sample.

Relationships to Other Rating Scales

Relationships will be presented with three other interview rating scales: the Hamilton Rating Scale for Depression [5], the Raskin Three Area Depression Scale [39], and the Brief Psychiatric Rating Scale (BPRS) [10]. A previous report [2] has described relationships of individual items of the scale to an interviewer clinical global impression of severity of illness. Relationships with a self-report symptom and mood scale [38] have also been reported previously [16, 22]. Correlations were significant but modest and there was evidence of systematic discrepancies attributed in part to self-report response sets.

Table 26.7 shows correlations of the Depression and Anxiety Total Scores from the Clinical Interview for Depression with total scores of other interview scales. These were derived from the three studies also shown in Table 26.5. The depression total showed moderately high correlations with the Hamilton Scale total score, the Raskin Three Area Total and a global clinical impression of severity of illness, but lower correlations with the BPRS total score, which has a wider content than depression. However, at least 50% of the variance was not in common with each of these scales.

Correlations of the anxiety total with other scales were lower, reflecting the difference of content in relation to depression scales or global measures in predominantly depressed patients. The anxiety total correlated to some extent with the Hamilton Depression Scale, reflecting the inclusion of several anxiety items in the latter.

Table 26.7. Correlations of Clinical Interview for Depression, total depression and anxiety scores with total scores of other interview scales

	Depression total			Anxiety total	
	Study 1 $N=214$	Study 2 $N=86$	Study 3 $N=46$	Study 1 $N=214$	Study 2 $N=86$
Hamilton Depression Scale (17-item total)	0.70***	0.63***	0.53***	0.36***	0.53***
Raskin Three Area Scale (Total score)	0.73***	0.69***	0.54***	0.18**	0.20*
BPRS (Total score)	0.53***	0.34***	0.59***	0.15*	0.27**
Global clinical impression of severity of illness (seven-point)	0.67***	0.62***	0.71***	0.25***	0.23*

* $P<0.05$;   ** $P<0.01$;   *** $P<0.001$

Uses

The instrument has been used extensively in a variety of different kinds of studies in the United States and Britain, primarily by the Yale, Boston and St. George's groups. In the United States these studies have included a survey study of treated depressives [20], a follow-up study of the same sample [15], the acute treatment phase [6] and maintenance treatment phase [26] of a study of recovering depressed women treated by drugs and psychotherapy, a study of suicide attempters [24], studies of depression in medical inpatients [9] and in a women's counselling centre [48]. The scale was used but the results were not reported in controlled trials in depressives of maprotiline [36] and of acute amitriptyline and psychotherapy [3], and in schizophrenics of amitriptyline-perphenazine combination [37]. In Britain the instrument has been used in a predictor study of response to phenelzine [29], in a controlled trial of phenelzine, amitriptyline and placebo in depressives and mixed anxiety-depressives [44], in a controlled service evaluation comparing community psychiatric nurse domiciliary care with standard outpatient psychiatric follow-up care in neurotic patients [19], in a descriptive and classificatory study of depressives in general practice [45], in controlled trials currently under way of a new antidepressant in outpatients and inpatients, of amitriptyline against placebo in general practice, and in biological studies under way in depressive inpatients. It was used, but not published, in a study of mild postpartum depression in the community [30].

In reports from these studies the instrument has been used successfully for a variety of different purposes: (a) *description of samples, including relationship to treatment setting, treatment received, ethnic status, personality, social adjustment, other phenomena* [7-9, 14, 20, 24, 27, 45-48]; (b) *outcome measure in controlled trials and follow-up studies* [6, 26, 29, 32, 33, 44]; (c) *classification, including the main data base for factor-analytic and cluster-analytic studies* [11-13, 17, 18, 21, 28]; (d) *predictor variables for predictor studies* [15, 23, 25, 29, 32, 34]; and (e) *studies of relationship to other rating scales* [2, 16, 22, 35].

Conclusion

This chapter describes and summarises work with an interview-rating scale, the Clinical Interview for Depression. The instrument is suitable for use by psychiatric and by non-medical interviewers. It covers comprehensively symptoms of depression and includes items covering anxiety and other neurotic symptoms. It is set out in the form of a semistructured interview with defined items, interview cues and seven-point rating scales with detailed anchor points. The scale has been shown to be reliable both with psychiatrists and with non-medical interviewers, to relate significantly to other depression scales, to be sensitive to change, to discriminate drug treatment effects, to form a suitable data base for classificatory analyses and to correlate with a variety of other data. It has been employed in many studies in Britain and the United States in samples ranging from severely ill inpatients to subjects in the community being treated by general practitioners or not receiving treatment. Scoring systems are described; the instrument has in addition a sufficiently wide item pool of symptoms for ad hoc use in special situations. It is useful as an instrument to assess depressives, particularly in qualitative descriptive studies, outcome studies, controlled trials of drugs and other therapies, and studies of classification and of prediction.

References

1. Bech, P., Bolwig, T.G., Kramp, P., and Rafaelsen, O.J. 1979. The Bech-Rafaelsen mania scale and the Hamilton Depression Scale. Acta Psychiatr. Scand. 59: 420-430.
2. Chipman, A., and Paykel, E.S. 1974. How ill is the patient at this time? Cues determining clinician's global judgements. J. Consult. Clin. Psychol. 42: 669-674.
3. DiMascio, A., Weissman, M.M., Prusoff, B.A., Neu, C., Zwilling, M., and Klerman, G.L. 1979. Differential symptom reduction by drugs and psychotherapy in acute depression. Arch. Gen. Psychiatry 36: 1450-1456.
4. Fava, G.A., Kellner, R., Munari, F., and Pavan, L. 1982. The Hamilton Depression rating scale in normals and depressives. Acta Psychiatr. Scand. 66: 26-32.
5. Hamilton, M. 1967. Development of a rating scale for primary depressive illness. Br. J. Soc. Clin. Psychol. 6: 278-296.
6. Haskell, D.S., DiMascio, A., and Prusoff, B. 1975. Rapidity of symptom reduction in depressions treated with amitriptyline. J. Nerv. Ment. Dis. 160: 24-33.
7. Klerman, G.L., and Paykel, E.S. 1970. Depressive pattern, social background and hospitalization. J. Nerv. Ment. Dis. 150: 466-478.
8. Klerman, G.L., Paykel, E.S., and Prusoff, B.A. 1973. Antidepressant drugs and clinical psychopathology, In: J.O. Cole, A. Friedhof, and A. Freedman (Eds.) Psychopathology and Psychopharmacology, pp. 172-188, Ch. 11. John Hopkins Press, Baltimore.
9. Moffic, S., and Paykel, E.S. 1975. Depression in medical inpatients. Br. J. Psychiatry 126: 346-353.
10. Overall, J.E., and Gorham, D.R. 1962. The brief psychiatric rating scale. Psychol. Rep. 10: 799-812.
11. Paykel, E.S. 1971. Classification of depressed patients: a cluster analysis derived grouping. Br. J. Psychiatry 118: 275-288.
12. Paykel, E.S. 1972. Depressive typologies and response to amitriptyline. Br. J. Psychiatry 120: 147-156.
13. Paykel, E.S. 1974. Recent life events and clinical depression. In: E.K. Gunderson and R.H. Rahe (eds.), Life Stress and Illness, pp. 134-163. Charles C. Thomas, Springfield, Illinois.
14. Paykel, E.S. 1977. Depression and appetite. J. Psychosom. Res. 21: 401-407.
15. Paykel, E.S., and Dienelt, M. 1971. Suicide attempts following acute depression. J. Nerv. Ment. Dis. 153: 234-243.
16. Paykel, E.S., and Prusoff, B.A. 1973. Response set and observer set in the assessment of depressed patients. Psychol. Med. 3: 209-216.
17. Paykel, E.S., and Henderson, A.L. 1977. Application of cluster analysis in the classification of depression: a replication study. Neuropsychobiology 3: 111-119.
18. Paykel, E.S., and Rassaby, E. 1978. Classification of suicide attempters by clusters analysis. Br. J. Psychiatry 133: 45-52.
19. Paykel, E.S., and Griffith, J.H. 1983. Community Psychiatric Nursing for Neurotic Patients: the Springfield Controlled Trial. Royal College of Nursing, London.
20. Paykel, E.S., Klerman, G.L., and Prusoff, B. 1970. Treatment setting and clinical depression. Arch. Gen. Psychiatry 22: 11-21.
21. Paykel, E.S., Prusoff, B.A., and Klerman, G.L. 1971. The endogenous-neurotic continuum in depression: rater independence and factor distributions. J. Psychiatr. Res. 8: 73-90.

22. Paykel, E. S., Prusoff, B. A., Klerman, G. L., and DiMascio, A. 1973. Self-report and clinician's assessments of depression. J. Nerv. Ment. Dis. 156: 166-182.
23. Paykel, E. S., Prusoff, B. A., Klerman, G. L., Haskell, D., and DiMascio, A. 1973. Clinical response to amitriptyline in depressed women. J. Nerv. Ment. Dis. 156: 149-165.
24. Paykel, E. S., Hallowell, C., Dressler, D. M., Shapiro, D. L., and Weissman, M. M. 1974. Treatment of suicide attempters: a descriptive study. Arch. Gen. Psychiatry 31: 487-491.
25. Paykel, E. S., Klerman, G. L., and Prusoff, B. A. 1974. Depressive prognosis and the endogenous-neurotic distinction. Psychol. Med. 4: 57-64.
26. Paykel, E. S., DiMascio, A., Haskell, D., and Prusoff, B. A. 1975. Effects of maintenance amitriptyline and psychotherapy on symptoms of depression. Psychol. Med. 5: 67-77.
27. Paykel, E. S., Klerman, G. L., and Prusoff, B. A. 1976. Personality and symptom pattern in depression. Br. J. Psychiatry 129: 327-334.
28. Paykel, E. S., Prusoff, B. A., and Tanner, J. 1976. Temporal stability of symptom patterns in depression. Br. J. Psychiatry 128: 369-374.
29. Paykel, E. S., Parker, R. R., Penrose, R. J., and Rassaby, E. 1979. Depressive classification and prediction of response to phenelzine. Br. J. Psychiatry 134: 572-581.
30. Paykel, E. S., Emms, E. M., Fletcher, J., and Rassaby, E. S. 1980. Life events and social support in puerpeval depression. Br. J. Psychiatry 136: 339-346.
31. Paykel, E. S., Mangen, S. P., Griffith, J. H., and Burns, T. P. 1982. Community psychiatric nursing for neurotic patients: a controlled trial. Br. J. Psychiatry 140: 573-581.
32. Paykel, E. S., Rowan, P. R., Parker, R. R., and Bhat, A. V. 1982. Response to phenelzine and amitriptyline in sub-types of neurotic depression. Arch. Gen. Psychiatry 39: 1041-1049.
33. Paykel, E. S., West, P. S., Rowan, P. R., and Parker, R. R. 1982. Influence of acetylator phenotype on antidepressant effects of phenelzine. Br. J. Psychiatry 141: 243-248.
34. Prusoff, B. A., and Paykel, E. S. 1977. Typological prediction of response to amitriptyline: a replication study. International Pharmacopsychiatry 12: 153-159.
35. Prusoff, B. A., Klerman, G. L., and Paykel, E. S. 1972. Concordance between clinical assessments and patient's self-report in depression. Arch. Gen. Psychiatry 26: 546-552.
36. Prusoff, B. A., Weissman, M. M., Tanner, J., and Lieb, J. 1976. Symptom reduction in depressed outpatients treated with amitriptyline or maprotiline: repeated measurement analysis. Compr. Psychiatry 17: 749-754.
37. Prusoff, B. A., Williams, D. H., Weissman, M. M., and Astrachan, B. M. 1979. Treatment of secondary depression in schizophrenia. Arch. Gen. Psychiatry 36: 569-575.
38. Raskin, A., Schulterbrandt, J., Reatig, N., McKeon, J. J. 1969. Replication of factors of psychopathology in interview, ward behaviour and self-report ratings of hospitalized depression. J. Nerv. Ment. Dis. 148: 89-98.
39. Raskin, A., Schulterbrandt, J., Reatig, N., and McKeon, J. 1970. Differential response to chlorpromazine, imipramine and placebo. A study of sub-groups of hospitalised depressed patients. Arch. Gen. Psychiatry 23: 164-173.
40. Rassaby, E., and Paykel, E. S. 1979. Factor patterns in depression: a replication study. J. Affective Disord. 1: 187-194.
41. Rosenthal, S. H., and Klerman, G. L. 1966. Content and consistency in the endogenous depressive pattern. Br. J. Psychol. 112: 471-484.
42. Rosenthal, S. H., and Gudeman, J. E. 1967. The self-pitying constellation in depression. Br. J. Psychiatry 113: 485-489.
43. Rosenthal, S. H., and Gudeman, J. E. 1967. The endogenous depressive pattern. Arch. Gen. Psychiatry 16: 241-249.
44. Rowan, P. R., Paykel, E. S., and Parker, R. R. 1982. Phenelzine and amitriptyline: effects on symptoms of neurotic depression. Br. J. Psychiatry 140: 475-483.
45. Sireling, L. I., Paykel, E. S., Freeling, P., and Rao, B. M. 1985. Depression in General Practice: Clinical features and comparison with outpatients. Br. J. Psychiatry 147: 113-119.
46. Tonks, C. M., Paykel, E. S., and Klerman, G. L. 1970. Clinical depression among negroes. Am. J. Psychiatry 127: 329-335.
47. Weissman, M. M., and Paykel, E. S. 1974. The Depressed Woman: A Study of Social Relations. University of Chicago Press, Chicago.
48. Weissman, M. M., Pincus, C., Radding, N., Lawrence, R., and Siegel, R. 1973. The educated housewife: mild depression and the search for work. Am. J. Orthopsychiatry 43: 565-573.

Chapter 27 Schedule for Affective Disorders and Schizophrenia: Regular and Change Versions

J. ENDICOTT

The Schedule for Affective Disorders and Schizophrenia (SADS) was developed in the mid-1970s in an effort to provide research investigators with a clinical procedure which would reduce information variance in both diagnostic and descriptive evaluations of subjects [2]. It was designed to accomplish these aims by providing for (1) a detailed description of the features of the current episode of illness when they were at their most severe; (2) a similar description of the major features during the week prior to the evaluation; (3) a series of questions and criteria which enable one to make diagnoses using the Research Diagnostic Criteria [7]; and (4) a detailed description of past psychopathology and functioning relevant to the evaluation of prognosis and overall severity of disturbance.

The Change Version of the SADS (SADS-C) was developed for use in those studies where the focus was upon an evaluation of the subject's symptoms and functioning during the past week only. The items are the same as the "past week" items in the regular SADS.

Coverage

The coverage of the SADS is broad enough to provide for evaluation of a wide variety of patients in a dimensional fashion (individual items and summary scale scores) in addition to typological (diagnostic) categories. This article will focus upon those measures of direct relevance to the evaluation of depressive mood and behavior and syndromes, as well as the diagnosis of depressive disorders.

Dimensional Measures of Depression

The SADS contains 30 items which can be used to describe various aspects of depressive mood, ideation, or syndromes which have characterized the current episode of illness. They are listed in Table 27.1. For the most part they are judged on 1-6 point scales with defined levels of severity (accompanied by examples). The past week items and those of the SADS-C are a subset of these (as noted in Table 27.1).

Table 27.1. SADS items descriptive of depression

Depressed mood[a]	Increased sleep
Brooding[a]	Insomnia[a]
Feelings of self-reproach/guilt[a]	Initial[a]
Feeling of inadequacy[a]	Middle[a]
Discouragement/pessimism[a]	Terminal[a]
Loss of appetite[a]	Suicidal tendencies[a]
Weight loss[a]	Number of attempts
Increased appetite	Seriousness of intent to die
Weight gain	Medical threat to life
Loss of interest or pleasure[a]	Distinct quality of mood[a]
Psychomotor agitation[a]	Lack of specific concerns
Psychomotor retardation[a]	Reactivity[a]
Lack of energy[a]	Worse in morning[a]
Indecisiveness	Worse in evening[a]
Difficulty concentrating	
Depressed appearance	

[a] Past week items and also SADS-C items

The SADS items are grouped in a variety of ways to derive composite additive summary scale scores of (a) depressive mood and ideation (5 items); (b) endogenous (i.e., melancholic, vital, or vegetative) features (13 items); (c) depressive syndrome of associated features (12 items); and (d) suicidal ideation and behavior (4 items). The past week or SADS-C items are scored to obtain summary scale scores of (a) depressive syndrome and (b) endogenous features.

In addition to these summary scores, a procedure was developed to "extract" Hamilton Depression Rating Scale Scores [6] for both the "past week" and "worst during episode" items of the SADS. The derivation and testing of the "Extracted HDRS" is described in detail elsewhere [4].

The reliability of the individual items and the summary scale scores have been assessed using both joint rater and test-retest procedures and have been found to be very high [2]. The intraclass correlation coefficients of reliability for the four summary scale measures of depression were all between 0.95 and 0.97. The test-retest reliability was somewhat lower, but still quite high (Cronbach's alpha range, 0.78-0.87). Other investigators who have assessed reliability with well-trained raters have reported similar values.

There is some evidence from a comparison study of the SADS-C and the Hamilton Depression Rating Scale (HDRS) that the use of items with 1-6 point defined levels of severity in the SADS improved the reliability over that of similar items in the HDRS [4]. A comparison of the reliability of the individual items included in both the SADS and the HDRS for the same group of 48 inpatients indicated that the absolute values of 12 of the reliability coefficients from the SADS items were higher than those of HDRS while six of the HDRS items were more reliable than SADS items. Furthermore, the Extracted HDRS scores were somewhat more reliable than were the Real HDRS scores [4].

Table 27.2. RDC diagnoses of depressive disorders covered by the SADS

For patients who ever met criteria for a major depressive syndrome
  Bipolar disorder with mania (bipolar I)[a]
  Bipolar disorder with hypomania (Bipolar II)[a]
  Unipolar major depressive disorder[a]
  Recurrent unipolar major depressive disorder[a]
  Schizoaffective disorder (depressed subtype)
  Depressive syndrome superimposed on residual schizophrenia
Subtypes of episodes of major depressive episode (more than one may apply)
  Primary
  Secondary
  Psychotic
  Incapacitating
  Endogenous
  Agitated
  Retarded
  Situational
  Simple
For patients who ever met criteria for a "non-major" depressive syndrome
  Minor depressive disorder
    Episodic
    Chronic
    With significant anxiety
  Intermittent depressive disorder
  Cyclothymic personality
  Labile personality
  Generalized anxiety disorder with significant depression

[a] Diagnoses are made for life time course. All other diagnoses are for episode

Categorical Measures of Depression

The SADS is organized so that one can make Research Diagnostic Criteria (RDC) diagnoses at the completion of the evaluation. The RDC disorders used to characterize subjects with a depressive syndrome are shown in Table 27.2. These diagnoses are made on an episode as well as on a lifetime basis. The reliability of diagnoses based upon SADS evaluations has been found to be very high in both joint rating and test-retest studies [7].

Measures of Other Variables of Relevance to an Evaluation of Depression

In addition to the measures of depressive features, the SADS has items and summary scales of importance in the description or subtyping of conditions characterized by prominent depression. For example, many investigators and clinicians are interested in particular types of delusions, hallucinations, or thought disorder that may have prognostic, familial, or diagnostic relevance in the study of affective disorders. The SADS has 27 items descriptive of such behaviors or beliefs.

Items descriptive of mood or behavioral changes often considered to be of relevance in the study of depression include those descriptive of hypomania/mania (18 items); anger/irritability (2 items); various types of anxiety such as phobias, panic attacks, obsessions, and compulsions (5 items); somatic complaints (2 items); and drug and alcohol abuse (2 items). Furthermore, the overall level of impairment in functioning during the current episode and past week is evaluated, as are many aspects of past functioning relevant to differential prognosis. While the coverage of the SADS-C is somewhat more limited, it also includes items measuring anxiety, delusions, hallucinations, hypomania/mania, and alcohol and drug abuse.

Validity

No procedure is valid or invalid. Rather it does or does not have demonstrated usefulness for certain tasks. The SADS items, scale scores, and diagnoses have been repeatedly demonstrated to have research and clinical usefulness for many purposes. Only a few examples from our own work will be noted here. Investigators considering the use of the SADS may wish to obtain a computer or library search of major publications in the field. There have been over 60 published reports to date.

Examples of ways in which the usefulness of the SADS has been demonstrated include the following:

1. The individual items and scale scores measuring depressive features have been found to be sensitive to differences in the depressive syndrome of patients with schizoaffective disorder, depressed subtype, and those with psychotic major depressive disorder (i.e., delusions and hallucinations but not of the particular type which defines schizoaffective disorder) [3].
2. They have also been shown to be sensitive to change in drug-placebo differences even among outpatients [8].
3. The prognostic significance of specific types of delusions, hallucinations, and thought disorder in a group of hospitalized patients with a major depressive syndrome has also been demonstrated [1].

Mechanics of Use of the SADS and SADS-C

There are two major ways in which the SADS and SADS-C can be used. The most common pattern of usage of the SADS (and the one the developers consider the most valid) allows the rater to use all sources of information in completing his or her evaluation. In many cases, this would include prior medical records, an admission note, nurses' observations, and information from the family or a previous therapist. After review of all available information, the rater would then use the interview guide in the SADS to conduct a clinical interview (if the patient were able to participate). Discrepancies between the information obtained during the interview and that recorded elsewhere would be clarified whenever possible, either during the interview itself or afterwards (for example, in consultation with the spouse). The SADS ratings would summarize the evaluator's best clinical judgment taking into account all of the information available to the evaluator.

The other manner in which the SADS is used limits the ratings to information obtained during a direct interview of the subject. This method of data collection is most suitable for those studies in which a "blind" evaluation of the patient is required. It is also of value in those settings where there are no prior records or other informants available. Since the SADS-C is frequently used in the evaluation of treatment (sometimes following an intake evaluation using the regular SADS) it is more frequently used in this "interview-only" mode. However, even in this case a rater with prior contact with a subject may use his or her knowledge of past symptoms (e. g., delusions of guilt) in exploring current beliefs.

The interview guide contained in the SADS and SADS-C is designed to be used as a guide, not as a questionnaire. This means that the person making the SADS evaluation is expected to be knowledgeable regarding the items to be judged and the diagnostic criteria to be used. This knowledge should further guide the interview to assure that needed discriminations are made whenever possible, for example, the differentiation between lack of energy and lack of interest.

After the SADS evaluation is completed, the diagnoses are made directly by the clinician. Since the forms are designed for computer analysis, most investigators use a standard computer program available from the author to "store" the SADS data and derive the various summary scale scores. Instructions are also available for investigators who do not have access to computer scoring so that the original scale scores may be derived by hand.

There is no computer program available to derive the RDC diagnoses. The developers' experience with computerized diagnosis [7] led to the conclusion that it was far better to collect the data in a systematic fashion and to let a well-trained clinician make the diagnostic summary. Although the individual items of information regarding diagnostic criteria are recorded, the more subtle aspects of a diagnostic evaluation having to do with the sequence of development of symptoms or the level of confidence of the evaluator regarding aspects of the criteria increase the likelihood that a well-trained clinician would be able to make a more valid RDC diagnosis than would a computer algorithm.

On the other hand, the availability of specific items judged at varying levels of severity will enable an investigator to return to the data and "score" it using diagnostic rules other than those contained in the RDC. The detailed nature of the coverage of the SADS encourages such re-scoring for use in biological studies and in attempts to replicate findings reported by other investigators.

Training in Use of the SADS

As is the case with all evaluation procedures, training improves both the reliability and the validity of data collection. Training makes it more likely that the user will understand the intent of the items and less likely that idiosyncratic definitions will be substituted for either the items themselves or the levels of severity.

The training materials available for the SADS include a manual of instructions and videotapes of SADS interviews accompanied by ratings of SADS items and an explanation of the reasoning behind such ratings when such may be unclear from the videotaped interview. A suggested training program using these materials as well as direct clinical interviews of subjects similar to those to be studied is described in detail elsewhere [5].

Availability of SADS and SADS-C Materials

Copies of the SADS, SADS-C, RDC, and training materials are available from the author at cost. Since new materials are under development, investigators who plan to use the SADS should avail themselves of those which are most recent.

The SADS has been translated into a number of different languages including Spanish, Japanese, French, and German. These translations have been made, with the permission of the authors of the SADS, by investigators who plan to use the procedure with subjects whose primary language is other than English. Since funds were not available for independent retranslation back to English, the adequacy of the various translations has not been evaluated by the developers.[1]

Discussion

There are a number of ways in which the SADS differs from most of the other commonly used procedures designed for the evaluation of depression. The most important of these are the broad coverage of many specific aspects of depressed mood, ideation, and associated clinical features, including hypersomnia and increased appetite. The format of the items as six-point scales with their five levels of severity has the effect of not only increasing the reliability of clinical judgments over that of

---

[1] If an investigator wishes to use a translated version of the SADS, the author encourages contact with investigators who have translated the SADS in the past. It has been our experience that some investigators prefer to make their own translations because of differences in the use of specific languages (for example, Spanish among Cubans, Mexicans, Puerto Ricans, and Argentinians). Investigators who plan to use translations of the SADS are urged to be in close contact with the author and her staff regarding the appropriate interpretations of the intent of the items to be judged.

dichotomized or trichotomized ratings, but also of providing more sensitive discrimination between subjects and in the same subject over time. The availability of an interview guide and training materials improves the comparability of data collection within studies as well as across studies in the same facility and in different facilities and even different countries. Any feature which improves the comparability of data collection also improves the generalizability of the results of specific studies and the likelihood that those results will be replicated elsewhere if the same procedures are followed. The separation of the SADS coverage into that for the past week, for the most severe manifestations of specific symptoms during the current episode, and for the time prior to the current episode, provides measures which are more descriptive of the overall clinical picture of psychopathology and course of symptoms than does a cross-sectional or total composite evaluation alone. The availability of the SADS-C encourages an investigator to obtain the more detailed evaluation at intake and to evaluate change over time using the past week subset of items. The comparability of coverage in the past week subset avoids the problem of comparability across procedures.

What are some of the consequences of these differences between the SADS procedure and other measures of depression? While some investigators find the detailed coverage of the SADS quite compatible with the needs of their studies, others find that the appropriate use of the procedure requires more time and a higher degree of professional competence on the part of the clinical evaluator than can be afforded. Such investigators often decide to use the SADS-C for all evaluations rather than the SADS as an initial evaluation (or prefer to use other procedures altogether).

If one can afford the luxury of such detailed data collection, there are many advantages for the investigator. One has a data base that is much more detailed than with the more commonly used Hamilton Depression Rating Scale. Having available HDRS scores at the same time allows comparison with the results of other studies in which the HDRS has been a measure of depression.

The availability of the other items in the SADS allows one to search for correlates of nondepressive clinical features which may not be possible in other studies. Clinical features of possible relevance for the study of the pathophysiology of depressive disorder, treatment response, and short and long-term outcome include panic attacks, anger, specific types of delusions and hallucinations or thought disorder, or signs of "bipolarity." Dependence upon measures of depression alone may fail to detect important differences among subgroups of patients with a major depressive syndrome. Furthermore, dependence upon current state measures alone will obscure important differences among patients related to their prior history. Before one can assume that two samples are similar because of similar means and standard deviation of depression scores, one would want to compare features of the past history known to be of relevance, for example, evidence of alcohol abuse, "bipolarity," hospitalization, or even treatment. Although the SADS does not include all possible items of information of relevance, most of those that have already been shown to be of importance are included.

The content of the SADS was selected on an atheoretical basis and primarily designed to be descriptive of the major phenomenological manifestations of affective disorders. The other, nondepressive, items are included because they are of importance in the differential diagnosis of depression for nondepressive disorders or because they are frequently associated with depressive disorders and have been found to be of potential importance in their study.

References

1. Coryell, W., and Lavori, P. 1984. Outcome in schizoaffective, psychotic and nonpsychotic depression: Course over a six to twenty-four month follow up. Arch. Gen. Psychiatry 41: 787-791.
2. Endicott, J., and Spitzer, R. L. 1978. A diagnostic interview: The Schedule for Affective Disorders and Schizophrenia. Arch. Gen. Psychiatry 35: 837-844.
3. Endicott, J., and Spitzer, R. L. 1979. Use of the Research Diagnostic Criteria and the Schedule for Affective Disorders and Schizophrenia to study affective disorders. Am. J. Psychiatry 136: 52-56.
4. Endicott, J., and Nee, J. 1981. Hamilton Depression Rating Scale extracted from Schedule for Affective Disorders and Schizophrenia and SADS-C. Arch. Gen. Psychiatry 38: 98-103.
5. Gibbon, M., and McDonald-Scott, P. 1981. Mastering the art of research interviewing: A model training procedure for diagnostic evaluation. Arch. Gen. Psychiatry 38: 1259-1262.
6. Hamilton, M. 1960. A rating scale for depression. J. Neurol. Neurosurg. Psychiatry 23: 56-62.
7. Spitzer, R. L., and Endicott, J. 1974. Constraints on the validity of computer diagnosis. Arch. Gen. Psychiatry 31: 197-203.
8. Stewart, J. W., and Nee, J. Detection of drug-placebo differences in depressed outpatients. In press.

Chapter 28   The Assessment of Depression in Children and Adolescents

M. STROBER and J. S. WERRY

Introduction

That there are significant differences between children and adults in the range, intensity, and comprehension of emotional states seems virtually unassailable. Hence, it is surprising that while the ontogeny of emotional expression has been a concern of psychoanalysis and developmental psychology for several decades, research in child psychiatry has only recently addressed itself to developing a theoretically sound and empirically validated understanding of affective disorders in children, their classification, and possible relation to adult psychopathology. Undoubtedly, there are many reasons for this neglect; (1) incompleteness of our knowledge of maturational and environmental influences that normally govern the elicitation, expression, and control of affective behavior in different natural settings through childhood, and the unknown influence of these processes on the triggering and phenomenology of emotional disorders; (2) psychoanalytic dictum that emotions in children are sometimes obscured by their tendency to blend with, modulate, amplify, or suppress each other [46, 15]; and (3) the intrinsically "unstable" nature of the child's affective systems, resulting from continuing shifts and transformations in the interpersonal, cognitive, and somatic domains, and the child's environment.

Reflecting these developmental considerations, psychiatric approaches to childhood depression have faced unique and challenging problems in regard to its proper denotation, measurement, and nosological classification. As the literature indicates, there has been a considerable divergence of approaches to these matters despite a consensus that depression in children is a legitimate clinical phenomenon that warrants more rigorous scientific scrutiny [4, 32, 39]. Thus, some workers argue that prototypic features of adult depression are rarely observable in children, that depressed children have variable and multiform symptomatologies, and that childhood depression cannot be comprehended from the vantage points of traditional descriptive nosology and diagnostic schemas, but must be inferred instead on the basis of other anomalous behaviors, such as truancy, delinquency, enuresis, eating disturbances, somatization of anxiety, boredom, and so on - so called "masking" or "equivalent" signs of depression. This view persists despite the obvious pitfalls and logical fallacies of an inferential diagnosis based on a wide assortment of behaviors commonly used to diagnose nonaffective emotional disorders and other handicapping conditions, and which often reflect a child's reaction to adverse life circumstances.

Critiques of the masked depression concept may be found in Gittelman [12], Graham [13], and Werry [47].

Others, such as Lefkowitz and Burton [23], have argued that any stipulation about the predictive validity of childhood depression may be premature in the light of the age-related incidence of putative symptoms of depression in epidemiological surveys of children. The authors suggest therefore that depressive behavior in children may, in the majority of cases, represent little more than benign and transitory developmental processes and, as such, is not validly assignable to categories of psychiatric illness.

Although knowledge of the broader epidemiological characteristics of depressive phenomena in childhood is incomplete, it is fair to say that a burgeoning clinical literature supports the view that depressive states do exist in children in a form that bears considerable phenotypic resemblance to the adult syndromes, and that adult diagnostic criteria (e.g., DSM-III, RDC) can be used reliably to identify major depression and certain of its more narrowly defined clinical subforms (e.g., endogenous, psychotic) in children and adolescents referred for psychiatric treatment [20, 32, 33, 4, 7].

This increasing reliance on adult criteria for the diagnosis of depression in juveniles is, no doubt, being encouraged with particular force by the expansion of specific pharmacological treatments of affective illness, and is an attempt to capitalize on recent advances in descriptive psychopathology, especially the refinements of methods for ascertaining and quantifying descriptive data and the development of rules for classifying syndrome entities by explicit and consensual criteria. At the same time, we cannot assume that clinical similarities between juvenile and adult depression imply a shared etiology or method of treatment. But in regard to these empirical questions, application of the better established adult criterion of major depression to juveniles has inherent heuristic and analytic advantages. First, the stipulation of inclusion and exclusion criteria avoids ambiguities generated by the previously widespread and indiscriminate use of such ambiguous diagnostic labels as masked depression; furthermore, by enhancing definitional clarity systematic comparisons across studies become more feasible. Along these lines it provides a unified diagnostic framework for necessary prospective follow-up research aimed at identifying continuities and discontinuities between childhood and adult depressive disorders. And last, the validity of this criterion in juveniles could be tested empirically by comparing index and control samples in terms of well-established external validating characteristics of adult depression. Recently published accounts of elevated familial prevalence of affective disorders, increased 24-h levels of corticosteroid excretion, and a failure of hypothalamic-pituitary-adrenal suppression by dexamethasone in endogenously depressed children and adolescents make a reasonable case that certain juvenile and adult depression do, in fact, share a common familial predisposition and deficits in neuroendocrine regulation [40, 34, 35, 31, 11, 37, 9].

With interest in juvenile depression increasing, a proliferation of self-report inventories, clinician rating schedules, and formalized interview measures has taken place [18, 19, 16]. These approaches vary considerably from each other in terms of theoretical orientation from which they are derived and extent of validation. An excellent discussion of the psychometric properties of these measures may be found in Kazdin and Petti [16]. We do not attempt to match the comprehensiveness of the Kazdin and Petti review here. Rather, we offer brief descriptions of existing assessments and summarize information concerning their reliability, sensitivity, and validity.

Structured Interview Measures

Kiddie-SADS (K-SADS) [8]

The K-SADS was developed by Puig-Antich and colleagues at the New York State Psychiatric Institute as a childhood version of the Spitzer and Endicott Schedule for Affective Disorders and Schizophrenia. It is a systematic structured interview designed to elicit objective and phenomenological information concerning the mode of onset, chronology, and character of the child's current and past episodes of depression and other major functional psychiatric illness, and permits assignment of categorical diagnoses using DSM-III criteria. The overall design and organization of the interview, item coverage, progression of questioning, and scoring of operationally defined gradients of severity of individual symptoms are analogous to the adult SADS. Item ratings and final diagnoses are based on information developed from separate interviews of the child and his or her primary caretaker. Administration of the K-SADS requires a reasonably seasoned professional with advanced knowledge of psychopathological concepts and basic principles of psychiatric interviewing. Reports indicate that the entire interview is generally accomplished in 45-90 min.

Interrater reliability of the K-SADS section on depression has been established by Puig-Antich's group by independent (test-retest) evaluations conducted on 52 children screened thus far in their ongoing validation study of prepubertal depressive illness (Puig-Antich 1983, personal communication). All but two items – excessive guilt and impaired concentration – have been found to have acceptable reliability with intraclass coefficients of item ratings ranging from 0.60 to 0.80. Internal consistency of items comprising the depressive syndrome global score (depressed mood, excessive guilt, psychomotor agitation, psychomotor retardation, insomnia, hypersomnia, anorexia, pervasive anhedonia, excessive appetite, impaired concentration, suicidal ideation, and fatigue) was likewise found to be high (Cronbach alpha, 0.80). The K-SADS has also been found to yield highly reliable retrospective assessments of depressive psychopathology in a diagnostically heterogeneous (depression, nonaffective psychiatric disorder, no detected psychiatric illness) subgroup ($N=17$) of these children, reinterviewed in an asymptomatic state 6 months to 2 years following their initial project evaluation [27]. All 11 of the children receiving initial project diagnoses of major depression were so diagnosed upon reinterview; sensitivity and specificity of the retrospective assessment of discrete symptoms (concordant judgment of the symptom's historical presence or absence) was also shown to be high for most items.

Thus far, construct validity of the K-SADS has been adduced from psychobiological investigations of depressed and nondepressed cohorts. To summarize briefly, prepubertal children diagnosed as primary major endogenous depressives on the basis of K-SADS interviews have been differentiated from nonendogenously depressed controls in terms of 24-h patterns of cortisol hypersecretion, hyposecretion of growth hormone to insulin-induced hypoglycemia, and increased familial prevalence of unipolar depressive illness ([32, 36], and Puig-Antich 1983, personal communication) - major validating characteristics of adult depressive illness. K-SADS summary ratings of depressive syndrome in nondelusional depressed subjects undergoing antidepressant therapy have also been shown to correlate strongly with steady-state plasma levels of drug achieved after 5 weeks of treatment [34, 35], suggesting the measure to be sensitive to biological indices of clinical change, although the absence of a double-blind protocol in this study is problematic.

Interview Schedule for Children (ISC) [17]

The ISC is a structured face-to-face clinical interview designed for psychiatric assessments of children aged 8-15 years. Its focus is on manifest psychopathology reflected in the 2-week period immediately preceding the interview. The ISC encompasses 43 major items which tap fundamental characteristics of depression and suicidal behavior, anxiety disorders, antisocial conduct, substance abuse, elimination disorders, and psychosis, and 12 ratings of behavioral abnormality/dysfunction observed during interview. The majority of items are rated for intensity and degree of functional impairment on a precoded nine-point scale following separate interviews of the parent and child. A final nine-point global rating of severity of the child's specific current condition is also entered upon completion of the interview pooling of all available information.

The depression item list is inclusive of the higher-order symptom cluster of adult depression as originally conceptualized by Beck [1]: (1) emotional (sadness, crying, a decreased hedonic tone, loss of affection, detachment); (2) cognitive (self-depreciation, hopelessness, pessimism, self-blame, negative self-evaluation); (3) motivation (withdrawal, diminished socialization, reduced volition, and avoidant tendencies); (4) vegetative (disturbed sleep, fatigue, diminished appetite); and (5) demeanor (altered postural, facial, and verbal behavior). Interrater reliability coefficients of these items, established through joint, but independent, evaluations of 46 child guidance patients examined as part of a prospective longitudinal follow-up study of childhood depression are all statistically significant ($P<0.001$), with the majority ranging from 0.75 to 0.95. Not surprising is the substantially lower concordance between parent and child interview ratings of depressive symptoms: for items comprising the affective symptom cluster, coefficients are in the range of 0.40; for cognitive symptoms, agreement is quite variable, with coefficients ranging from 0.06 (pessimism, $P=$ NS) to 0.56 (impaired concentration, $P<0.05$); and among vegetative symptoms the range is from 0.25 (fatigue, $P=$ NS) to 0.46 (reduced appetite, $P<0.05$).

There are as yet only limited data available concerning validity of the ISC, although these are instructive. In an initial principal components' analysis performed on ratings obtained from 39 child guidance clinic patients and 20 age-matched controls (no history of psychiatric assessment or treatment), five interpretable factors were identified, including a clearly recognizable depression factor consisting of items measuring motivational, affective, and psychomotor accompaniments of depression. Of course it will be necessary to pursue testing of the ISC in a wider variety of subgroups if the factorial validity of these items is to be established more firmly.

Diagnostic Interview for Children and Adolescents (DICA) [14]

The DICA is a structured psychiatric interview for children between the ages of 6 and 17 years. It is administered in separate but parallel forms to mother and child and covers the diagnostic categories of depression, mania, substance abuse, conduct disorder, phobic and anxiety disorders, obsessions and compulsions, Briquets syndrome, dissociative states, and psychosis. It differs from the ISC and K-SADS in two major ways: items are rated on a dichotomous yes/no basis and the interview is intended for use by paraprofessional technicians participating in clinical and epidemiological investigations of childhood psychopathology.

As the DICA is currently undergoing extensive pilot testing and methodological refinement, data concerning the reliability of its measurement of depression are sparse. However, preliminary indications are that *kappa* coefficients of concordance between parent and child interview ratings of symptoms from the section on depression fall considerably below the minimum acceptable level of interrater agreement, ranging from 0.09 to 0.38, although the authors note that interrater agreement averaged across all items on the child interview alone is 85%. Regrettably, specific concordance coefficients for individual depression items are not indicated.

Schedule for Affective Disorders and Schizophrenia (SADS) [10]

Suitability of the regular adult version of the Schedule for Affective Disorders and Schizophrenia (SADS) for formal psychiatric assessment of adolescents has been examined by Strober and colleagues at the UCLA Neuropsychiatric Institute, in an ongoing program of research on the genetic, neuroendocrine, and longitudinal characteristics of juvenile affective disorders.

Since 1977, the SADS has been administered to several hundred psychiatrically hospitalized adolescents who range in age from 13 to 17 years. Interrater agreement for the diagnostic classification of major affective disorder by DSM-III criteria, based on independent evaluation of SADS interviews conducted by two experienced clinicians, was found to be very satisfactory (*kappa* = 0.75) [41].

To determine reliability of individual items comprising the depression section of the SADS, independent evaluations were carried out subsequently on 40 patients with a final hospital diagnosis of major depression [42]. Intraclass coefficients for the 30 items were, by and large, high (ranging from 0.51 to 0.95), with 25 of the 30 coefficients (83%) above 0.60, often taken as the minimum acceptable level of interrater agreement. Items that proved less reliable ($r < 0.60$) included lack of specific concern, indecision, mood worse in morning, nonreactivity, and mood worse in evening. The more variable judgments of the raters on these items may be due to their low rate of occurrence as well as difficulty experienced by young adolescent patients in discriminating certain particularly subtle aspects of their current affective state.

As a group, the 40 patients showed considerable affective morbidity, with a high proportion of patients ($>50\%$) scoring positively on subjective dysphoria, loss of interest, impaired concentration, suicidality, loss of appetite, sleep disturbance, low self-esteem, lack of specific focus of depressed mood disturbance, and discouragement. Contrariwise, symptoms rated less frequently ($<20\%$) were retardation, mood-congruent psychotic features, agitation, and worsening of mood in the evening. The frequency of occurrence of *individual symptoms* comprising the SADS Summary Scale of Endogenous Features were as follows: loss of interest, 70%; loss of appetite, 68%; middle or terminal insomnia, 43% and 25% respectively; lack of specific concern, 58%; self-reproach, 55%; weight loss, 50%; distinct quality of mood, 50%; mood worse in morning, 35%; nonreactivity, 35%; motor retardation, 18%; and agitation, 10%. With respect to mood-congruent psychotic symptoms, five patients (13%) were grossly delusional at the time of examination with classically depressive themes of guilt about sexual misconduct, punishment, fears of impending disaster, and bodily illness. In addition, four of the five patients experienced auditory hallucinations of self-condemning voices concurrent with their delusions. Also noteworthy is the fact that syndromal forms of depression rarely ascribed to adolescents - i.e., endogenous, retarded, psychotic - did, in fact, occur in this cohort and were classified according to RDC criteria with very satisfactory reliability; *kappa* = 0.74, 0.70, and 0.82, respectively. Because the SADS is sufficiently inclusive, it allows for the grouping of certain individual symptoms into more global dimensions of depressive psychopathology. Using item assignments described in Endicott and Spitzer [10], summary scale scores have been calculated thus far for 65 major depressive probands and assessed for internal reliability using Cronbach's alpha [40]. Reliabilities proved satisfactory: depressive mood and ideation, 0.81; endogenous features, 0.71; depressed-associated features, 0.69; suicidal ideation and behavior, 0.74; delusions and hallucinations, 0.82.

Validity of the SADS in this population has been investigated through predicted associations between hospital diagnoses and expected familial and neuroendocrine validating features of depressive disorder. A summary of this work may be found in Strober [40]. Briefly, family psychiatric histories obtained blindly on first- and second-degree relatives of depressed, antisocial, and schizophrenic teenage probands revealed a statistically significant aggregation of secondary cases of affective illness only among relatives of depressed probands; rates of schizophrenia and antisocial disorder in these relatives did not deviate significantly from general population prevalence figures. With respect to neuroendocrine findings, failure to suppress serum cortisol upon dexamethasone challenge was observed in 9 of 18 (50%) probands meeting RDC criteria for primary endogenous depression, compared with 2 of 11 (18%) nonendogenous major depressions and 1 of 9 (11%) secondary depressives. Diagnostic sensitivity and specificity of cortisol suppression abnormality is currently being analyzed on a much larger series of probands.

Thus, overall implication of findings analyzed to date is that SADS can provide a reliable description of depression in young, psychiatrically hospitalized adolescents and, when used in conjunction with operational diagnostic criteria, permits the differentiation of depressive syndromes from other forms of mental disorder affecting this population.

Clinician Rating Scales

Children's Depression Rating Scale (CDRS) [30]

The CDRS was developed as a childhood version of the Hamilton Rating Scale for Depression and is intended for use with elementary school-age children. It is composed of 15 items (depressed mood, weepiness, irritability, self-esteem, morbid thoughts, suicidal behavior and ideation, school performance, capacity to have fun, social withdrawal, reduced expressive communication, sleep disorder, disruption of eating, somatic complaints, fatigue, and hypoactivity), rated on operationally defined scale points for degree of severity. The CDRS is completed during the course of a semistructured clinical interview, with final item ratings determined by the evaluator's review of all supplementary information available on the child, e.g., parent, teacher, and therapist report.

The initial testing of the CDRS was undertaken with a small ($N=30$) sample of children who were inpatients on the pediatric ward of a university teaching hospital. Each child was seen simultaneously by two psychiatrists using the interviewer/observer format. Evidence of reliability was examined chiefly through item-total correlations computed for each set of ratings, and agreement between raters in the total CDRS score. These homogeneity coefficients ranged from 0.38 (weeping) to 0.88 (depressed mood, capacity to have fun) for scores given by rater 1, and from 0.32 (weeping) to 0.92 (capacity to have fun) for scores given by rater 2. Overall, individual item ratings by the two raters show a very similar degree of correlation with the total score. Interrater agreement for sum scores was very high, $r=0.96$.

Evidence for concurrent validity of the measure was obtained from correlations between items and an independent global severity rating of depression made by the observing psychiatrist. These validity coefficients ranged from 0.27 (weeping) to 0.94 (depressed mood). Items showing the highest correlation with the independent global depression rating were hypoactivity, somatic complaints, expressive communication, social withdrawal, capacity for fun, decreased school work, irritability, and depressed mood.

A more recent report [29] has examined the psychometric utility of the CDRS in a small ($N=30$) residential psychiatric sample of children ranging in age from 6 to 12 years. Item-total score correlations were found to range from 0.13 (sleep) to 0.90 (depressed mood). The interrater agreement for total CDRS score was satisfactory, $r=0.80$. Items showing the strongest ($r>0.80$) association with total score were depressed mood, anhedonia, and expressive communication. Item correlations with the independent global severity rating of depression ranged from 0.04 (irritability) to 0.96 (depressed mood). Items correlating highly ($r = 0.80$) with this clinical rating were depressed mood and anhedonia.

Several methodological issues complicate evaluation of the CDRS. First, information on the short-term temporal stability of item ratings and interrater agreement for individual items is lacking. And second, since CDRS and global depression ratings were made by each psychiatrist, it is conceivable that the correlations reported are influenced by halo effects and response bias. Also noteworthy is the fact that patterns of item-total and item-global depression score correlations in the pediatric and psychiatric samples differ to some degree, suggesting that homogeneity of the CDRS is not constant across populations.

Bellevue Index of Depression (BID) [20]

The BID is a 40-item questionnaire completed by a clinician by pooling information obtained from the child, parents, and other adults who can provide details concerning the child's general emotional and behavioral functioning. It is intended for use with children aged 6 to 13 years. The 40 items encompass ten symptom categories and are each rated on a four-point scale for severity. The ten categories are dysphoric mood, self-deprecation, aggression, sleep disturbance, diminished school performance, diminished socialization, changing attitude toward school, somatic complaints, loss of energy, and weight loss or appetite change. To be classified as depressed the child must obtain at least one positive symptom rating from the categories dysphoric mood and self-deprecation, and receive a minimum total score of 20.

Initial testing of the BID was carried out on 73 psychiatrically hospitalized children ranging in age from 6 to 12 years. Concurrent validity was ascertained by comparing classification agreement between the BID criterion and a clinician's independent judgment of the presence or absence of depression in the child. This agreement was 83%. However, general psychometric characteristics of the BID remain unknown. Lacking are data on the scale's homogeneity and stability of scores, evidence of interrater agreement for quantifying individual items and total score, and data about crucial aspects of its construct validity.

Children's Affective Rating Scale (CARS) [25]

The CARS was designed as a quantitative measurement of depression in children for use in an ongoing study of developmental psychopathology in the offspring of unipolar and bipolar depressive illness. The scale contains only three items—mood and behavior, verbal expression, and fantasy. Each is dimensionalized on a ten-point continuum with implied deviant characteristics given as examples for low-, moderate-, and high-severity ratings. Ratings are made following a structured interview designed to elicit information concerning history of symptoms of mood disorder, content of fantasy, feelings of self-worth, and evidence of general psychopathology.

The CARS has been applied to a sample of 30 children who are offspring of 14 patients hospitalized for unipolar or bipolar illness. Interrater reliabilities are reported to range from 0.71 to 0.95. As of yet, no further data are available on internal consistency or validity.

Self-Report Inventories

Children's Depression Inventory (CDI) [20, 21]

The CDI is a 27-item self-report questionnaire designed for use with children between the ages of 8 and 13 years. It was modelled after the adult BDI, although preliminary field testing has led to modifications in design and item coverage appropriate for a juvenile population. Each item presents three alternative responses, graded 0 to 2 for increasing severity of disturbance. Instructions to the child specify that he/she rate each item on the basis of feelings and thoughts during the past 2 weeks.

A preliminary 20-item version of the CDI was studied in 39 child guidance clinic patients ranging in age from 8 to 13 years and 20 controls with no reported history of psychiatric contacts. Mean CDI score of clinic children was found to be nearly double that of controls, although several items had surprisingly high rates of endorsement in control subjects; between 35% and 50% of controls admitted to the presence of symptoms of sadness, suicidal wish, indecisiveness, and school difficulty. By way of contrast, relatively few controls endorsed items concerning feelings of failure, loneliness, and social withdrawal. Comparison of endorsement rates across the two samples suggested that the items feelings of failure, irritability, and being friendless were most discriminative of clinic group membership. Total CDI score correlated 0.55 ($P<0.001$) with an independent global rating of depression severity. Concerning reliability, Kuder-Richardson 20 coefficients of internal consistencies were 0.85 and 0.78 in the clinic and nonclinic samples, respectively. Item-total score correlations for the combined sample ranged from 0.34 ($P<0.01$) to 0.65 ($P<0.001$).

More recently, evidence of criterion-related validity and construct validity of the CDI has been presented by Carlson and Cantwell [6] and Cantwell and Carlson [5], who have studied the dimensional structure of the CDI and the relation between CDI scores and independent psychiatric diagnosis in 102 children aged 7 to 17 years who were undergoing inpatient or outpatient psychiatric treatment. It was found that patients with higher self-rated depression on the CDI received higher global severity ratings of depression on the basis of a semistructured interview administered without knowledge of the patients' CDI score, and were more likely to receive a formal diagnosis of major depressive disorder. A principal component factor analysis on CDI scores of these 102 patients yielded four interpretable factors. The first factor, which accounted for 26% of the variance, consisted of eight items and was labelled dysphoria and poor self-image. The second factor explained 7% of the variance and was characterized by fatigue, indecisiveness, crying spells, self-accusation, and sense of failure. Factor 3 accounted for 6% of the variance, consisting of somatic preoccupation and sleep disturbance. The fourth factor consisted of weight loss and anorexia, and accounted for 4% of the variance. Factor scores derived for factors 1 and 2 were found to discriminate significantly patients diagnosed as depressed from those patients with nonaffective psychiatric illness. Discriminant function analysis correctly classified 81% of the cohort.

The current 27-item version of the CDI is still undergoing psychometric evaluation in various psychiatric and control samples. Recent data reviewed by Kovacs [18, 19], based on administration of the inventory to 875 Canadian schoolchildren between 10 and 17 years of age, suggest satisfactory internal consistency (coefficient alpha = 0.86; item-total coefficients ranging from 0.31 to 0.54) and temporal stability ($r = 0.72$).

Children's Depression Scale (CDS) [22]

The CDS contains 66 items, of which 48 are statements of depression and 18 are positively oriented statements of self-worth or perceptions of competency. The two item clusters are scored separately. Each of the 66 items is printed on separate cards and is presented to the child, who is instructed to place the card in one of five boxes – labelled "very wrong" to "very right" – which best approximates the statement's fit with his or her experience.

Scale items were developed in accordance with the author's conceptualization of childhood depression as a syndrome characterized by affective change, negative self-concept, decrease in mental productivity and drive, psychosomatic complaints, preoccupation with death, and aggressivity. Specific content of items was formulated by inspecting psychotherapy transcripts and projective test protocol of allegedly depressed school phobic children. The Depression Scale is broken down into five component subscales, including affective response (e.g., "I feel life is not worth living"; "Sometimes I don't know why I cry"); social problems (e.g., "Often I feel lonely"); self-esteem (e.g., "Often I feel I'm not worth much); preoccupation with sickness and death (e.g., "I feel tired most of the time when I'm at school"; "Often I feel dead inside"); and guilt (e.g., "Often I feel like I'm letting my mother/father down"). Nine nonclustered items are grouped together and scored as "miscellaneous." The CDS has an adult companion form which is designed for use with parents, teachers, other family members, etc., who can provide information about the child's behavior.

The CDS was first administered to a sample of 96 children aged 9 to 16 years, including 40 with severe school refusal, 37 with no evidence of psychological illness, and 12 receiving treatment for a variety of emotional problems, excluding school refusal. Adult CDS ratings were obtained from a total of 130 parents. Statistically significant differences between the "depressed" and control subjects were noted for 35 of the 48 depressive items; when CDS ratings made by mothers were examined, 47 of the 48 items proved to be discriminating. However, a factor analysis failed to extract dimensions equivalent to the originally specified depression subscales, suggesting that any assumption about construct validity of the CDS subscales is premature.

A variety of investigators around the world have engaged the CDS for use in clinical and epidemiological research. Preliminary data from these studies have been reviewed by Tisher and Lang [45]. Subscale reliabilities are reported to range from 0.54 to 0.77, with internal consistency of the full CDS estimated to be 0.92. A test-retest coefficient of 0.74 has been reported over a 7- to 10-day period.

Face Valid Depression Scale (FVDS) [26]

The FVDS is comprised of 35 items selected from the full Minnesota Multiphasic Personality Inventory (MMPI) which are purported to reflect essential characteristics of adolescent depression. Five clinicians, working independently, selected items according to a proposed definition of adolescent depression which included such features as garrulousness alternating with withdrawal and apathy, anger and rage, sadness, feelings of insufficiency, ambivalence over independence, sensitivity to criticism, somatic complaints, and so on. The final criterion of an item's inclusion in the scales was selection by at least four of the five judges.

The resulting 35-item FVDS was applied to MMPI protocols of 212 ambulatory and hospitalized adolescent patients. A target-depressive subsample was demarcated on the basis of a patient's scoring at least one standard deviation above the mean on the scale. There was a significant difference in sex distribution between the depressive and nondepressive sample so defined, with a female predominance in the FVDS-positive group. Items endorsed most frequently (90% or greater) by the FVDS-positive subgroup included feeling unhappy, feeling useless, feeling no good, feeling life is a strain, wanting to leave home, death wishes, lacking self-confidence, sleep loss, lacking understanding from others, and feeling blue. The full FVDS had a Kuder-Richardson reliability of 0.93 and correlated 0.71 with the MMPI Standard Depression Scale score. A factor analysis of the 35 items suggested six factors, labelled lack of self-confidence, social abandonment, loss of interest, sadness, somatic symptoms, and acting out. Twenty-five of the 35 items were found to have significant factor loadings with no item loading on more than one factor, suggesting a satisfactory degree of simple structure.

Beck Depression Inventory (BDI) [2]

Utility of the standard 21-item BDI with psychiatrically hospitalized adolescents has been reported by Strober et al. [43]. Testing was completed on 78 consecutively admitted patients, aged 13-17 years, representing a range of diagnostic categories.

No significant difference between sexes in total BDI score was found, nor did scores correlate with age or IQ. The coefficient alpha estimate of internal reliability was 0.79. Further evidence of the homogeneity of the scale was demonstrated by statistically significant item-total score product-moment correlations obtained for all but one (somatic preoccupations) of the 21 items. These coefficients ranged from 0.22 to 0.86, the average being 0.68 ($P < 0.001$). Test-retest reliability, determined by readministering the BDI to all 78 patients after 5 days, indicated total scores to be highly correlated across this time period, $r(76) = 0.69$, $P < 0.001$. On clinical diagnostic grounds, it is noteworthy that this stability coefficient was greater in patients with major depression than in patients with nonaffective diagnoses, $r(18) = 0.74$, $P < 0.001$, and $r(55) = 0.51$, $P < 0.05$, respectively. Although the difference between these correlations does not reach statistical significance, this finding is in keeping with the invariant quality of mood disturbance typically associated with major depressive disorder.

The Pearson correlation between BDI score and a global clinical rating of depression was highly significant, $r = 0.67$, $P < 0.001$, which is of the same order as values obtained by Beck et al. [2] in a psychiatrically hospitalized adult population. Applying Beck's recommended cutoff score of 16 and above to designate moderate to severe clinical depression permitted correct classification of 81% of the sample (14% of the total sample were false positives and 5% were false negatives). A Kruskall-Wallace analysis of variance indicated further that BDI scores varied significantly across the four degrees of depression categories, $H(3) = 17.53$, $P < 0.001$; pairwise comparison of scores by the Nemenyi procedure indicated that differences were significant between patients in nonadjacent categories.

Patients with a diagnosis of major depression differed from nondepressed patients in total BDI score, 23.68 versus 13.36, respectively, $P < 0.001$, and endorsed higher severity ratings on 17 of the 21 inventory items. The four nondifferentiating items were sense of failure, self-hate, irritability, and somatic preoccupations. The point-biserial correlation between total BDI score and hospital diagnosis treated as a dichotomous variable (major depression versus nondepressive diagnosis) was highly significant, $r(76) = 0.72$, $P < 0.001$.

Psychometric performance of the BDI has also been studied in a large sample of 14- to 17-year-old high school students in Vermont [44]. The correlations of each item with total score ranged from 0.27 to 0.62, with a mean of 0.49. Coefficient alpha for the entire sample was 0.87, indicating the scale's high level of internal consistency when applied to this population.

Principal components analysis applied to the 21 items suggested factorial heterogeneity, with Varimax extraction of four factors accounting for 47% of the total variance: Factor 1, labelled general depression, included the items feeling sad, discouragement, fear of failure, guilt, need for punishment, disappointment, self-blame, impaired decision-making, feelings of unattractiveness; Factor 3, labelled psychomotor retardation and reduced tolerance, accounted for 7% of the variance and was a vegetative symptom factor including the items weight loss and diminished appetite. Nonetheless, in the absence of cross-validation, there is no guarantee of the generalizability of these factors, or similar factorial composition in adolescent psychiatric patients.

Construct validity was further suggested by the finding that more females than males had total scores at least one standard deviation in excess of the sample mean – consistent with the observed sex-ration disparity in depression – and that significantly higher scores were obtained by subjects with failing grade averages and students not living with their natural parents.

The Depressive Self-Rating Scale [3]

The original version of the Depressive Self-Rating Scale (DSRS) consisted of 35 items believed representative of the characteristic symptoms and behavioral maladjustment of depressive disorder in prepubertal children. The items cover affective change (e.g., "I feel like crying, " "I am moody and bad tempered," "I feel so sad I can hardly stand it"); guilt and self-denigration (e.g., "I feel as though I am a bad person," "I blame myself a lot for things," "I think other children don't like me"); disturbed concentration and school performance (e.g., "I find it hard to keep my mind on school work," "I worry about going to school"); decreased socialization (e.g., "I feel lonely," "I like talking to my family," "I feel like running away"); irritability and aggressiveness (e.g., "I fight with people more than I used to," "I get angry at people"); diminished drive and capacity for pleasure (e.g., "I feel very bored," "I don't look forward to things as much as I used to"); fears and worries (e.g., "I have horrible dreams," "I get frightened in the dark," "I worry about death and dying"); somatic complaints (e.g., "I get headaches"); and changes in vegetative and motoric functioning (e.g., "I get very tired," "I sleep very well," "I have lots of energy"). Each item is scored on a three-point scale in the direction of increasing disturbance, based on the child's experiences during the past week. To avoid an acquiescent response bias, items were keyed both positively and negatively and distributed randomly through the inventory.

As a second step in the construction of the scale, the original 37 items were administered to four groups of children: 17 psychiatric clinic patients with a diagnosis of depressive disorder according to specified operational criteria; 17 nondepressed emotionally disturbed children attending the same clinic; 20 children in residence at a school for the emotionally disturbed; and 19 nondisturbed children. As a group, the children ranged in age from 7 to 13, the mean being 10.5 years.

Next, an analysis of variance was conducted to identify those items which statistically discriminated the children with depressive disorder from the three other groups. Eighteen items were identified and retained in the final version of the scale. Inspection of the distribution of scores within each of the four cohorts suggests that a cutoff of 12 correctly classifies 77% of the depressives and results in a 12% false-positive classification of depressive disorder among the nonaffective, emotionally disturbed children. Test-retest reliability was assessed only within the residential school population and was found to be 0.80. The final scale is reported to have a split-half reliability of 0.86, although the reference group for this figure is not specified.

Naturalistic Measures

Peer Nomination Inventory of Depression (PNID) [24]

A unique approach to the quantification of depression in children, the PNID is a sociometric device which has been used as a method of assessment of various childhood behavior. Starting from a working definition of childhood depression as a state marked by reduced ebullience and capacity for pleasure, 20 items were formulated – 14 pertaining to depressive traits (e.g., "who plays alone?"; "who doesn't have fun?"), four measuring happiness (e.g., "who is often cheerful?"; "who often smiles?"), and two measuring popularity (e.g., "who would you like to have for your best friend?"; "who would you like to sit next to in class?").

A total of 944 fourth- and fifth-grade students attending New York City schools stratified with respect to socioeconomic level participated in the psychometric evaluation of the PNID. These students were randomly assigned to either a standardization or cross-validation sample. The PNID was administered by having the children of each class simply indicate the names of all classmates for whom each question was most relevant. This procedure yielded two scores; (1) an item score, which amounted to the sum of nominations by all other children in the class and (2) a total score for the entire item set. Evidence for concurrent and construct validity was obtained from correlations with other established self-report measures of depression and self-esteem and teacher ratings of depression, school achievement, and work study habits.

The depression items showed a coefficient alpha of 0.85; item-total score correlations for these items ranged from 0.34 to 0.71. For the happiness items, item-total correlations ranged from 0.63 to 0.78 with a coefficient alpha of 0.88. Two-month test-retest stability coefficients for the depression and happiness items were 0.79 and 0.74 respectively.

Evidence for concurrent validity was obtained from correlations with modified versions of the CDI and Zung Self-Rating Scale for Depression. Though statistically significant, the magnitude of these coefficients is not substantial – 0.23 and 0.14 for the CDI and Zung, respectively. This would seem to be due to the fact that the PNID is not oriented towards description of behavior pathology or dysfunction and is devoid of items representing somatic or vegetative symptoms of depressive disorder. PNID score did, however, correlate more strongly with teacher ratings of depression, $r = 0.41$.

With respect to construct validity, higher PNID scores were found to correlate with lower test scores in reading and maths, poorer social adjustment, external locus of control, poor work study habits, and lower family income. A multiple regression analysis showed four variables to be significantly correlated with PNID: teacher-rated depression, social achievement, self-rating of depression, and days absent from school. The multiple correlation between these variables and PNID score was 0.51, accounting for 26% of the common variance. It is noted, however, that magnitudes of the significant correlations between PNID and the construct-validating measures are not great, ranging from 0.07 to 0.27. Factor analysis of thirteen depression and four happiness items suggested four interpretable factors, which together accounted for 54% of the variance. These were labelled loneliness, inadequacy, dejection, and happiness.

Concluding Remarks

This brief review of instruments for the assessment of depression in children and adolescents is intended to be complementary to that of Kazdin and Petti [16] and shows, if nothing else, that there is a great deal of activity in this area. This should not, however, obscure some very real problems relating to the measurements of depression in children and adolescents, many of which are discussed in greater detail in Cantwell [4], Graham [13], Kazdin and Petti [16], and Werry [48].

Multiplicity of Instruments

This review cites a number of measures but these are only those which have been published and the subject of at least *some* psychometric study. The authors are aware of several others currently under study or in press. Most notable of these is the US National Institute of Mental Health DISC (Diagnostic Interview Schedule for Children), a structured interview method rather similar to the SADS, which comes in two forms, one for child and one for parent interviews. It is based on and yields DSM-III diagnoses (including depressive disorders). Since it is "official" and is to be the subject of a nationwide epidemiological survey in the United States, it is likely to supplant many of those discussed above.

Suffice it to say that the choice of an instrument to measure depression in children at this point in time presents some difficulty.

Reliability

Further data are needed on the interrater agreement and test-retest ability of many of the inventory measures reviewed here. A further neglected issue is the extent to which clinical ratings of depression in children are influenced by the setting, procedure, and context surrounding the construction and the testing of the measurement device.

Convergent and Discriminant Validity

There is a particular need for the application of more complex strategies designed to explicate interrelationships among various measures of depression and other psychopathological disorders in juveniles. In this regard, we underscore the recommendation of Kazdin and Petti [16] that future research in this area should be directed towards investigating convergent and discriminant validity within a multitrait multimethod framework. In short, the need is for replication studies involving larger samples of children drawn from a variety of settings to determine the extents and limits to which measures contribute to description, diagnosis, and differential diagnosis of depression in this age group.

Generalizability

Practically all the work described in this review has originated from the United States. We sought, through correspondence, to ascertain the state of thinking about depression and its measurement in children in non-English-speaking countries. Unfortunately, replies to our queries were disappointingly few, but such as we had suggest that work and interest in the United States is considerably more intensive and advanced than in the majority of other English- and non-English-speaking countries. Though data are sketchy, such as there are suggest that rates of depression reported for children in the United States are higher than those in other countries [48]. A similar state of affairs has obtained in the past with respect to Attention Deficit Disorder with Hyperactivity (minimal brain dysfunction), where attempts to replicate work in the United States have failed [38]. As Werry [48] asks: Is the rate of depressive disorder in children in the United States really higher than was previously thought or is it simply a case of overdiagnosis based on popular trends of the moment? Thus, we urge caution in the application of these instruments outside research settings and outside the United States.

Predictive Validity

As already pointed out in the review, most instruments lack anything other than pilot studies attesting to their longitudinal, biological, demographic, genetic, clinical, and, above all, therapeutic predictions. The latter is particularly difficult since there is already a substantial body of literature in pediatric psychopharmacology which shows that other disorders such as attention deficit disorder with hyperactivity and possibly conduct disorders and certain anxiety disorders may respond to the use of antidepressants in children [48]. Unless the instruments purportedly defining depression in children can meet the acid test of predictive validity the existence of the syndrome must remain in doubt. It is important in this respect to note that there are discrepancies between child self-reports, parental reports, and structured interview methods so that psychiatric interview diagnosis cannot be used as the ultimate validating criteria [48].

Classification of Depression

Much of the recent work in the study of affective disorders in adults has been concerned with subcategorization into such epidemiologically, therapeutically, and biologically discreet categories as unipolar major depression; bipolar major depression; "neurotic," atypical, or reactive depression (in the DSM-III, dysthymic disorder); and depressive symptoms occurring in other disorders. While there are important exceptions, there is still a regrettable tendency in child psychiatry to talk about depression and to develop instruments which ignore these critical subcategorizations. It belittles a generation of serious research in affective disorders in adults to talk about depression as if it were a homogeneous entity. Nowhere is the problem of subcategorization of depression more critical and perplexing than in prepubertal children. There seems little doubt that major affective disorder often begins in adolescence, particularly the bipolar type, but as far as prepubertal children are concerned Graham's [13] admonition of a decade ago remains as cogent as ever [48]. He pointed out then that adult-type depression seemed rare in children but that transitory dysphoric states were common in stress and in other childhood psychiatric disorders [13].

Clearly child psychiatry cannot stand aside and ignore one of the more significant developments in adult psychiatry; it would be fair to say that juvenile depression is an idea whose time has clearly come. We simply urge that its study be prosecuted with the utmost of scientific rigor. Some of the assessment instruments described here will be helpful in this quest but they are not yet robust enough to be used as the only method of clinical assessment.

References

1. Beck, A.T. 1967. Depression: Clinical, Experimental, and Theoretical Aspects. Harper and Row, New York.
2. Beck, A.T., Ward, C., Mendelson, M., Mock, J., and Erlbaugh, J. 1961. An Inventory for measuring depression. Arch. Gen. Psychiatry 4: 53–63.
3. Birleson, P. 1981. Validity of depressive disorder in childhood and the development of a self-rating scale: A research report. J. Child Psychol. Psychiatry: 73–88.
4. Cantwell, D.P. 1982. Childhood depression. In: B.B. Lahey and A.E. Kazdin (eds.), Advances in Clinical Child Psychology, pp. 39–95, Vol. 5. Plenum Press, New York.
5. Cantwell, D.P., and Carlson, G.A. 1981. Factor analysis of a self-rating depressive inventory for children: Factor structure and nosological utility. Paper presented at the annual meeting of the American Academy of Child Psychiatry, Dallas, Texas, October 1981.
6. Carlson, G.A., and Cantwell, D.P. 1979. Survey of depressive symptoms in a child and adolescent psychiatric population. J. Am. Acad. Child Psychiatry 18: 687–599.
7. Carlson, G.A., and Strober, M. 1979. Affective disorders in adolescence. In: H.S. Akiskal (ed.), Psychiatric Clinics of North America, pp. 511–526, Vol. 2 (3). Saunders, Philadelphia.

8. Chambers, W., Puig-Antich, J., and Tabrizi, M. A. 1978. Ongoing development of the Kiddie-SADS. Presented at the annual meeting of the American Academy of Child Psychiatry, San Diego, California.
9. Crumley, F. E., Clevenger, J., Steinfink, D., and Oldham, D. 1982. Preliminary report on the dexamethasone suppression test for psychiatrically disturbed adolescents. Am. J. Psychiatry 139: 1062–1064.
10. Endicott, J., and Spitzer, R. L. 1978. A diagnostic interview: The Schedule for Affective Disorders and Schizophrenia. Arch. Gen. Psychiatry 35: 837–844.
11. Extein, I., Rosenberg, G., Pottash, A. L., and Gold, M. S. 1982. The dexamethasone suppression test in depressed adolescents. Am. J. Psychiatry 139: 1617–1619.
12. Gittleman, R. 1977. Definitional and methodological issues concerning depressive illness in children. In: J. G. Schulterbrandt and A. Raskin (eds.), Depression in Childhood: Diagnosis, Treatment, and Conceptual Models, pp. 69–80. Raven Press, New York.
13. Graham, P. 1974. Depression in prepubertal children. Dev. Med. Child. Neurol. 16: 340–349.
14. Herjanic, B., and Reich, W. 1982. Development of a structured psychiatric interview for children: Agreement between child and parent on individual symptoms. J. Abnorm. Child Psychol. 10: 307–324.
15. Izard, C. E. 1977. Human Emotions. Plenum Press, New York.
16. Kazdin, A. E., and Petti, T. A. 1982. Self-report and interview measures of childhood and adolescent depression. J. Child Psychol. Psychiatry 23: 437–457.
17. Kovacs, M. 1978. The Interview Schedule for Children, 10th Ed. University of Pittsburgh School of Medicine, Pittsburgh, Pennsylvania.
18. Kovacs, M. 1981. The Interview Schedule for Children: A semistructured psychiatric interview for the initial and follow-up assessment of youngsters. Presented at the Annual Meeting of the American Academy of Child Psychiatry, Dallas, Texas.
19. Kovacs, M. 1981. Rating scales to assess depression in school aged children. Acta Paedopsychiatr. (Basel) 46: 305–315.
20. Kovacs, M., and Beck, A. T. 1977. An empirical-clinical approach towards a definition of childhood depression. In: J. G. Schulterbrandt and A. Raskin (eds.), Depression in Childhood: Diagnosis, Treatment, and Conceptual Models, pp. 1–25, Raven Press, New York.
21. Kovacs, M., Betof, N. G., Celebre, J. E., Mansheim, P. A., Petty, L. K., and Raynak, J. T. 1977. Childhood depression: Myth or clinical syndrome. Unpublished manuscript. University of Pittsburgh. Pittsburgh, Pennsylvania.
22. Lang, M., and Tisher, M. 1978. The Children's Depression Scale. The Australian Council for Educational Research, Victoria, Australia.
23. Lefkowitz, M. M., and Burton, N. 1978. Childhood depression. Psychol. Bull. 85: 716–726.
24. Lefkowitz, M. M., and Tesiny, E. P. 1980. Assessment of childhood depression. J. Consult. Clin. Psychol. 48: 43–50.
25. McKnew, D. H. Jr., Cytryn, L., Efron, A. M., Gershon, E. S., and Bunney, W. E. Jr. 1979. Offspring of patients with affective disorders. Br. J. Psychiatry 134: 148–152.
26. Mezzich, A. C., and Mezzich, J. E. Symptomatology of depression in adolescence. J. Pers. Assess. 43: 267–275.
27. Orvaschel, H. O., Puig-Antich, J., Chambers, W., Tabrizi, M. A., and Johnson, R. Retrospective assessment of child depression with the Kiddie-SADS-E. J. Am. Acad. Child Psychiatry. In press.
28. Petti, T. 1978. Depression in hospitalized child-psychiatry patients. J. Am. Acad. Child Psychiatry 17: 49–59.
29. Poznansky, E. O., Cook, S. C., and Carroll, B. J. 1979. A depression rating scale for children. Pediatrics 64: 442–450.
30. Poznansky, E. O., Carroll, B. J., Banegas, M. C., Cook, S. C., and Gross, J. A. 1982. The dexamethasone suppression test prepubertal depressed children. Am. J. Psychiatry 139: 321–324.
31. Poznansky, E. O., Cook, S. C., Carroll, B. J., and Corzo, H. 1982. The Children Depression Rating Scale: Its performance in a residential psychiatric population. Unpublished manuscript. University of Illinois, Chicago, Illinois.
32. Puig-Antich, J. 1980. Affective disorders in childhood. In: B. Blinder (eds.), Psychiatric Clinics of North America, pp. 430–424, Vol. 3. Saunders, Philadelphia.

33. Puig-Antich, J. 1982. The use of RDC criteria for major depressive disorder in children and adolescents. J. Am. Acad. Child Psychiatry 21: 291-293.
34. Puig-Antich, J., Chamber, W., Halpern, F., Hanlon, C., and Sachar, E. 1979. Cortisol hypersecretion in prepubertal depressive illness: A preliminary report. Psychoneuroendocrinology 4: 191-197.
35. Puig-Antich, J., Perel, J.M., Lupatkin, W., Chambers, W., Shea, C., Tabrizi, M.A., and Stiller, R.L. 1979. Plasma levels of imipramine and desmethylimipramine and clinical response in prepubertal major depressive disorder. J. Am. Acad. Child Psychiatry 18: 616-627.
36. Puig-Antich, J., Tabrizi, M.A., Davies, M., Coetz, R., Chambers, W.J., Halpern, F., and Sachar, E.J. 1981. Prepubertal endogenous major depressives hyposecrete growth hormone in response to insulin induced hypoglycemia. J. Biol. Psychiatry 16: 801-818.
37. Robbins, D.R., Alessi, N.E., Yanchyshyn, G.W., and Colfer, M.V., 1982. Preliminary report on the dexamethasone suppression test in adolescents. Am. J. Psychiatry 139: 942-943.
38. Sandberg, S.T., Wieselberg, M., and Shaffer, D. 1980. Hyperkinetic and conduct problem children in a primary school population: Some epidemiological considerations. J. Child Psychol. Psychiatry 21: 293-311.
39. Schulterbrandt, J.G., and Raskin, A. (eds.). 1977. Depression in Childhood: Diagnosis, Treatment and Conceptual Models. Raven Press, New York.
40. Strober, M. 1983. Clinical and biological perspectives on depressive disorders in adolescence. In: D.Cantwell and G.Carlson (eds.), Affective Disorders in Childhood and Adolescence. Spectrum, New York, pp. 97-105.
41. Strober, M., Green, J., and Carlson, G. 1981. Reliability of psychiatric diagnosis in hospitalized adolescents. Arch. Gen. Psychiatry 38: 141-145.
42. Strober, M., Green, J., and Carlson, G. 1981. Phenomenology and subtypes of major depressive disorder in adolescence. J. Affective Disord. 3: 281-290.
43. Strober, M., Green, J., and Carlson, G. 1981. Utility of the Beck Depression Inventory with psychiatrically hospitalized adolescents. J. Consult. Clin. Psychol. 49: 482-484.
44. Teri, L. 1982. The use of the Beck Depression Inventory with adolescents. J. Abnorm. Child Psychol. 10: 277-284.
45. Tisher, M., and Lang, M. 1983. The Children's Depression Rating Scale: Review and recent development. In: D.P.Cantwell and G.A.Carlson (eds.), Affective Disorders in Childhood and Adolescence. Spectrum Publications, New York.
46. Tomkins, S.S. 1962. Affect, Imagery, Consciousness: The Positive Affects. Springer, New York Heidelberg Berlin.
47. Werry, J. 1976. Commentary on C.K.Conners, Classification and treatment of childhood depression and depressive equivalents. In: D.M.Gallant and G.M.Simpson (eds.), Depression: Behavioural, Biochemical, Diagnostic, and Treatment Concepts, pp. 196-199. Spectrum Publications, New York.
48. Werry, J.S. 1982. Major depressive disorder in prepubertal children. Symposium in honour of Professor L.G. Kiloh, Sydney, Australia.

Chapter 29 Instruments Used in the Assessment of Depression in Psychogeriatric Patients

T. HOVAGUIMIAN

Introduction

Depression is the most common psychiatric problem from which an aging individual is liable to suffer. Between 5% and 20% of elderly citizens in industrialized societies are estimated to present some degree of clinical depression [16] and up to 30% of the patients admitted to a geriatric service seem to be affected by a severe form of the illness [23].

While depression increases in frequency and depth in later life and tends to become resistant to therapy, its clinical manifestations are not radically different from those observed in younger people. Some of the general depression scales seem therefore to have the potential to assess virtually all the major dimensions displayed in old age. The first section of this chapter examines the suitability of using with elderly patients a number of depression assessment instruments developed with a younger population.

There remain, however, a number of characteristics or problems which are specific to old-age depression. Cognitive symptoms, for instance, though observed in adult depressive states, may become so prominent in the elderly that they induce a "pseudo-dementia" [29, 32]. Some somatic symptoms, which are valuable diagnostic aids in rating depression in young individuals, lose their specificity as they become normal or common accompaniments of aging (e.g., late insomnia, decline of sexual function, constipation, aches and pains).

There are also special considerations for the proper assessment of an older person. Age-related factors, such as a more defensive attitude towards psychiatric investigation, fatigue, and deficits of recent memory, can alter the properties of a scale if the formulation and design of questions and time period covered are not appropriate.

In order to respond to the special aspects of the measurement of depression in old age a number of instruments have been developed specifically for elderly patients. These are reviewed in the second section of this chapter. The last part of this section examines the so-called Life-Satisfaction Scales, which are constructed to assess the older person's attitude towards life. These instruments can reflect and measure a particular form of depression in the elderly, referred to as demoralization. This concept has been defined as a persistent trait, not characteristically associated with the somatic or biological symptoms, nor the perceptual or thinking distortions included in the depressive syndrome [17].

Nongeriatric Depression Scales Suitable for Use in the Elderly

Salzman et al. [55] reviewed all the major depression inventories (not specifically designed for the elderly), with particular reference to their suitability for psychotropic drug research in the field of aging. None was considered quite optimal. The shortcomings did not only relate to the lack of evidence on sensitivity to drug effects in old age, but also to the acceptability of the scales by elderly people and to the doubtful geriatric relevance of some dimensions or the absence of others. Format which in some instances made the rating difficult with an older patient was criticized.

Other subsequent reviews of the depression-rating scales proposed primarily for adults [34, 42] confirmed again their rather limited applicability in old age. In spite of these limitations, certain general depression scales have been quite extensively used with elderly people. These geriatric applications are reviewed in this section.

The Zung Self-Rating Depression Scale [68]

The Zung scale, described in Chap. 21 of this book has probably been most widely used with the elderly. Its popularity is mainly due to the fact that it is one of the rare depression scales with published normative data for aged individuals. Normal samples of elderly subjects were consistently found in several studies to have higher depressive scores on the Zung scale than younger normative groups [69, 70, 72]. Depressive symptom levels on the Zung scale were also reported more recently by Freedman et al. [10] in successive old-age groups ranging from 60 to 80 years and above. The data gathered by these authors in 166 family practice patients living in the community, all without previously diagnosed psychiatric impairment, indicated globally a borderline symptom level with a curvilinear relationship between depressive symptom und aging: women showed peak symptom level in the 65 to 69-year age group and men in the 70 to 74-year age group.

The reliability of the scale in older subjects was established in a study by Morris et al. [44]: two factors identified in the data gathered from 89 aged inpatients (agitation and self-satisfaction) had high internal consistency.

Some qualitative normative data on the Zung scale are also available for the elderly, as several studies reported on distinct symptom clusters between young and old-age groups [3, 10, 72]. Loss of self-esteem seems to be the factor accounting for higher depressive baselines in the elderly.

The Zung scale has the advantage of being brief and easy to read and understand. A certain degree of intellectual impairment does not seem to preclude its use; Heidell and Kidd [26] used the scale with 120 nursing home residents, many of whom had intellectual impairment. However, their results suggested that a number of patients judged "senile" by the staff were actually unrecognized depressives, who scored higher than those with depression without cognitive impairment.

The observer-rated analogue of the Zung Self-Rating Depression Scale [71] can be useful when self-rating is beyond the patient capacity or when an evaluator's judgment is sought.

Besides these advantages, a number of limitations in the use of the Zung scale in the elderly were also reported through the numerous studies for which it was used. Salzman et al. [55] pointed to the complexity of the four possible response formats and deplored the lack of a "not applicable" position regarding some of the items, which decreased the accuracy of the answers and the subject's collaboration.

Kochansky [34] noted that the scale does not sufficiently stress a relevant dimension of depression in the elderly, which is the area of somatic complaints and dysfunctions. However, the loading of physical symptoms is a difficult problem in assessing depression in the elderly. Some somatic symptoms of depression in the young can be related to physiological changes or medical illness in the aged.

In a recent study [63] the relationship between the Zung scale somatic symptoms index [3], depression as measured by the total scale score, and physical status based on medical examination was explored among a group of 60 elderly depressed patients in relatively good physical health. While there was a significant relationship between the physician's ratings of health and the self-reported somatic symptoms, the total depression score did not correlate with the objectively diagnosed physical status. The authors suggested that these data should "lessen the concern ... that health as a confounding variable obscures the measurement of depression in the elderly."

The Zung scale was used with the elderly as a diagnostic tool as well as in outcome research.

Outcome studies were reviewed by McNair [42], who summarized the data of a number of psychopharmacological trials that used the Zung scale with aged patients. Some of these studies could not establish the sensitivity of the scale to drug effects in the aged as no significant treatment result occurred; but others reported the scale to be sensitive to even moderate effects of active drugs [56, 73].

Among the recent studies using the Zung scale as a screening device with the elderly is the work of Kitchell et al. [33]. She and her associates evaluated the performance of the Zung scale and the Popoff Index of Depression [50] in detecting affective disorders in 42 medical inpatients aged 60 years or more. Compared with interview diagnosis the Zung scale correctly classified 74% of the patients as being depressed or not. In comparison, the Popoff index correctly identified 66% of the patients. The authors concluded that "although performance on both scales is reduced compared with that of younger depressed patients, these self-rating scales appear to be useful aids for the detection of depression in geriatric medical patients."

In another study [52] a geriatric population discharged from a general hospital was screened and followed up with the Zung scale: a large number of unrecognized relapses of depressive episodes were detected. This study implied that, in a number of cases, the Zung scale might have tended to overestimate, at a level of a major depressive relapse, experiences that the clinical interview showed to be instead depressive dysphoria impairing the quality of life. In contrast with other opinions on the scale loading of somatic symptoms [34], these authors suggested that "the Zung scale may be vulnerable to overestimating syndrome depression in the elderly because of its emphasis on physical aspects of depression."

The Hamilton Rating Scale for Depression [22]

The Hamilton scale, described in Chap. 14 of this book, has been used in a number of studies of aged depressives. There are no formal normative data available for this scale in old age. Some indications about norms in aging can be found, however, in studies comparing depression at different life stages. Hodern et al. [28], for instance, assessed with the Hamilton scale a sample of 137 female depressive patients about to receive a tricyclic antidepressant. The size of the sample was sufficient to allow comparison of results in three groups: young (up to 49 years), middle aged (50–59 years), and elderly (60–70 years). The mean overall severity scores at baseline assessments were not significantly different between young and elderly patients; however, a number of individual symptoms explored in the scale showed significant age-related differences: agitation, delayed insomnia, loss of weight, and depressed mood were more severe in the elderly, while the severity of genital symptoms prevailed in the young patients.

A factorial structure of the Hamilton scale in old-age depression has been described by Sarteschi et al. [57]. These authors performed a cross-sectional evaluation of the depressive symptomatology obtained by using the Inpatient Multidimensional Psychiatric Scale (IMPS) of Lorr et al. [40] and the Hamilton Depression Scale in 807 patients in two age groups under and over 60 years. Symptoms of somatization/hypochondriasis, insomnia, anxiety, and agitation mainly distinguished older from younger patients in both endogenous and neurotic depressive subgroups.

The Hamilton scale has mainly been used in the elderly to assess treatment effects.

Kochansky [34] reviewed three psychotropic drug studies [4, 28, 53] and one other outcome study of the therapeutic effects of sleep deprivation [6] all using the Hamilton scale with elderly patients. He concluded that the validity of this scale in its sensitivity to treatment or drug effects in the elderly population "seems tentatively established."

Following this review at least two further studies used the Hamilton Rating Scale in conjunction with other depression inventories for the assessment of antidepressant drug treatment in geriatric depressions [11, 14]; both reported sensitivity of the Hamilton scale to drug effects.

The Profile of Mood States (POMS) [43]

Four geriatric applications of this scale [37, 54, 60] were traced in a review chapter by its developer [42], who found in these studies a good acceptability of the scale by elderly subjects and a sensitivity to active drug effects in this age group.

More recently, POMS scores were also reported in 44 elderly patients (involved in a study of response to the Dexamethosone Suppression Test [61]) with a mean age of 71 years who met the DSM-III diagnostic criteria for major depression.

The Depression Scale of the MMPI [25]

This scale has published evidence of validity and reliability of use in an elderly male population, where it has been found to record higher mean levels of depressive symptoms [35].

It was criticized because of its length, a specially impeding feature with the poorly motivated or impaired geriatric patients [55].

The depression scale has 60 items; Harmatz and Shader [24] found significant age-related differences in the responses to nearly 50% of these items.

McNair [42] reviewed two psychotropic drug studies using the MMPI Depression Scale in elderly patients [56, 60]; his conclusions suggest that the norms require further revision to make them appropriate for the elderly.

The Present State Examination (PSE) [64]

The PSE, a semistructured interviewing schedule that enables a standardized rating to be made of nearly 140 psychopathological items, can elicit depressive symptoms experienced in the previous month and grade their severity in terms of intensity and persistence. The instrument was used in at least two studies, both by Murphy, with elderly populations.

In the first study [46] a group of 119 elderly depressed patients were compared with matched age groups of normal subjects living in the community. Of the 200 subjects who constituted the original community sample 70% were found to be normal on the basis of the PSE interview. The remaining 30% had positive ratings of psychiatric symptoms. These were classified on the basis of the PSE assessment and clinical judgment: 13% were considered as "borderline," as their psychiatric symptoms were not severe enough to warrant a case diagnosis, while the others were cases of first onset of depression ($N=19$), chronic depression ($N=8$), depression and anxiety ($N=2$), anxiety ($N=2$), and alcohol abuse ($N=1$).

Thus most psychiatric disturbance detected by the PSE in this community sample of elderly subjects was of the affective kind.

In the comparison between the community sample and the depressed patients referred to a hospital an association was found between severely adverse life events, major social difficulties, poor physical health, and the onset of depression.

The second study [47] used the PSE to assess the initial depressive illness and follow up the outcome of 124 ambulatory and hospitalized elderly patients. All were consecutive referrals to a psychiatric service who were included in the study whenever they met the Feighner research criteria for primary depression [9].

An impressive proportion of the sample was found at initial assessment to be suffering from symptoms described in the literature as characteristic of psychotic or endogenous depression (such as distinct quality of depression, guilt feelings, early morning wakening, and in some cases depressive delusions). When the sample was considered as a whole (i.e., "neurotic" and "psychotic" depression together) no particular symptom was found to be associated with poor outcome. However, a high

PSE score (which is derived in this multiple psychopathology rating schedule by summing up the number of psychiatric symptoms scored as present) appeared to be the most important discriminant variable predicting bad prognosis of depression in old age. Poor somatic health also had the same prognostic value.

Depression Scales Specifically Designed for the Elderly

Most geriatric depression scales are included in instruments developed to assess multiple psychopathology in the elderly or in the psychiatric section of multidimensional batteries. Only one of the instruments reviewed here (the Geriatric Depression Scale [67]) measures solely depression.

Schwab's Depression Scale [58]

This scale has been developed with and applied to an elderly population; it is part of a structured interview used in a study of mental health and aging [58]. The questions relate more or less evenly to physical and mood depression symptoms rated on a four-position format according to their frequency from "most of the time" to "never." Cognition is not assessed in the depression section.

A shortened version of ten items of the scale was validated in a comparative study [12] of 45 elderly inpatient depressives age-matched with 45 controls living in the community. The scale was found to differentiate between groups of elderly depressives and controls. Repeated assessment of the case from admission to discharge indicated that the scale was sensitive to change and reflected behavioral differences within the depression sample.

The Sandoz Clinical Assessment Geriatric Scale (SCAG) [59]

This scale is intended mainly for psychopharmacological studies in the elderly. It covers 18 symptom areas relevant to senile dementia and depressive states rated on a seven-point format and dealing with mood, cognition, motivation and initiative, sociability and cooperativeness, self-care, and physical symptoms.

The SCAG was administered by its developers to 51 volunteers and hospitalized subjects aged 65 years and above who were classified as healthy, depressed, and mildly or severely demented. Depressed inpatients differed from demented inpatients on 7 of the 18 symptom dimensions of the scale. The authors concluded that the SCAG can help to differentiate between early senile deterioration and depressive disorders.

A review article by Hughes et al. [30] critically examined several clinical investigations which used this instrument to assess a cognitive-acting alkaloid in the treatment of dementia. Sensitivity of the SCAG to active drug treatment effects on condition and/or mood was repeatedly reported across these studies.

Kochansky [34] in a critical review of psychiatric-rating scales for the elderly summarized the few available data on the validity, reliability, and factorial composition of the SCAG and commented favorably on its use in geriatric psychopharmacological studies.

The Geriatric Mental State (GMS) [7]

This instrument is an old-age adaptation of the Present Status Examination [64] and the Mental Status Schedule [62]. It is a semistructured interviewing guide and an inventory of items constructed for eliciting and recording psychopathology in elderly psychiatric patients. Nearly 500 items are scored on the basis of information obtained by a highly trained interviewer during a single session of less than 1 h. One hundred items cover observed behavior.

Fifty-one items of the GMS relate to depression, which emerged as one of the 21 factors when the data gathered from geriatric hospitalized patients of a United States/United Kingdom diagnostic project were factor analyzed [16].

The capacity of the GMS to detect change in depression over time and to discriminate between patients with organic brain symptoms and functional psychiatric patients (most of whom were suffering from a mood disorder) was established in a study of 100 older patients admitted to a geriatric hospital [19].

No cross-validation studies were conducted, to the present author's knowledge, between the depression measurement of the GMS and other depression scales. However, some data in this regard can be found in a study of Jacoby and Levy [31]; these authors compared computed tomography data of 41 depressed elderly patients with their clinical symptoms as measured with a battery of tests including the GMS, the Hamilton Depression Scale, and the Newcastle Depression Scale. In their results, they reported a subgroup of nine patients with enlarged ventricles who differed from normals in being significantly older and having higher scores in the Newcastle Depression Scale. Depression in the enlarged ventricle subgroup was not detected by the GMS nor by the Hamilton Scale.

The Comprehensive Assessment and Referral Evaluation (CARE) [20]

This semistructured interviewing guide is described as an inventory of defined ratings covering the patient's functioning in the psychiatric, medical, nutritional, economic, and social fields. The CARE contains probably more information of relevance to the psychiatric realm than other multidimensional instruments.

In particular it contains a depression scale with a cutoff point that was validated to differentiate between elderly who would probably be clinically assessed as suffering from some degree of depression and those who would not [21].

The CARE was used in a study of hearing impairment in relation to mental state of elderly residents in London [27]. Of the 235 respondents who completed the full depression scale a particularly high proportion (35%) scored above the depression cutoff point. The author partly explained this finding of a higher prevalence figure of depression than those reported in other community studies by the predominance of women of advanced age in their sample. This study found a significant relation between deafness and depression which was independent of age and socioeconomic status.

Golden and his associates [13] have recently developed, on the basis of items selected from the CARE, two indicator scales for detection of dementia and depression in elderly subjects living in the community. They assumed that "a more promising approach to a detection of depression or dementia cases results from considering the information from both these domains." Dementia items and depression items which were selected from the CARE were those regarded to have face and statistical validity for either or both of these conditions; the scales were constructed with these items so as to meet specified criteria regarding content and construct validity and internal consistency.

Using data collected in two large surveys with the CARE of elderly living in London and New York City, the authors reported only three misclassifications with their dementia and depression scale out of 138 cases.

The Geriatric Depression Scale (GDS) [67]

This recently developed rating scale aims primarily at screening depression in the elderly. Its design takes into account the special problems reported in the assessment of psychopathology and particularly of mood in the aged.

The GDS includes 30 dichotomous items which can be either rated by the patient or read to him and rated by the evaluator. These items were derived from a selection of 100 questions regarded by specialists in geriatric psychiatry to have potential for distinguishing older depressives from normals. Thus the scale covers areas of particular geriatric relevance such as cognitive complaints, self-image, and losses. A careful distinction is made between the physical symptoms and their affective repercussions.

The developers found the GDS to be a reliable screening test because it discriminated well between groups of normals and depressives of different severity in one validation study. Two other studies suggested that the scale capacity to differentiate depressed from nondepressed was also satisfactory in a population of physically ill elderly and a population of demented elderly [67]. As the GDS is quite recent, studies determining its sensitivity to measuring change in depression over time and following treatment are still lacking.

The scale was nevertheless positively commented upon and regarded as a promising tool in a paper presented at the US National Institute of Aging Conference on Assessment [15].

The Life Satisfaction Scales

These instruments stem from relatively long-standing research that has been attempting since the 1950s to establish an operational definition of well-being in late life and a measure of successful aging. The instruments used in this approach assess behavioral variables, such as the activities of older subjects and their social participation and/or inner states such as subjective opinion about life progression, self-esteem, energy, and happiness.

The various instruments measuring life satisfaction, adjustment, and morale which have been developed over the past 3 decades have a lot in common. Lohman [39] reported the correlations between seven of the most frequently used measures of life satisfaction [the Cavan Adjustment Scale [5], the Kutner Morale Scale [36], the Dean Scale [8], the Life Satisfaction Indexes A and B [48], the Philadelphia Geriatric Centre Morale Scale [38], and a global measure [51]] and modified versions of three of these instruments [1, 44, 65]. Except for the global measure (a single question on "how satisfied are you with your life"), which correlated poorly, she found all the other scales to have a high level of correlation, "suggesting that many of these measures are directed toward a common underlying construct."

While these instruments are not designed to map the features of depression as a clinical syndrome, they might reflect, as suggested by Gurland [17], a depressive attitude with scattered symptoms. This possible entity seems to have an age distribution pattern distinct from those of neurotic or psychotic depression [16].

Others, however [2], have seriously queried the face validity of these "contentment scales" and considered them as unsatisfactory research tools.

Conclusions

The problems which researchers faced when they used depression scales developed for young subjects with elderly subjects led to recent efforts to design old-age specific assessment instruments.

Some time will have to elapse before enough experience is gathered with tools such as the Geriatric Depression Scale (see p. 350), which looks quite promising but still needs complete standardization. On the other hand, certain general depression scales, such as the Zung scale (see p. 221), have already been used quite extensively with elderly subjects; some further adaptation of their norms might make such scales sufficiently appropriate for the assessment of the aged.

The question then arises as to whether future research in this field should continue to promote a separate development of an instrumentarium for the measurement of depression in the elderly; or whether the experience that will be gained with certain well-designed old-age-specific scales should be used to adapt general depression scales so as to cover depression in old age.

The latter approach, which allows direct comparisons between depression in the various life stages, offers in the present author's opinion some advantages for the understanding of the phenomenology of depression in a developmental perspective.

Nevertheless some special purpose assessment tools will always be needed in gerontopsychiatry. Depression in demented patients, for instance, has to be approached with instruments having items for the assessment of both conditions, such as the indicator scales derived recently from the Comprehensive Assessment and Referral Evaluation (see p. 350).

Epidemiological and pharmacological research have so far been the main fields of application of standardized assessment of depression in the elderly. Today, when increasing numbers of aged cases are seen and managed by nonpsychiatric physicians, a simple and reliable tool to assess old-age depression is needed in everyday practice. While it is obvious that no rating scale can ever replace clinical judgment and experience, it should be remembered that a good assessment instrument, in skillful hands, can become part of the therapeutic process and improve the difficult relationship with an old and depressed patient.

References

1. Adams, D. L. 1969. Analysis of a life satisfaction index. J. Gerontol. 24: 470–474.
2. Bloom, M. 1975. Discontent with contentment scales. Gerontologist 15: 99.
3. Blumenthal, M. D. 1975. Measuring depressive symptomatology in a general population. Arch. Gen. Psychiatry 32: 971–978.
4. Burt, C. G., Gordon, W. F., Holt, N. F., and Hodern, A. 1962. Amitryptiline in depressive states: a controlled trial. J. Ment. Sci. 108: 711–730.
5. Cavan, R. S., Burgess, E. W., Havieghurst, R. J., et al. 1949. Personal adjustment in old age. Science Research Associates, Chicago.
6. Cole, M. E., and Miller, H. F. 1976. Sleep deprivation in the treatment of elderly depressed patients. J. Am. Geriatr. Soc. 24: 308–313.
7. Copeland, J. R. M., Kelleher, M. J., Kellet, J. M., et al. 1976. A semi-structured clinical interview for the assessment of diagnosis and mental state in the elderly: The Geriatric Mental State Schedule. I. Development and reliability. Psychol. Med. 6(8): 439–449.
8. Cumming, E., Dean, L. R., and Newell, D. S. 1958. What is "morale"? A case history of a validity problem. Human Organization 17: 3–8.
9. Feighner, J. P., Robins, E., Guze, S. B., et al. 1972. Diagnostic criteria for use in psychiatric research. Arch. Gen. Psychiatry 26: 57–73.
10. Freedman, N., Bucci, W., and Elkowitz, E. 1982. Depression in a family practice elderly population. J. Am. Geriatr. Soc. 30(6): 372–377.
11. Georgotas, A., Friedman, E., McCarthy, M., et al. 1983. Resistant geriatric depressions and therapeutic response to monoamine oxidase inhibitors. Biological Psychiatry 18(2): 195–205.
12. Gilleard, C. J., Willmott, M., and Vaddadi, K. S. 1981. Self-report measures of mood and morale in elderly depressives. Br. J. Psychiatry 138: 230–235.
13. Golden, R. R., Teresi, J. A., and Gurland, B. J. 1982-1983. Detection of dementia and depression cases with the comprehensive assessment and referral evaluation interview schedule. Int. J. Aging Hum. Dev. 16(4): 241–254.
14. Goldstein, S. E., Birnbom, F., and Laliberte, R. 1982. Nomifensine in the treatment of depressed geriatric patients. J. Clin. Psychiatry 43(7): 287–289.
15. Granick, S. 1983. NIA Conference on assessment: Psychologic assessment technology for geriatric practice. J. Am. Geriatr. Soc. 31(12): 728–742.

16. Gurland, B.J. 1976. The comparative frequency of depression in various adult age groups. J. Gerontol. 31: 283-292.
17. Gurland, B.J. 1980. The assessment of the mental health status of older adults (Depression). In: J.E. Birren and R.B. Sloan (eds.), Handbook of Mental Health and Aging, pp. 682-684. Prentice-Hall, Englewood Cliffs.
18. Gurland, B., Copeland, J., Sharpe, L., and Kelleher, M. 1976. The geriatric mental status interview (GMS). Int. J. Aging Hum. Dev. 7(4): 303-311.
19. Gurland, B.J., Fleiss, J.L., Goldberg, K., et al. 1976. A semi-structured clinical interview for the assessment of diagnosis and mental state in the elderly: the geriatric mental state schedule. II, A Factor analysis. Psychol. Med. 6: 451-459.
20. Gurland, B.J., Kuriansky, Y., Sharpel, L., et al. 1977. The comprehensive assessment and referral evaluation (CARE). Rationale, development and reliability. Int. J. Aging Hum. Dev. 8: 9-42.
21. Gurland, B.J., Sharpe, L., Simon, R., et al. 1981. A cross-national comparison between New York and London of the frequency, management and outcome of psychiatric, medical and social problems among the elderly living in the community. Haworth Press, New York.
22. Hamilton, M. 1960. A rating scale for depression. J. Neurol. Neurosurg. Psychiatry 23: 56-62.
23. Hamilton, M. 6983. Problems of depression in the elderly. Psychiatry in the 80's, pp. 1-8, Vol. 1, No. 1. Excerpta Medica, Amsterdam.
24. Harmatz, J.S., and Shader, R.I. 1975. Psychopharmacologic investigations in healthy elderly volunteers: MMPI depression scale. J. Am. Geriatr. Soc. 23: 350-354.
25. Hathaway, S.R., McKinley, J.D. 1951. Minnesota multiphasic personality inventory: Manual. Psychological Corporation, New York.
26. Heiddel, E.D., and Kidd, A.H. 1975. Depression and senility. J. Clin. Psychol. 31: 643-645.
27. Herbst, K.H., and Humphrey, C. 1980. Hearing impairment and mental state in the elderly living at home. Br. Med. J. 281/6245: 603-905.
28. Hodern, A., Holt, N.F., Burt, C.E., et al. 1963. Amitryptiline in depressive states: phenomenology and prognostic considerations. Br. J. Psychiatry 109: 815-825.
29. Hovaguimian, T. 1982. Démence tardive ou dépression grave? Un guide pour le diagnostic. Médicine et Hygiène 40: 4057-4061.
30. Hughes, J.R., Williams, J.G., and Currier, R.D. 1976. An ergot alkaloid preparation (Hydergine) in the treatment dementia: critical review of the clinical literature. J. Am. Geriatr. Soc. 24: 490-497.
31. Jacoby, R.J., and Levy, R. 1980. Computed tomography in the elderly. 3. Affective disorders. Br. J. Psychiatry 136(3): 270-275.
32. Kiloh, L.E. 1961. Pseudodementia. Acta Psychiatr. Scand. 37: 336-351.
33. Kitchell, M.A., Barnes, R.F., Veith, R.C., et al. 1982. Screening for depression in hospitalized geriatric medical patients. J. Am. Ger. Soc. 30(3): 174-177.
34. Kochansky, G.E. 1979. Psychiatric rating scales for assessing psychopathology in the elderly: a critical review. In: A. Raskin and L.F. Jarvik (eds.), Psychiatric Symptoms and Cognitive Loss in the Elderly, pp. 125-156. John Wiley and Sons, New York.
35. Kornetsky, C. 1983. Minnesota multiphasic personality inventory: results obtained from a population of aged men. In: J.E. Birren (ed.), Human Aging, pp. 217-253. PHS Publ., Washington D.C.
36. Kutner, B., Fanshel, D., Togo, A.M., et al. 1956. Five hundred over sixty. Russel Sage Found, New York.
37. Laforet, E.G., Sidd, J.J., and Waterman, W.E. 1974. The relationship of heart to mood in patients with heart block: effect of pacing. J. Gerontol. 29: 643-644.
38. Lawton, M.P. 1972. The dimensions of morale. In: D. Kent, R. Kastenbaum, and S. Sherwood (eds.), Research Planning and Action for the Elderly: The Power and Potential of Social Science. Behavioural Publications, New York.
39. Lohman, N. 1977. Correlations of life satisfaction, morale, and adjustment measures. J. Gerontol. 32: 73-75.
40. Lorr, M., McNair, D.M., Klett, C.J., et al. 1966. Inpatient multidimensional psychiatric scale. Consulting Psychologist Press, Palo Alto.
41. Maroney, R., Gurel, L., and Davis, J. 1969. Patient's perception of nursing home placement. Geriatrics 24: 119-124.

42. McNair, D. M. 1979. Self-rating scales for assessing psychopathology in the elderly. In: A. Raskin and L. F. Jarvik (eds.), Psychiatric Symptoms and Cognitive Loss in the Elderly, pp. 157-168. John Wiley and Sons, New York.
43. McNair, D. M., Lorr, M., and Droppleman, L. F. 1971. Profile of Mood States: Manual. Educational and Industrial Testing Service, San Diego.
44. Morris, J. N., and Sherwood, S. 1975. A retesting and modification of the Philadelphia Geriatric Centre Morale Scale. J. Gerontol. 30: 77-84.
45. Morris, J. N., Wolf, R. S., and Klerman, L. V. 1975. Common themes among morale and depression scales. J. Gerontol. 30: 209-215.
46. Murphy, E. 1982. Social origins of depression in old age. Br. J. Psychiatry 141: 135-142.
47. Murphy, E. 1983. The prognosis of depression in old age. Br. J. Psychiatry 142: 111-119.
48. Neugarten, B., Havighurst, R., and Tobin, S. 1961. The measurement of life satisfaction. J. Gerontol. 16: 134-143.
49. Pierce, R. C., Clark, M. M. 1973. Measurement of morale in the elderly. Int. J. Aging Hum. Dev. 4(2): 83-101.
50. Popoff, L. 1969. A simple method for diagnosis of depression by the family physician. Clin. Med. 76: 24.
51. Rose, A. M. 1955. Factors associated with life satisfaction of middle class, middle aged persons. Marriage and Family Living 17: 15-19.
52. Sadavoy, J., Reiman-Sheldon, E. 1983. General hospital geriatric psychiatric treatment: A follow-up study. J. Am. Geriatr. Soc. 31(4): 200-205.
53. Sakalis, G., Gershon, S., and Shopsin, B. 1974. A trial of Gerovital-H3 in depression during senility. Current Therapeutic Research 16: 59-63.
54. Salzman, C., and Shader, R. I. 1973. Methodology of the evaluation of psychotropic agents for geriatric patients. In: F. G. McMatron (ed.), Principles and Techniques of Human Research and Therapeutics, Vol. III, Psychopharmacological Agents. Futura, Mt. Kisco, New York.
55. Salzman, C., Kochansky, G., Shader, R., and Cronin, D. 1972. Rating scales for psychotropic drug research with geriatric patients. II mood ratings. J. Am. Geriatr. Soc. 20: 215-221.
56. Salzman, C., Shader, R. I., Harmatz, J., and Robertson, L. 1975. Effects of Diazepam in males. J. Am. Geriatr. Soc. 23: 451-457.
57. Sarteschi, R., Cassano, G. B., Gastrogiovanni, P., et al. 1973. The use of rating scales for computer analysis of the affective symptoms of old age. Compr. Psychiatry 14: 135-141.
58. Schwab, J. J., Holzner, C. E., and Warheit, G. J. 1973. Depressive symptomatology and age. Psychosomatics 14: 135-141.
59. Shader, R. I., Harmatz, J. S., and Salzman C. 1974. A new scale for clinical assessment in geriatric populations: Sandoz Clinical Assessment Geriatric (SCAG). J. Am. Geriatr. Soc. 12(3): 107-113.
60. Shader, R. I., Harmatz, J. S., Kochansky, G. E., et al. 1975. Psychopharmacologic investigations in healthy elderly volunteers: Effects of pipradol-vitamin (Alertonic) elixir and placebo in relation to research design. J. Am. Geriatr. Soc. 23: 277-279.
61. Spar, J. E., and La Rue, A. 1983. Major depression in the elderly: DSM-III criteria and the dexamethasone suppression test as predictors of treatment response. Am. J. Psychiatry 140(7): 844-847.
62. Spitzer, R. L., Fleiss, J. F., and Burdock, E. I. 1964. The mental status schedule: rationale, reliability and validity. Compr. Psychiatry 5: 384-395.
63. Steuer, J., Bank, L., Olsen, E. J., and Jarvik, L. F., 1980. Depression, physical health and somatic complaints in the elderly: a study of the Zung Self Rating Depression Scale. J. Gerontol. 35(5): 683-688.
64. Wing, J. K., Cooper, J. E., and Sartorius, N. 1974. The Measurement and Classification of Psychiatric Symptoms. Cambridge University Press, London.
65. Wood, V., Wylie, M., and Sheafer, B. 1969. An analysis of a short self-report measure of life satisfaction: Correlation with rater judgments. J. Gerontol. 24: 465-469.
67. Yesavage, J. A., Brink, T. L., Rose, T. L., et al. 1983. Development and validation of a geriatric depression screening scale: A preliminary report. J. Psychiatr. Res. 17(1): 37-49.
68. Zung, W. W. K. 1965. A self-rating depression scale. Arch. Gen. Psychiatry 12: 371-379.
69. Zung, W. W. K. 1967. Depression in the normal aged. Psychosomatics 8: 287-292.

70. Zung, W. W. K. 1970. Mood disturbances in the elderly. The Gerontologist 10: 2-4.
71. Zung, W. W. K. 1972. The depression status inventory: An adjuvent of the self-rating depression scale. J. Clin. Psychol. 28: 539-543.
72. Zung, W. W. K., and Green, R. L. 1973. Detection of affective disorders in the aged. In: C. Eisdorfer and W. E. Fann, (Eds.), Psychopharmacology and Aging. Plenum Press, New York.
73. Zung, W. W. K. Gianturco, D., Pfeiffer, E., et al. 1974. Pharmacology of depression in the aged: evaluation of Gerovital-H3 as an antidepressant drug. Psychosomatics 15: 127-131.

Chapter 30 Self-Report and Clinical Interview in the Assessment of Depression

E. S. PAYKEL and K. R. W. NORTON

This chapter will compare clinical interview and self-report methods of assessment of depressed patients. The two methods overlap to some extent, but each has particular advantages and disadvantages.

Spitzer and Endicott [43] have enumerated five major modes of psychiatric rating: (1) The patient may fill out a self-report questionnaire; (2) a relative or other informant may fill out a questionnaire reporting on the patient; (3) a professional, most commonly a nurse, may observe the patient in a naturalistic setting, such as a hospital ward; (4) a professional may interview an informant; and (5) a professional may interview the patient and rate both what the patient tells him and what he has observed.

The major division is between the first method, the self-report questionnaire, and the remaining methods, which depend on an outside observer: a relative, nurse, or psychiatrist at interview. Most studies in depression have, in fact, contrasted the self-report method with the interview, incorporating verbal material and observed behaviour, the usual method of the psychiatrist-administered rating scale.

Sources of Discrepancy

There are easily identifiable sources of potential discrepancy both in self-report and in interview scales. First some aspects of psychopathology cannot readily be assessed by the self, since they are mainly apparent to others. These include purely observational elements such as appearance of depression and psychomotor retardation. The extent to which this gap in assessment actually matters will depend on the extent to which the observational elements behave differently to subjective feelings. In addition, self-report scales cannot tap fully those aspects, such as delusions, hallucinations, and hypochondriacal overconcern, into which the patient does not have insight. Carefully framed questions can elicit some aspects of the phenomena, without clearly distinguishing the reality-based from the delusional.

A possibility which has tended to be neglected is the presence in self-report symptom questionnaires of pencil-and-paper answering habits or response sets which may distort answers. One such set is acquiescence or yea-saying [10] – the tendency to respond affirmatively to all questions, irrespective of content. Another response set, social desirability [16], involves the tendency to select a socially acceptable response rather than the true one.

An extensive literature exists regarding these response sets in personality questionnaires but few similar investigations have been carried out on symptom scales. Some studies using the Multiple Affect Adjective Checklist, a self-report mood scale, have shown evidence of acquiescence, but other studies have failed to do so [47]. Social desirability has been shown to affect interview responses to questioning regarding mental illness in epidemiological field studies [33, 14]. In one study [33] subjects' evaluations of what was socially undesirable in an inventory varied with their social status and whether they had experienced the symptom. There is evidence [15] that the items in the Minnesota Multiphasic Personality Inventory (MMPI) depression scale are heavily biased towards social undesirability.

Langevin and Stancer [22] hypothesized that, because the low self-esteem of depressed patients implies attributing socially undesirable qualities to the self, depression scales might in fact mainly measure social undesirability. In a small study correlations of the Edwards Social Desirability Scale with the Beck Depression Inventory, Carroll Self-Rating Depression Scale, and MMPI Depression Scale were between 0.8 and 0.9. Student raters rated most items on the Beck and Carroll scales as increasing in undesirability with increasing severity. These findings would suggest that the low self-esteem of depression and social undesirability may be indissolubly bound together.

Social desirability is not the only possible response set related to content. We have hypothesized [29] that some subjects may have a specific tendency to give responses indicative of presence and severity of symptoms. Such a tendency might be labelled "sick set". It is certainly consistent with long-standing psychiatric views that some patients, including hysterics and some other neurotics, tend to exaggerate their symptoms [24]. On the other hand it has been postulated [27] that some subjects may show another response set, a tendency not to give away information about themselves, or defensiveness.

The above might imply that psychiatrists' ratings are necessarily more accurate. Such a one-sided interpretation would oversimplify. The psychiatrist does have a background in a spectrum of depression from the most mild to the most severe which the patient usually lacks, and which may enable him to put the illness more accurately into context. Moreover, he has observational cues of appearance and posture which are not accessible to the patient. However, his contact with the inner world of the patient may be limited, particularly at first acquaintance. In those aspects which depend on patient report at interview, it is quite possible that the questionnaire response sets already mentioned may also carry over to interview and colour the information volunteered.

Moreover, psychiatrists may have their own rater sets. These have not been well studied. Most raters tend to prefer middle points in scales and to avoid extremes. Raters are liable to halo effects, forming a general impression and rating specific items in accordance with preconceptions based on it. Nonpsychiatrists and those less experienced in ratings tend to rate psychopathology higher than do psychiatrists and other experienced raters who have encountered many of the phenomena previously [9, 46, 12].

Raters may have additional biases. Psychiatrists are notoriously unsympathetic to patients with hysterical personalities and may be unwilling to accept that they are seriously depressed but expressing their symptoms differently [24]. On the other hand presence of such psychotic features as delusions will usually lead psychiatrists to the conclusion that the patient is seriously depressed. The process of rating by the psychiatrist involves an interaction with the patient and the qualities and results of that interaction may be affected by features both of psychiatrist and patient.

It is apparent that where discrepancies between interview and self-report ratings are found it is not necessarily easy to say which set of ratings is at fault. Validation of self-report scales against interview-rating scales or global judgments based on interview is limited in that it accepts the interviewer's viewpoint. There are some more objective external validating criteria, such as ability to differentiate different kinds of patients, to change with improvement and to distinguish between treatments. To some extent, however, both forms of assessment need to be regarded as potentially valid, alternative views sampling different aspects of the phenomena.

Empirical Comparison of Self-Report and Interview Ratings

One of us carried out several studies with colleagues at Yale University into the relationship between the two types of scales [29, 34, 35, 31]. Two instruments were used: the Clinical Interview for Depression [30], Chap. 26, this volume, an interview-rating scale with seven-point scales rating a comprehensive range of depressive symptoms and observed behaviour; and a composite self-report symptom and mood inventory [32].

The two scales were administered to 207 depressed patients spanning a wide range of severities and treatment settings. Correlations between parallel items were mostly significant, but not very high, ranging from 0.17 to 0.64 (34, 35). General factors measuring severity were obtained from the two instruments and the correlation between them found to be 0.27, relatively low.

The magnitude and direction of the discrepancy between the two severity measures were then related to other data. Patients rating themselves low on self-ratings compared with the interview ratings tended to be more severely depressed, more often psychotically depressed, and with more evidence of obsessional personalities on self-report [23] and informant ratings. Patients rating themselves as more severely ill in relation to the clinician ratings were younger and less severely and more neurotically depressed, showing hysterical and oral-dependent personalities on the personality scales and higher neuroticism scores on the Maudsley Personality Inventory [17]. A direct rating by the psychiatrist of the patient's tendency to exaggerate symptoms did not correlate with the discrepancy between the two types of assessment.

Findings suggested the presence of both a response set in certain types of patients (to exaggerate symptoms) and of an observer set in raters tending to underrate some patients such as hysterical personalities while perceiving others, such as those with delusions, as severely ill. Direct testing of the self-report response set could not be carried further, but it did not appear to be a simple yea-saying since it did not produce positive responses on all the items in the personality questionnaires. It appeared to be related to content, possibly to social desirability but more probably to a specific tendency to give responses indicating presence and severity of symptoms. Neither of the rating methods was necessarily in itself more valid than the other, although in this study the interview assessments did appear more closely to reflect expected characteristics in relation to other data such as treatment setting and classification.

Subsequently, a second sample of 190 depressed women was studied [31]. The findings of the first study were replicated. In addition, ratings were repeated after 4 weeks. The correlation between general pathology scores on the two scales was 0.48 initially and 0.72 after 4 weeks. The correlation between subtraction change scores was 0.45, relatively low. The same general tendency for correlations between self-report and interview scales to be substantially higher on repeated rating after improvement has been found in a number of other studies described below. The explanation is not fully clear. It might reflect practice effects producing more valid ratings particularly with the self-report scale; statistical effects related to range of scores, which tends to be lower when all patients are ill than on repeated ratings, when most patients have improved and some have not; greater validity on one or both types of scale in the lower range; or greater concordance in the limited contrast between being relatively well and ill than in degrees of illness in the higher range. Several of these reasons probably contribute.

Comparisons of Other Scales

A number of other studies have compared the two methods of assessment, most commonly using the Hamilton Rating Scale for Depression [19] as the interview scale. Several studies have compared it with the Beck Depression Inventory [4]. Schwab et al. [38] found that the total scores on the two measures correlated 0.75 with one another. When individual items of the two scales were examined, high correlations were found particularly to involve two items of the Hamilton Scale – suicide and somatic anxiety. The authors commented on the differing item content of the two scales. The Hamilton Scale is heavily orientated to somatic symptoms, the Beck to cognitive elements such as pessimism and guilt. In another study [45], a correlation of 0.82 was found.

Bech et al. [3] found Hamilton and Beck total scores correlated 0.72, although change scores after improvement showed a lower correlation. On plotting scores against global assessments of severity both scales differentiated poorly between moderate and severe depression, although in another study [21] the Hamilton Scale appeared adequate in this regard.

Bailey and Coppen [2] also compared the two scales in depressed inpatients. On admission the correlation between total scores was only 0.33. After a week it reached 0.71 and thereafter rose a little higher to 0.79. When successive rating pairs in individual patients were correlated only about two-thirds of the patients showed correlations of satisfactory magnitude. The authors examined severity of depression and personality inventory scores as possible explanations of the absence of correlation in some patients, but failed to find any differences on these measures.

Carroll et al. [7] compared the Hamilton and Beck scales in inpatients with a range of diagnoses. Total scores correlated 0.60 while another self-rating scale, the

Carroll Rating Scale, modelled on the item content of the Hamilton Scale, correlated 0.71 with it. In a study in outpatients [18] the Hamilton Scale correlated 0.68 with a self-rating visual analogue scale and 0.75 with the Carroll Self-Report Scale. The Hamilton Scale had a slightly higher correlation with a global severity rating than did either self-report scale, suggesting better validity, but possibly merely reflecting common ground between interviewer global and specific assessments.

Correlations between the Hamilton Scale and the Zung Self-Rating Depression Scale [48] have also been reported. Zung [49] reported a correlation of 0.56 in an English sample. Carroll et al. [6] found that total scores only correlated 0.41, with higher correlation in general practice patients than psychiatric inpatients or day patients (consistent with the general trend for correlations to be higher with milder illness). When correlations between individual parallel items were examined they were moderate for suicide, insomnia, work and interests, gastrointestinal symptoms and weight loss; significant but low for depression and psychic anxiety; and not significant for agitation, somatic anxiety and general somatic symptoms. In a test of validity, the Zung Scale failed to differentiate between patients in different treatment settings, while the Hamilton Scale was able to do so.

Biggs et al. [5] found a correlation of 0.45 between the two scales on initial assessment, rising to 0.76 after 2 weeks of treatment. Correlations were highest when Hamilton scores were below 20. The Zung Scale was less sensitive than the Hamilton in differentiating severity levels based on a global rating by treating physicians.

Overall correlations between the Zung and Hamilton Scales appear lower than those between the Beck and Hamilton Scales. It is possible that part of this is due to the hybrid nature of the Beck Inventory, which strictly speaking is administered by an interviewer reading out the questions and possible responses. Even the correlations found with this inventory, around 0.7, leave half of the variance not shared between the scales. The Zung Scale has also been found [1] to correlate poorly with another interview instrument, the Cronholm-Ottosson scale, with correlations rising over time in successive ratings.

The CES-D (Center for Epidemiologic Studies Depression Scale), a self-report depression scale intended for epidemiological studies, has been reported [44] to show correlations in different psychiatric samples, ranging from 0.49 to 0.85 with the Hamilton Scale and from 0.28 to 0.79 with another interview assessment, the Raskin Three Area Depression Scale. The lowest correlations were in acute depressives, the highest in schizophrenics and alcoholics, suggesting higher correlations in the lower ranges of depression.

Snaith et al. [40] devised a self-report scale for depressive symptoms, the Wakefield Inventory, and showed a correlation of 0.87 between total scores on this scale and ratings on the Hamilton Depression Scale, somewhat inflated by selecting ratings from different stages of illness to cover a wide range of severity. In subsequent development the scale was expanded by ten items and renamed the Leeds Scale [41]. In patients with depression and anxiety a total score from this scale correlated 0.85 and 0.83 respectively with subscales from the observer-rated Hamilton Depression Scale and Hamilton Anxiety Scale. In a later study [42] using a revised self-assessment scale by the same group, a depression subscore correlated 0.75 with the subscale from the Hamilton Depression Scale, while an anxiety subscore correlated 0.70 with the subscale from the Hamilton Anxiety Scale.

Craig and van Natta [11] compared interview ratings with self-report information on four scales. Patients covered a spectrum of diagnoses but numbers were low. Correlations between self-report and observer ratings were highest in a mixed "other diagnoses" group, chiefly of situational and character disorders, and lowest in schizophrenics. They were a little lower in depressive neuroses than affective psychoses but probably not significantly so.

Chesney et al. [8] compared scores in mixed outpatients on factors derived from the self-report Hopkins Symptom Checklist with ratings, primarily made by medical students, but checked by physicians, on dimensions corresponding to the factors. Correlations were highest for depression and sleep difficulty but only moderate (0.49), and were lowest for anger/hostility and sleep difficulty. Ratings did not differ in level for depression but patients tended to rate themselves higher than did the rater on anger hostility, phobic anxiety, obsessive-compulsive symptoms and sleep difficulty. Patients rated themselves lower on somaticism. Neurotic patients tended to rate themselves higher than physicians, psychotic patients lower, confirming our own findings [29]. In another study [28] of anxious patients using a modification of the Hopkins Symptom Checklist rated both by doctor and patient together with an anxiety scale and a rating of global improvement, correlations between patient and doctor measures were low at initial interview, rising progressively with time.

The above studies measured correlations and sometimes differences in level between self-reports and interview ratings of similar qualities. Another approach is to examine the internal structure of assessments. In a novel study Leff [25] used the Osgood Semantic Differential to elicit concepts of anxiety, depression, and irritability on 22 constructs, from psychiatric patients and psychiatrists. The psychiatrists produced highly differentiated concepts of the three emotions; in particular there was no correlation between the constructs of depression and anxiety. The patients produced concepts of the three emotions overlapping to a considerable degree, most so for depression and anxiety. Somatic symptoms did not distinguish anxiety and depression in the patients' concepts, but did differentiate anxiety and irritability. This study suggests that symptom assessments based on self-report will be more global and less differentiated than those based on interview ratings by psychiatrists.

Some confirmation comes from factor analyses of self-report and doctor ratings in neurotic outpatients on the Hopkins Symptom Checklist [13]. On the doctor ratings five well-differentiated factors were obtained, each accounting for 8.2%–14.1% of the variance. On the patient ratings, however, there was a tendency for a general neurotic factor to emerge, accounting for 26.6%–33.8% of the variance in different samples, and tending to fuse separate factors from the doctor ratings for depression and irascibility.

A similar trend was seen in a factor analysis of an expanded derivative of this scale [36].

Psychiatrist ratings produced six well-differentiated factors accounting for 11.8%–8.5% of the variance. Patient self-rating produced a first large general factor accounting for 33% of the variance; the next factor accounted for only 8.3%. However, good differentiation was obtained on self-report factors in a replication study using a larger sample [37], and in a comparison of the Hamilton Depression Scale and the self-report Carroll Rating Scale for Depression [39] factors explaining similar proportions of variance were obtained from the two instruments.

The most crucial questions concern the more objective aspects of validity such as discrimination between different kinds of patients and treatments. Here the existing literature is not explicit and few direct comparisons have been reported. In our own work interview assessments have tended to appear more valid in differentiating between patient types and severities and, somewhat marginally, different treatments. However, in one study [32] a self-report scale was able to distinguish between drug and placebo in mild persisting depression and relapses related to drug withdrawal when an interview scale failed to do so.

There has been little study of assessment instruments for childhood depression. Kadzin and Petti [20] have reviewed the topic. The distinction between interview and self-report assessments is somewhat blurred, since many self-report inventories are routinely presented to children orally by the clinician to ensure comprehension. There is some evidence of discrepancies between self-reports and ratings by parents or clinicians. The extent to which depression occurs in young children, or can be recognised and portrayed by them, is not clear.

In summary, empirical studies suggest: 1. Correlations between self-report and interview measures are not high, indicating that to some extent the two measure different phenomena. 2. Correlations tend to be higher for aspects such as verbal rather than observational, which are shared between self-report and interview scales. 3. Correlations tend uniformly to be lower at the height of illness, prior to treatment, than they are on repeated ratings after improvement. It is not clear which of several possible factors, previously referred to, is responsible for this effect. 4. The discrepancies are not random, but show systematic elements suggesting self-report response sets and observer-rating sets. In particular severely ill and psychotic depressives appear to underrate themselves in comparison with psychiatrists' interview ratings, while neurotic patients overrate themselves. There are also personality influences. 5. Self-report ratings of emotional states and symptoms tend to be more global with undifferentiated reflections of feeling pleasant or unpleasant than are psychiatrists' ratings based on interview.

Choice of Rating Method

Table 30.1 summarizes the main features of comparison between the two kinds of scales, which have emerged in this discussion. Self-report and clinical interview differ in the areas they can assess. Self-reports cannot tap observable behaviours apparent only to others, or aspects requiring considerable insight. Both types can record verbal reports by the patient of symptoms. Self-reports may provide better access to subjective feelings and moods.

Empirical work suggests that self-report scales, because of higher correlations between items, are more global in their assessments while psychiatrist ratings, with background of training and education in psychiatric concepts and the terms used to describe emotions, are more specific. In severely ill, retarded and psychotic depressives self-ratings tend to be less satisfactory, diverging considerably from interviewer ratings and failing to reflect apparent severity. Self-ratings are more dependent

Table 30.1. Comparison of clinical interview and self-report assessments in depression

	Self-report	Clinical interview
Areas assessed		
Subjective feelings/ moods	Yes	Less well
Verbal reports of symptoms	Yes	Yes
Observable behaviours	No	Yes
Judgments depending on insight	No	Yes
Specificity	More global	More specific
Range of severity	Less useful with severe depression, major retardation or psychotic features	Can be used over whole range. May be less sensitive in mild depression
Circumstances	Requires patient cooperation, motivation and ability to concentrate and read	Can be completed with minimal patient cooperation
Costs	Brief, easy, cheap in professional time	Longer. Requires professional rater
Potential biases	Pencil-and-paper response sets. Complaining (sick) sets	Rater sets and bias

on such patient features as cooperation, motivation, concentration and ability to read and understand the questions which may be impaired in severe depression and in other circumstances. On the other hand, interviewer-rating scales, and particularly the Hamilton Depression Scale, tend to be weighted towards the features of severe and endogenous depression. In the milder depressions where subjective moods and negative thought content are more important than somatic disturbances the self-report scales may have advantages. Self-report mood checklists [26, 36] may be particularly valuable to measure feelings: the Beck Inventory measures depressed thought content particularly well.

The major advantage of self-report scales lies in their reduced cost in terms of research effort, time and professional expertise which are required. Most self-report scales are brief and, while some supervision is required in their completion, this can be done without involving the psychiatrists or clinical psychologists, whose time is very expensive. Interview assessments take longer and usually require professionals as raters and special additional training for reliability.

A last comparative feature concerns potential biases. Here there is little to choose: both patients and professional raters have preconceived sets and biases which will obtrude in the rating process.

The choice of instruments for any particular study depends on a number of factors. One is the purpose of the study – is the instrument required as a first-stage screen to identify depression, for which a self-report may be highly suitable and economical? Is it required to make a diagnosis, in which case interview and professional judgment will be required? Is it required to be sensitive to change and to distinguish between treatments? Choice will also depend on the nature of the population to be studied. Severely depressed inpatients are best rated on interview scales such as the Hamilton Scale; general practice patients and general population subjects are likely to be mildly depressed and self-reports may be more useful. Choice inevitably also depends on the resources and personnel available.

As a general rule we believe that it is best to use several different measures, preferably of different types, in most studies. This particularly applies to controlled trials of drugs and other treatments. The effort and time involved in collecting subjects in clinical studies is usually very large; the time required to administer an additional assessment is usually small. Any rating scale may behave idiosyncratically or fail to live up to its record in some situations, which are not always easily predictable. It is best to use both an interview and a self-report measure with, for inpatients, a nurses' observational assessment as well. Studies should not depend on single-assessment scales, particularly self-reports.

Given that several assessment instruments of different types are used, it is also important that findings be examined on each separately rather than combining elements from each into a single score. Since the discrepancies between clinical interview and self-report are non-random, combining results from the two kinds of instrument may cancel out real findings of importance. With this proviso, use of multiple assessment measures is strongly recommended, combined with a critical attitude to any face value interpretations of findings.

References

1. Arfwidsson, L., d'Elia, G., Laurell, B., Ottosson, J.O., Perris, C., and Persson, G. 1974. Can self-rating replace doctor's rating in evaluating antidepressive treatment? Acta Psychiatr. Scand. 50: 16-22.
2. Bailey, J., and Coppen, A. 1976. A comparison between the Hamilton rating scale and the Beck inventory in the measurement of depression. Br. J. Psychiatry 128: 486-489.
3. Bech, P., Gram, L.F., Dein, E., Jacobsen, O., Vitger, J., and Bolwig, T.G. 1975. Quantitative rating of depressive states. Acta Psychiatr. Scand. 51: 161-170.
4. Beck, A.T. 1967. Depression: Clinical, Experimental and Theoretical Aspects. Harper & Row, New York.
5. Biggs, J.T., Wylie, L.T., and Ziegler, V.E. 1978. Validity of the Zung self-rating depression scale. Br. J. Psychiatr. 132: 381-385.
6. Carroll, B.J., Fielding, J.M., and Blashki, T.G. 1973. Depression rating scales: a critical review. Arch. Gen. Psychiatry 28: 361-366.
7. Carroll, B.J., Feinberg, M., Smouse, P.E., Rawson, S.G., and Greden, J.F. 1981. The Carroll Rating Scale for Depression I. Development, reliability and validation. Br. J. Psychiatry 138: 194-200.
8. Chesney, A.P., Larson, D., Brown, K., and Bunce, H. 1981. A comparison of patient self-report and physicians' observations in a psychiatric outpatient clinic. J. Psychiatr. Res. 16: 173-182.
9. Copeland, J., Kelleher, M.J., Gourlay, A.J., and Smith, A.M.R. 1975. Influence of psychiatric training, medical qualification and paramedical training on the rating of abnormal behaviour. Psychol. Med. 5: 89-95.
10. Couch, A., and Kenison, K. 1960. Yeasayers and naysayers: agreeing response set as a personality variable. J. Abnormal. Soc. Psychol. 60: 151-174.
11. Craig, T.J., and van Natta, P.A. 1976. Recognition of depressed affect in hospitalized psychiatric patients: staff and patient perceptions. Diseases of the Nervous System 37: 561-566.

12. Cranach, M. von, and Cooper, J. E. 1972. Changes in rating behaviour during the learning of a standardized psychiatric interview. Psychol. Med. 2: 373-380.
13. Derogatis, L. R., Lipman, R. S., Covi, L., and Rickels, K. 1971. Neurotic symptom dimensions as perceived by psychiatrists and patients of various social classes. Arch. Gen. Psychiatry 24: 454-464.
14. Dohrenwend, B. P. 1966. Social status and psychiatric disorder: an issue of substance and an issue of method. Am. Sociol. Rev. 31: 14-34.
15. Edwards, A. L. 1957. The Social Desirability Variable in Personality Assessment and Research. Holt Rinehart Co., New York.
16. Edwards, A. L. 1959. Social Desirability and Personality Test Construction. In: B. M. Bass and I. A. Berg (eds.), Objective Approaches to Personality, pp. 101-116. van Norstrand, New York.
17. Eysenck, H. J. 1959. The Manual of the Maudsley Personality Inventory. University of London Press, London.
18. Feinberg, M., Carroll, B. J., Smouse, P. E., and Rawson, S. G. 1981. The Carroll Rating Scale for Depression III. Comparison with other rating instruments. Br. J. Psychiatry 138: 205-209.
19. Hamilton, M. 1967. Development of a rating scale for primary depressive illness. Br. J. Soc. Clin. Psychol. 6: 278-296.
20. Kazdin, A. E., and Petti, T. A. 1982. Self-report and interview measures of childhood and adolescent depression. J. Child Psychol. Psychiatry 23: 437-457.
21. Knesevich, J. W., Biggs, J. T., Clayton, P. J., and Ziegler, V. E. 1977. Validity of the Hamilton Rating Scale for Depression. Br. J. Psychiatry 131: 49-52.
22. Langevin, R., and Stancer, H. 1979. Evidence that depression rating scales primarily measure a social undesirability response set. Acta. Psychiatr. Scand. 59: 70-79.
23. Lazare, A., and Klerman, G. L. 1966. Oral, obsessive and hysterical personality patterns. Arch. Gen. Psychiatry 14: 624-630.
24. Lazare, A., and Klerman, G. L. 1968. Hysteria and depression: the frequency and significance of hysterical personality features in hospitalized depressed women. Am. J. Psychiatry 124: 48-56.
25. Leff, J. P. 1978. Psychiatrists' versus patients' concepts of unpleasant emotions. Br. J. Psychiatry 133: 306-313.
26. Lubin, B. 1967. Manual for the Depression Adjective Checklists. Educational and Industrial Testing Service, San Diego.
27. Mann, A., and Murray, R. 1979. Measurement in psychiatry, Chap. 4, pp. 77-98. In: P. Hill, R. Murray, and A. Thorley (eds.), Essentials of Postgraduate Psychiatry. Academic Press, London.
28. Park, L. C., Uhlenhuth, E. H., Lipman, R. S., Rickels, K., and Fisher, S. 1965. A comparison of doctor and patient improvement ratings in a drug (meprobamate) trial. Br. J. Psychiatry 111: 535-540.
29. Paykel, E. S., and Prusoff, B. A. 1973. Response set and observer set in the assessment of depressed patients. Psychol. Med. 3: 209-216.
30. Paykel, E. S., Klerman, G. L., and Prusoff, B. A. 1970. Treatment setting and clinical depression. Arch. Gen. Psychiatry 22: 11-21.
31. Paykel, E. S., Prusoff, B. A., Klerman, G. L., and DiMascio, A. 1973. Self-report and clinician's assessments of depression. J. Nerv. Ment. Dis. 156: 166-182.
32. Paykel, E. S., DiMascio, A., Haskell, D., and Prusoff, B. A. 1975. Effects of maintenance amitriptyline and psychotherapy on symptoms of depression. Psychol. Med. 5: 67-77.
33. Phillips, D. L., and Clancy, K. J. 1970. Response biases in field studies of mental illness. Am. Sociol. Rev. 35: 503-515.
34. Prusoff, B. A., Klerman, G. L., and Paykel, E. S. 1972. Concordance between clinical assessments and patients self-report in depression. Arch. Gen. Psychiatry 26: 546-662.
35. Prusoff, B. A., Klerman, G. L., and Paykel, E. S. 1972. Pitfalls in the self-report assessment of depression. Can. Psychiatr. Assoc. J. 17: 101-107.
36. Raskin, A., Schulterbrandt, J., and Reatig, N. 1967. Factors of psychopathology in interview, ward behaviour and self-report ratings of hospitalized depressives. J. Consult. Psychol. 31: 270-278.
37. Raskin, A., Schulterbrandt, J., Natalie, M. S., Beatig, B. A., and McKeon, J. J. 1969. Replication of factors of psychopathology in interview, ward behaviour and self-report ratings of hospitalized depressives. J. Nerv. Ment. Dis. 148: 87-98.

38. Schwab, J.J., Bialow, M.R., and Holzer, C.E. 1967. A comparison of two rating scales for depression. J. Clin. Psychol. 23: 94–96.
39. Smouse, P.E., Feinberg, M., Carroll, B.J., Park, M.H., and Rawson, S.G. 1981. The Carroll Rating Scale for Depression II. Factor analyses of the feature profiles. Br. J. Psychiatr. 138: 201–204.
40. Snaith, R.P., Ahmed, S.N., Mehta, S., and Hamilton, M. 1971. Assessment of the severity of primary depressive illness. Psychol. Med. 1: 143–149.
41. Snaith, R.P., Bridge, G.W.K., and Hamilton, M. 1976. The Leeds Scale for the self-assessment of anxiety and depression. Br. J. Psychiatry 128: 156–165.
42. Snaith, R.P., Constantopoulos, A.A., Jardine, M.Y., and McGuffin, P. 1978. A clerical scale for the self-assessment of irritability. Br. J. Psychiatry 132: 164–171.
43. Spitzer, R.L., and Endicott, J. 1975. Psychiatric rating scales. In: A.M. Freedman, H.I. Kaplan, and B.J. Sadock (eds.), Comprehensive Textbook of Psychiatry. Vol. 11, 2nd Ed. Williams and Wilkins, Baltimore.
44. Weissman, M.M., Sholomskas, D., Pottenger, M., Prusoff, B.A., and Locke, B.Z. 1977. Assessing depressive symptoms in five psychiatric populations: a validation study. Am. J. Epidemiol. 106: 203–214.
45. Williams, J.G., Barlow, D.H., and Agrass, W.S. 1972. Behavioural measurement of severe depression. Arch. Gen. Psychiatry 27: 330–333.
46. Wing, J.K., Henderson, A.S., and Winckle, M. 1977. The rating of symptoms by a psychiatrist and a non-psychiatrist: a study of patients referred from general practice. Psychol. Med. 7: 713–715.
47. Zukerman, M. 1969. Response set in a checklist test: a sometimes thing. Psychol. Rep. 25: 773–774.
48. Zung, W.W.K. 1965. A self-rating depression scale. Arch. Gen. Psychiatry 12: 63–70.
49. Zung, W.W.K. 1969. A cross-cultural survey of symptoms in depression. Am. J. Psychiatry 126: 116–121.

Chapter 31 Sensitivity to Treatment Effects of Evaluation Instruments Completed by Psychiatrists, Psychologists, Nurses, and Patients

A. RASKIN

Introduction

There is a widespread belief that psychiatric patients make unreliable informants, especially when it comes to rating the presence and severity of their psychiatric symptoms. Hence it is felt that symptom-rating scales completed by patients are likely to be less accurate and therefore less sensitive to treatment effects than comparable scales completed by psychiatrists or psychologists [1]. (Henceforth, psychiatrist or psychologist-rated scales will be referred to as doctor-rated scales.)

A similar view is also held with regard to the value of nurse ratings compared with doctor ratings. It is felt that psychiatric nurses are more likely either to miss important signs of psychopathology or to attribute too much importance to minor signs of mental illness because they have not had the extensive training in diagnosing psychiatric illness and in the meaning of signs and symptoms of psychopathology given to psychiatrists and psychologists [39].

This chapter will examine the bases for and against these beliefs. More importantly, an effort will be made to spell out the necessary ingredients for sensitivity in any assessment instrument, whether completed by doctors, nurses, or patients. The term scale sensitivity in this chapter refers to the "... ability of a scale to discriminate the effects of different treatments upon important aspects of the patient's clinical condition" [40]. Other authors have used the term sensitivity to characterize a scale's ability to distinguish various degrees of severity of illness [37].

Key Ingredients in Scale Sensitivity

Relevance of Scale Items to Population Sampled and Anticipated Treatment Effects

The appropriateness of the rating scale to the patient population sampled or for the behavioral or pharmacologic treatments to be evaluated is basic to any discussion of scale sensitivity. This issue first surfaced in the early 1960s with the pioneering studies undertaken to assess the value of psychotherapy and of chemotherapy in psychiatric populations. In these early studies, investigators used instruments such as the Wechsler-Bellevue Intelligence Scale and subscales of the Minnesota Multiphasic Personality Inventory (e.g., Taylor Manifest Anxiety Scale) to assess treatment effects because these scales were in popular usage at the time. However, it soon became apparent that these scales were measuring enduring character traits that would not be expected to show much change over a relatively brief time span, such as 3-6 months, regardless of the treatment offered. As a consequence we now have rating scales that distinguish, for example, between trait and state anxiety [38], the former being more enduring and the latter more tied to immediate events.

However, the issue of the appropriateness of the rating scale to the patient population sampled has not disappeared completely with the emergence of new rating scales. For example, the use of the Zung Self-Rating Depression Scale [43] in older depressed patients has been criticized because a number of the indicators of depression such as sleep disturbance, weight loss, decreased appetite, confusion, decreased libido, and hopelessness are very common in normal elderly persons and tend to elevate total depression scores in this age group [2].

Evaluation instruments also need to be sensitive to changes in the patient's condition over time. Most symptom-rating scales are designed to assess the more severe forms of psychopathology and are therefore most effective in the acute phase of an illness. As patients improve, their sensitivity in distinguishing mild forms of psychopathology diminishes. Hence, a scale that includes items to assess mild as well as severe forms of psychopathology and may even include positive signs of mental health is better suited to measure changes in patients over time than one that focuses almost exclusively on severe forms of mental illness.

Observer-rated scales may also provide false impressions about a patient's clinical status over time. For example, when a patient is mute or unresponsive to an observer's questions, the patient may show less psychopathology on a symptom-rating scale than when he or she becomes more responsive and can tell the observer that he or she has hallucinations and/or delusions [10].

Matching the Rating Source to the Information Desired

The debate over the value of doctor ratings to patient self-report ratings or doctor ratings to nurse ratings often loses sight of the fact that each of these rating sources is best suited to rate certain behaviors and is poorly suited to rate others. The patient is the best source for rating his or her own inner feelings or mood states. Hence, instruments such as adjective checklists or mood scales are best completed by the patient. On the other hand, patients often have difficulty distinguishing anxious behaviors from depressed behaviors or stress-related somatic complaints, such as headaches and heart racing or pounding, from nonstress-related physical complaints. Hence, a symptom checklist containing a variety of psychic and somatic complaints should probably be completed by a psychiatrist rather than the patient, especially if one wishes to obtain separate anxiety and depression factor scores [33, 34]. Finally, if one wishes to assess the patient's behavior on the ward and interaction with other patients, the nurse who is with the patient for extended periods has the best opportunity to observe the patient on the ward and a ward behavior rating scale completed by a nurse is the preferred source for these ratings.

Support for this view may be found in a study by Raskin et al. [31] of antidepressant drug effects in hospitalized depressed patients. In this study an adjective checklist (The NIMH Mood Scale) showed a greater number of statistically significant treatment effects than a comparable scale rated by study nurses. However, a checklist of psychic and somatic complaints (the Inventory of Psychic and Somatic Complaints) was more sensitive and showed more significant treatment effects in the hands of doctors than the same instrument completed by the patients. A ward behavior rating scale completed by study nurses also proved to be very sensitive to treatment effects, especially the sedative-hypnotic effects of the drugs.

Literature Review

General Comments

The ideal studies to review for determining the differential sensitivity of doctor-rated, nurse-rated and patient-rated evaluation instruments would be studies that include two or more rating sources and provided sufficient data to permit comparisons of their relative sensitivity in detecting treatment effects. For this purpose one would want to rule out studies where the treatments themselves appeared to be ineffective, where rater reliability was in question, and where the evaluation instruments were flawed because they failed to meet criteria previously specified for scale sensitivity such as the item content of the instrument and were inadequate to describe the patient population sampled or the expected treatment effects. A number of authors have attempted a review of studies meeting part or all of the criteria outlined above and came to the conclusion that they were too few in number to adequately address the issue of differential sensitivity of observer-rated and self-rated scales [19, 20, 28, 40].

There have been quite a few studies that have correlated doctor-rated and self-rated scales and have reported low correlations between these scales especially when patients were acutely ill [6, 12, 30]. Most of these authors have concluded that the presence of these low correlations indicated that the patient self-report measures were doing a poorer job of assessing patient psychopathology than the doctor-rated measures. However, the presence of low correlations between these rating sources does not necessarily imply that one source is more sensitive to treatment effects than another.

Doctor-rated and patient-rated evaluation instruments have also been compared on their ability to discriminate levels of severity of illness. In general, doctor-rated instruments have fared better in this regard. For example, in one study of a doctor-rated instrument, the total score on the Hamilton Rating Scale for Depression [15], was superior to the total score on the Zung Self-Rating Depression Scale [43] in its ability to discriminate patients in inpatient, day hospital, and general practice settings [6]. Presumably patients in inpatient settings should be rated as more severely ill than those in outpatient or general practice settings. However, the ability of a scale to discriminate levels of severity of illness need not be equated with its ability to detect treatment effects. For example, the Hamilton Rating Scale for Depression referred to above has been criticized as being too heavily loaded with items indicative of severe forms of depression such as endogenous depression. Hence, this may be a poor instrument to use with milder forms of depression such as dysthymic disorder. This scale as well as other scales which emphasize severe forms of psychopathology may also lose sensitivity to treatment effects as patients begin to show signs of improvement and move into the moderate to mild range of severity of illness.

Self-Report Measures

The advantage of self-rating scales cited by Arfwidsson et al. [1] is that they are time-saving, economical, independent of theoretical frame of reference, not influenced by rater bias and that they permit comparisons between treatment sites and doctors. The rater bias issue refers to the fact that psychiatrist ratings of patient psychopathology in drug trials have been shown to be influenced by factors that could break the double-blind conditions such as the sedative effects of the drugs. Fisher [8], for example, noted a trend among psychiatrists to rate greater patient improvement in patients who showed sedation or complained of drowsiness on the assumption that this was a sign the patient was on an active treatment rather than a placebo and therefore would be expected to show improvement.

The treatment site comparison issue refers to the fact that when comparisons are made of treatment effects in collaborative studies involving two or more sites there appears to be greater concordance in treatment effects on the patient self-report measures than on the doctor-rated measures. On the other hand, doctor-rated measures agree more with each other within certain sites than patient-rated measures. Hence, it appears that certain biases regarding the rating of psychopathology or the evaluation of treatment effects are operating among doctors within sites that tend to reduce agreement across sites.

Snaith [37] noted that self-assessment scales suffered from the following deficiencies; they can be used only by cooperative patients who are also literate and not too ill, and they must not suffer from a condition where noncomprehension (e.g., senile dementia) or falsification (e.g., anorexia nervosa) of the scale responses would be likely to occur.

As noted by Snaith [37], the greatest failing of self-assessment scales is that the patients must be cooperative and not too confused or inattentive to complete the forms. However, self-report forms have been used with success in hospitalized depressed patients [35] as well as early senile dementia of Alzheimer's type (SDAT) cases [36]. In most instances it is recommended that a mental health professional be with the patient while the form is being completed to offer reassurance and assistance as needed. It is also recommended that the patient's level of cooperation and comprehension be assessed by the mental health professional on a scale such as the Task Behavior Rating Scale [9]. Test forms completed by patients rated poorly on level of comprehension or cooperation can then be discarded but the items on the Task Behavior Rating Scale could still be used as measures of patient pathology.

Snaith [37] also makes reference to issues such as patient falsification. This is a complex issue having to do with patient test-taking behaviors and attitudes. Scales have been constructed to control for some of these behaviors. For example, there is a Lie Scale on the Minnesota Multiphasic Personality Inventory. A Social Desirability Scale has also been created to measure a patient's tendency to give socially desirable responses. Reference has also been made to a "sickset", defined as patients' attempts to present themselves as very sick to their psychiatrist or to the test examiner. Patients operating under this set indiscriminately check all or most items in the "sick" direction whether the item applies to them or not. Although the development of scales measuring test-taking behavior and attitudes provides a means of identifying and possibly controlling some of these sources of test unreliability, an investigator is well advised not to rely wholly on these scales to assure that the test responses are reasonable and seem truthful. It is suggested that an investigator also examine the individual forms to ensure that the patient has complied with the instructions and answered the items truthfully.

The point was made previously that the patient was the best source for rating inner feelings and moods. However, it has been suggested that the patient's inner feelings and moods are not the proper subject matter for evaluating treatment effects, particularly the effects of psychoactive drugs [6]. One reason cited for this attitude is that these feeling states are not sufficient for purposes of defining a disease entity or for differential diagnosis. However, it is interesting that some of these same authors have also been critical of symptom-rating scales for this same reason and advise that they should not be used for diagnostic purposes. Mood scales or adjective checklists describing feelings such as depressed or anxious mood or feelings of hostility and aggression have been able to detect drug effects and have also been effective in profiling or discriminating the effects of different drugs within a drug class, such as different antidepressants [31].

McNair [28] undertook a survey of self-report scales and their sensitivity to drug effects. However, he excluded from his survey adjective checklists and mood scales because they had not been used extensively in drug trials. McNair concluded that self-report forms are more sensitive to drug effects if they include inpatients, fixed or mixed dosage schedules, no placebo washout period, several evaluation periods, and groups of more than 30 subjects.

Kellner and his associates [19, 20, 21, 22] have written a number of articles detailing steps they had taken to improve the sensitivity of a number of self-rating scales that they developed. They were able to show that when attention was paid to item content, the time focus for making ratings, and the cues for rating symptom intensity, the self-rating scales included in their study significantly discriminated the effects of chlordiazepoxide and of a placebo [23]. Significant drug-placebo differences emerged on 11 subscales as well as on the total pathology scores derived from these instruments. In contrast, a doctor-rating scale, the Hamilton Anxiety Scale, did not discriminate between the effects of chlordiazepoxide and of a placebo.

Nurse-Rating Scales

Perhaps the single most important advantage of nurse-rating scales over doctor-rating scales or patient self-report scales, is that they provide objective assessments of the patient's competence in social and interpersonal relationships and ability to perform essential activities of daily living, such as the ability to care for personal hygiene. These are often the critical behaviors that will determine whether a patient can be discharged. The nurse or aide generally spends more time with the patient than the psychiatrist or psychologist and is therefore in a better position to observe any small changes in behavior, especially of mute and very withdrawn patients and of very hostile patients who may refuse to talk to hospital personnel. Similarly the nurse and psychiatric aide have an advantage over the psychiatrist or psychologist in rating certain forms of psychopathology, such as sleep and appetite disturbances, which they can observe at first hand.

One of the major shortcomings of many of the nurse- and psychiatric aide-rating scales is the 1-week observational period specified for making ratings. In the course of a week the patient may show considerable variability in behavior, which complicates the nurse's task in deciding how to rate the patient. The recent trend toward shorter ward-behavior-rating scales that can be rated twice a week, or even daily, should minimize the problems associated with variability in patient behavior over time. As is true of other mental health professionals, the psychiatric nurse or psychiatric aide also brings with him or her certain attitudes about mental illness that can bias ratings of patient behavior. For example, Stoffelmayr [39] found that on a ward for chronic psychotic patients the prevailing view of the nurses was that the severely ill patients were not the more withdrawn and socially isolated patients but rather the patients who spend a long time in dressing, washing, or shaving. In other words, the nurses on this ward were more attuned to behavior that had a direct impact on ward management than to other signs and symptoms of psychopathology.

A number of nurse- or psychiatric aide-rating scales have been developed to measure patient ward behavior, and the more popular of these, such as the various versions of the Nurses' Observation Scale for Inpatient Evaluation (NOSIE [17], the Ward Behavior Rating Scale (WBRS [4], and the Psychotic Inpatient Profile (PIP [27], have been able to detect treatment effects.

The NOSIE-30 [18] was able to demonstrate statistically significant improvement or worsening on at least one of the seven derived scores in 87 of 129 drug studies with acute or chronic schizophrenic patients [16]. The scale has also had limited usage in evaluating treatment effects with other patient groups. Geriatric patients treated with beer showed marked improvement in all areas [25]; underweight geriatric patients treated with deprivation reduced social interest and social competence in normal males [24]. The results cited with geriatric patients and other nonschizophrenic samples are interesting but should be regarded as tentative pending replication.

In studies with both schizophrenic and depressed patients the Wittenborn Psychiatric Rating Scale (WBRS) has proven to be a very sensitive instrument in detecting psychoactive drug effects [11, 31]. It has also proven effective in evaluating an intensive treatment program with geriatric patients [3].

The Psychotic Inpatient Profile (PIP) has shown sensitivity to the effects of antipsychotic drugs in two studies with chronic schizophrenics [7, 13]. Sensitivity data of a similar nature are also available for the PIP's predecessor, the Psychotic Reaction Profile [5, 14, 26, 29, 41].

A study referred to previously did look at the sensitivity to drug effects of nurse ratings as compared with doctor and patient ratings [31]. In that study nurses completed a mood scale as well as two ward behavior scales. The mood scale completed by the nurses was less sensitive to treatment effects than a similar mood scale completed by the patients themselves. On the other hand, the two ward behavior rating scales, the Ward Behavior Rating Scale and the Global Ward Behavior Scales, proved very effective in detecting antidepressant drug effects. These ward behavior scales were especially helpful in detecting the sedative-hypnotic effects of the study drugs.

These results support some of the comments made previously about rating scales completed by nurses. First, they indicate that nurses make good observers of patient behavior on the ward and should be called on to complete ward behavior rating scales rather than interview-oriented symptom-rating scales or mood scales. Second, these results also indicate that the nurses are probably the best persons to rate certain signs of psychopathology or drug effects such as sleep disturbances and the sedative-hypnotic effects of drugs.

Doctor-Rating Scales

Most authors who have written on the subject seem to feel that psychiatrists and psychologists are the best persons to rate psychopathology and that scales designed for use by psychiatrists and psychologists are most sensitive to treatment effects. The advantages of doctor-rated scales are obvious. Psychiatrists and psychologists are generally skilled in interviewing patients and in asking appropriate questions to elicit signs and symptoms of psychopathology. They have received training in the meaning of psychiatric symptoms and in making diagnoses so that they know what symptoms to probe for during the interview based on their assumptions regarding the patient's diagnosis. The training in psychiatry and psychology also permits them to make distinctions among symptoms, for example, distinguish signs of anxiety from signs of depression, that patients generally cannot distinguish. They do not have the patient's emotional involvement with his or her illness and so can be more objective and accurate in rating psychiatric symptoms, particularly negative symptoms such as signs of hostility.

The deficiencies of observer- or doctor-rated scales are less obvious but can be quite serious if not recognized and not corrected. Some of these deficiencies were noted in a review article on rating scales by Snaith [37].

The main drawback is that of rater bias, that is the user is influenced in his or her scoring by a general expectation of how ill the patient "ought" to be; for instance, it is generally recognized that patients are more ill before they commence on a drug trial than they are at the end of it. A second drawback is that raters are influenced in their scoring of severity by their general experience with patients suffering from the disorder; while the experience of one rater may be confined to mild cases in the community another rater may have a long acquaintance with severe cases in hospital [37], p. 512).

Reference was made previously in this chapter to other sources of doctor bias which affect their ratings such as assuming the patient is on an active and effective treatment if the patient complains of feeling drowsy. Biases associated with the types of patients seen within a specific treatment setting and with treatment practices within a setting were also discussed. What has not been discussed at any length is the need to train psychiatrists and psychologists in the use of doctor- or observer-rating scales. Their extensive training in psychopathology and in making psychiatric diagnoses does not guarantee competence in interviewing patients for the purpose of completing symptom-rating scales. Some of these scales, such as the Brief Psychiatric Rating Scale (BPRS [29], make fine distinctions such as distinguishing tension from anxiety or distinguishing apathy from withdrawal. If a scale makes these distinctions, raters schould be clear and in agreement about the meaning of these terms. Some observer-rating scales are also best completed as the interview progresses and observers are encouraged to ask the patient direct questions about the items covered. Other scales encourage the observer to conduct a "normal" clinical interview and to make the ratings when the interview has been completed. Training in the use of scales is vital to assure interrater agreement or reliability. Where there is poor interrater agreement, there is little likelihood of demonstrating treatment effects.

Conclusion

When used appropriately, doctor-, nurse-, and patient-rating scales have all demonstrated good sensitivity to treatment effects. However, each rating source has distinctive advantages as well as disadvantages. Hence, it makes sense to include ratings from as many sources as possible. In this regard an interesting approach that one can use is to perform a "super" factor analysis in which test scores derived from doctor-, nurse-, and patient-rating forms are included in a single factor analysis. When performed appropriately, with steps taken to minimize the emergence of instrument factors, one can derive factors representing the major forms of psychopathology under investigation that cut across the source of the rating [32]. Hence, a depression super factor will include simple factors or items from scales completed by doctors, nurses, and patients. These super factors appear to be both more reliable and more sensitive to treatment effects than simple factors from each rating source. The super factors have the added advantage of reducing the total number of measurement variables that need to be entered into the statistical analyses.

Although this chapter has dealt almost exclusively with the literature on scale sensitivity in drug trials, the issues discussed and the conclusions reached have equal relevance for the assessment of psychosocial treatments. For example, an investigator interested in evaluating various forms of psychotherapy would also be encouraged to include ratings by the therapist, by an observer, and by the patient.

This investigator should also be aware of the advantages as well as the disadvantages of each rating source and make efforts to minimize the disadvantages by techniques such as training sessions in scale use and requiring patients to complete scales designed to measure test-taking behaviors and attitudes.

References

1. Arfwidsson, L., d'Elia, G., Laurell, B., Ottossen, O., Perris, C., and Persson, G. 1974. Can self-rating replace doctor's rating in evaluating antidepressive treatment. Acta Psychiatr. Scand. 50: 16-22.
2. Blumenthal, M. D. 1975. Measuring depressive symptomatology in a general population. Arch. Gen. Psychiatry 37: 971-978.
3. Burdock, E. I., Elliott, H. E., Hardesty, A. S., O'Neill, F. J., and Sklar, J. 1960. Biometric evaluation of an intensive treatment programme in a state mental hospital. J. Nerv. Ment. Dis. 130: 271-277.
4. Burdock, E. I., Hardesty, A. S., Hakerem, G., and Zubin, J. A. 1960. A ward behaviour rating scale for mental patients. J. Clin. Psychol. 16: 246-247.
5. Caffey, E. M., Jr., Diamond, L. S., Frank, T. V., Grasberger, J. C., Herman, L., Klett, C. J., and Rothstein, C. 1964. Discontinuation or reduction of chemotherapy in chronic schizophrenics. J. Chronic Dis. 17: 347-358.
6. Carroll, B. J., Fielding, J. M., and Blashki, T. J. 1973. Depression rating scales: A critical review. Arch. Gen. Psychiatry 28: 361-366.
7. Dehnel, L. L., Vestre, N. D., and Schiele, B. C. 1968. A controlled comparison of clopenthizal and perphenazine in a chronic schizophrenic population. Current Therapeutics Research 10: 169-176.
8. Fisher, S. 1976. Measurement of anxiety in outpatient trials: Detection of bias in patient and doctor ratings. Psychopharmacol. Bull. 12: 17-18.
9. Friedhoff, A. J., and Alpert, M. 1960. The effect of chlorpromazine on the variability of motor task performance in schizophrenics. J. Nerv. Ment. Dis. 130: 110-116
10. Gernor, R. H., Catlin, O. H., Gorelick, D. A., Hui, K. K., and Li, C. H. 1980. B-Endorphin. Arch. Gen. Psychiatry 37: 642-645.
11. Goldberg, H. L., Finnerty, R. J., LaBrie, R., and Rickels, K. 1978. A study of concordance between observer and patient rating scales. Psychopharmacol. Bull. 14: 7-10.
12. Goldberg, S. C., Klerman, G. L., and Cole, J. O. 1965. Changes in schizophrenic psychopathology and ward behaviour as a function of phenothiazine treatment. Br. J. Psychiatry 111: 120-133.
13. Hall, W. B., Vestre, N. D., Schiele, B. C., and Zimmerman, R. 1968. A controlled comparison of haloperidol and fluphenazine in chronic treatment-resistant schizophrenics. Diseases of the Nervous System 29: 405-408.
14. Hanlon, T. E., Nussbaum, K., Wittig, B., Hanlon, D. D., and Kurland, A. A. 1964. The comparative effectiveness of amitriptyline, perphenazine and their combination in the treatment of chronic psychotic female patients. Journal of New Drugs 4: 52-60.
15. Hamilton, M. 1960. A rating scale for depression. J. Neurol. Neurosurg. Psychiatry 23: 56-62.
16. Honigfeld, G. 1974. History and current status of its use in pharmacopsychiatric research. Mod. Probl. Pharmacopsychiatry 7: 238-263.
17. Honigfeld, G., and Klett, C. J. 1965. The nurses' observation scale for inpatient evaluation: a new scale for measuring improvement in chronic schizophrenia. J. Clin. Psychol. 21: 65-71.
18. Honigfeld, G., Gillis, R. D., and Klett, C. J. 1966. NOSIE-30: A treatment sensitive ward behaviour scale. Psychol. Rep. 19: 180-182.
19. Kellner, R. 1971. Part 1. Improvement criteria in drug trials with neurotic patients. Psychol. Med. 1: 416-425.
20. Kellner, R. 1972. Part 2. Improvement criteria in drug trials with neurotic patients. Psychol. Med. 2: 73-80.

21. Kellner, R., Simpson, G. M. and Sheffield, B. F. 1977. The value of self-rating scales in drug trials. Psychopharmacol. Bull. 13: 42–43.
22. Kellner, R., Sheffield, B. F., and Simpson, G. M. 1977. Comparative value of self-rating scales in drug trials. Psychopharmacol. Bull. 13: 12–13.
23. Kellner, R., Rada, R. T., Anderson, R., and Pathak, D. 1979. The effects of chlordiazepoxide on self-rated depression, anxiety and well-being. Psychopharmacology 64: 185–191.
24. Kollar, E. J., Pasnav, R. O., Rubin, R. T., Naitch, P., Slater, G. G., and Kales, A. 1979. Psychological, psychophysiological, and biochemical correlates of prolonged sleep deprivation. Am. J. Psychiatry 126: 488–497.
25. Konik, D. S., Paolino, A. F., Friedman, I., and Hinko, E. M. 1967. Beer and geriatrics, an objective study. Washington Brewers Institute. Unpublished manuscript.
26. Lasky, J. J., Klett, C. J., Caffey, E. M., Bennett, J. L., Rosenblum, M. P., and Hollister, L. E. 1962. Drug treatment of schizophrenic patients. Diseases of the Nervous System 23: 698–706.
27. Lorr, M., and Vestre, N. D. 1968. Psychotic Inpatient Profile Manual. Western Psychological Services, Los Angeles.
28. McNair, D. M. 1974. Self-evaluation of antidepressants. Psychopharmacologia 37: 281–302.
29. Overall, J. E., and Gorham, D. R. 1960. The brief psychiatric rating scale. Psychol. Rep. 10: 799–812.
30. Prusoff, B. A., Klerman, G. L., and Paykel, E. S. 1972. Concordance between clinical assessments and patients' self-report in depression. Arch. Gen. Psychiatry 26: 546–552.
31. Raskin, A., and Crook, T. H. 1976. Sensitivity of rating scales completed by psychiatrists, nurses and patients to antidepressant drug effects. J. Psychiatr. Res. 13: 31–41.
32. Raskin, A., and McKeon, J. J. 1971. Super factors of psychopathology in hospitalized depressed patients. J. Psychiatr. Res. 9: 11–19.
33. Raskin, A., Schulterbrandt, J., Reatig, N., and Rice, C. E. 1967. Factors of psychopathology in interview, ward behaviour and self-report ratings of hospitalized depressives. J. Consult. Psychol. 31: 270–278.
34. Raskin, A., Schulterbrandt, J., Reatig, N., and McKoon, J. J. 1969. Replication of factors of psychopathology in interview, ward behaviour and self-report ratings of hospitalized depressives. J. Nerv. Ment. Dis. 1: 87–98.
35. Raskin, A., Schulterbrandt, J. G., Reatig, N., and McKeon, J. J. 1970. Difference response to chlorpromazine, imipramine and placebo. Arch. Gen. Psychiatry 23: 164–173.
36. Raskin, A., Gershon, S., Crook, T. H., Sathananthan, G., and Ferris, S. 1978. The effects of hyperbaric and normobaric oxygen on cognitive impairment in the elderly. Arch. Gen. Psychiatry 35: 50–56.
37. Snaith, P. 1981. Rating scales. Br. J. Psychiatry 138: 512–514.
38. Spielberger, C. D., Gorsuch, R. L., and Lushene, R. 1968. Self-evaluation questionnaire. Consulting Psychologists Press, Palo Alto.
39. Stoffelmayr, B. E. 1973. The relationship between nurses' ratings of patient behaviour and observed patient behaviour. Soc. Psychiatry 8: 37–40.
40. Uhlenhuth, E. H., Glass, R. M., Haberman, S. J., and Kellner, R. 1982. Relative sensitivity of clinical measures in trials of antianxiety agents. In: E. I. Burdock, A. Sudilousky, and S. Gershon (eds.), The Behaviour of Psychiatric Patients – Quantitative Techniques for Evaluation, pp. 393–410. Marcel Dekker, New York.
41. Vestre, N. D. 1966. Validity data on the Psychotic Reaction Profile. J. Consult. Psychol. 30: 84–85.
42. Wolpert, A., Sheppard, C., and Merlis, J. 1967. Method for evaluation of behavioural changes in aged hospital patients during anabolic steroid therapy. J. Am. Geriatr. Soc. 15: 470–473.
43. Zung, W. W. K. 1965. A self-rating depression scale. Arch. Gen. Psychiatry 12: 63–70.